JEWISH MEDICAL ETHICS

JEWISH MEDICAL ETHICS

A COMPARATIVE AND HISTORICAL STUDY
OF THE JEWISH RELIGIOUS ATTITUDE
TO MEDICINE AND ITS PRACTICE

By Rabbi Dr.
IMMANUEL JAKOBOVITS

PHILOSOPHICAL LIBRARY
New York, N. Y.

Printed in the United States of America

DEDICATED

To the Memory of My Sainted Father

RABBI DR. JULIUS JAKOBOVITS
(1886-1947)

AS THE FIRST FRUITS
OF HIS FIRST-BORN

PREFACE

Moral autonomy or moral automation—between these alternatives lies the most fateful choice confronting mankind today. As long as the moral law reigns supreme, the spectacular advances in science and technology will be effectively controlled by the overriding claims of human life and dignity. Man will be safe from the menace of his own productions. But when the quest for knowledge and power is unhemmed by moral considerations, and the fundamental rights of man, as conferred and defined by his.Creator, are swept aside in the blind march to mechanical perfection, the ramparts protecting mankind from self-destruction are bound to crumble. Today the contest between science and religion is no longer a competitive search for the truth as in other former times. It is a struggle between excesses and controls, between the supremacy of man's creations and the supremacy of man himself.

In the past, the human inventive genius served mainly to aid nature in the amelioration of life. Now it bids fair to supplant nature, replacing it by an artificial, synthetic existence in which the deepest mysteries of creation are not only laid bare but subjected to the arbitrary whims of mechanised man. The push of one button can now exterminate life by the million; psychologically waged advertising campaigns can determine the eating habits of whole nations; chemical drugs can curb or release human emotions at will, and break down the most determined will-power to extract confessions. The control over man's conscience, over procreation and extinction, over human existence itself is being wrested from

God and nature and surrendered to scientists and technicians.

In this new dispensation the physician, too, is playing an ever more vital role. Human life, which he can artificially generate out of test-tubes and terminate out of syringe-needles, is now at his bidding. Psychiatry can help him to bring even human behaviour under his sway, almost like a robot plane guided by a remote radio operator. But who will control the physician and the growing army of other scientists?

There can be little doubt that, of all practical sciences, it is pre-eminently medicine with which Judaism, historically and intellectually, enjoys a natural kinship, and to which Jewish law is best qualified to address its reasoned, pragmatic rules of morality. For many centuries rabbis and physicians, often merging their professions into one, were intimate partners in a common effort for the betterment of life. The perplexities of our age challenge them to renew their association in the service of human life, health and dignity. Indeed they challenge Judaism itself to reassert its place as a potent force in the moral advancement of humanity.

*   *

*

This work is a modest attempt at helping to meet that challenge. The opinions recorded in it are founded on the premise that the consciences of scientists and doctors cannot replace religion as a guide to moral conduct. They assume that the physician must turn to competent experts for the solution of moral or religious complications arising in his practice, just as a general practitioner will consult a medical specialist when he meets a problem which is outside the scope of his general training and competence.

The following chapters, while they may serve as a guide to the sources and principles governing the religious attitude to medico-moral problems, constitute a mainly historical study. As such, the decisions featured in it cannot be used as practical directives, whether by doctors, patients or theologians, except when endorsed by qualified scholars in each individual case. No religious rulings on medical procedures of any kind should therefore be made simply on the basis of this work. Our principal object has been, rather, to provide an introduction to the considerations involved, and to survey the development of views and teachings in an area where the three most vital disciplines of human life—religion, law and medicine—meet and often overlap.

*   *

*

It lies in the nature of an enquiry of such diversified scope that it should include many technical details and apparent minutiae. The range of the sources drawn upon is inevitably vast and heterogeneous, covering the whole gamut of the history of medicine, of rabbinic literature, and of numerous other historical, theological and legal writings. To facilitate the reader, references to the Bible and to the frequently quoted clauses of the Shulhan 'Arukh, the last authentic code of Jewish law, have been included in the text itself. All other sources, and often their amplification, are given in the rather copious notes. For the sake of convenience, many abbreviations (mainly as used in rabbinic works) and shortened book- and article-titles are used in the notes; their full version appears in the list of abbreviations and the bibliography at the end of the volume.

*   *

*

This treatise, in a somewhat larger format, was originally presented to the University of London as a thesis for the Doctorate of Philosophy in 1955. In rewriting it for publication, I have acted on the many invaluable suggestions given to me by Prof. Charles Singer, Rabbi Dr. I. Epstein and Dr. S. Stein. To their personal kindness, and to their front-rank scholarship in their respective fields of medical history, rabbinics and Hebrew literature, I owe much for the completion of my first literary enterprise in book-form. My abiding gratitude is particularly expressed to Dr. Epstein, Principal of Jews' College, London, at whose feet I was privileged to study for many years, and to Dr. Singer, who guided me in the early stages of my research and without whose encouragment and advice I could not have undertaken this work. I am grateful, too, for the facilities so helpfully extended to me at the libraries of the Royal College of Physicians, Dublin, of Jews' College and the British Museum, London, of the Bibliothéque Nationale, Paris, and especially of Trinity College, Dublin, and the Wellcome Historical Medical Library, London. Of the numerous individuals who have freely given me the benefit of their specialised knowledge and counsel—among them rabbinical scholars, several Catholic and Protestant theologians, doctors, lawyers and historians—I must make special mention of Dr. Cecil Roth (Oxford), Dr. E. Solomons (New York, formerly Dublin) and my brother, Dr. Joseph Jakobovits (London). To all of them I tender my most profound thanks.

My specially grateful acknowledgement is reserved for my revered father-in-law, Rabbi Dr. E. Munk, not only for the thoughtful Foreword with which he has graced this book, but even more for his untiring and helpful interest in the progress of its composition. The ties of affinity disqualify me from testifying to his share in the realisation of my project through the gift of his great learning as well as the supreme gift of his eldest daughter as my treasured helpmate.

This publication is made possible by a grant from

the Claims Conference obtained for this purpose through the Union of Orthodox Hebrew Congregations in London, thanks largely to the efforts of its Director, Rabbi Dr. A. Spitzer, to whom I am much obliged.

Dublin.

I. J.

CONTENTS

FOREWORD

By RABBI DR. ELIE MUNK, Ph.D. (Paris)

Medical science has made such far-reaching mechanical and technical progress since the beginning of the century, and especially since 1920, that the uneasiness experienced amongst the elite of our thinkers at seeing the moral principles on which medical practice is based being swept aside by the torrent of medical progress seems to be increasingly justified. The current tendency in medicine to use modern techniques of growing complexity, and to socialize medical practice, replacing the personal relationship between doctor and patient based on the respect of medical ethics, are becoming rapidly prevalent. The technical perfections and the complexity of our civilization in its various spheres, the specialization of knowledge, the fragmentation of science into so many distinct sectors, each composed of further divisions, the abuse of the analytical spirit, all these result in the loss of a synthetic view of the whole, lead to a disregard for the basic laws which govern the life of society, develop a spirit of short-sighted utilitarianism and, finally, obscure the essential moral laws. And as a consequence, a serious crisis arises in the medical, as well as in all other domains, only to be followed by the destruction of those civilizations which have forgotten the fundamental laws governing the life of human society.[1]

Thus, it is more important than ever to safeguard medical ethics and to give it the place of honour it merits in medical practice. The present work of our author, whose purpose is a detailed treatment of "Jewish Medical Ethics", is, therefore, a timely work. Keeping theoretical speculation to a minimum, he records the great problems of medical practice by analyzing the position of the Jewish doctrine with regard to them. Each subject is introduced by a historical and comparative study in order to permit the solutions inspired by Jewish ethics to appear in their true light. Thus, the vast subjects of medico-moral conflict (such as euthanasia, dissection, abortion, the problems of eugenics and legal medicine, as well as many others), which have not ceased, over the generations, to beset the moral conscience of humanity, are treated in the light of the eternal truths whose authentic source is the biblical revelation. The positions taken are clear; they are not the result of personal, logical or sentimental considerations, always subject to caution, nor of systematic philosophy, a product of the human spirit and, consequently, always relative in value; they are based, in the final analysis, on the solid foundations of universal morality whose charter is contained in the Decalogue. In practical life, man, faced with a crisis of conscience, can give it his confidence. It is the wisdom of Israel, derived from the most venerable sources of the history of our civilization, which raises its voice in the midst of the mental confusion of our epoch, an epoch of which Paul Valery said:

"We no longer know how to collect all our gains in the lottery of experience. All the results speak at once. And the mental confusion confounds itself with the confusion of reality."

In giving his book the sub-title: "A Comparative and Historical Study of the Jewish Religious Attitude to Medicine and its Practice," the author has desired to limit his field of research. He develops the principles, methods and problems of the medical art within the tradition of the Jewish religion, especially in a historical perspective with particular reference to their embodiment in the framework of Jewish law. A presentation of the characteristic traits of Jewish medicine in general is beyond the limits of this study, and it is perhaps useful to recall at least those traits, a knowledge of which might aid in a better understanding of certain positions of Jewish medical ethics.

1. In the first place, it is worth emphasizing the essentially prophylactic nature of Jewish medicine. While modern medicine is above all therapeutic in its aims, Hebrew medicine received, at its origin, a different orientation by this biblical verse: "If thou wilt diligently hearken to the voice of the Lord thy God, and wilt do that which is right in His sight, and wilt give ear to His commandments, and keep all His statutes, I will put none of these diseases upon thee, which I have brought upon the Egyptians, for I am the Lord that healeth thee". (Exodus xv, 26) This declaration has the value of a veritable program. With this declaration as their basis, many Jewish thinkers who are considered authorities recognized and demonstrated the prophylactic effect of a series of religious laws of primary importance, such as, notably, those concerning food and the purity of conjugal life.[2] Whatever the profound causes or other motives for the origin of these laws, it is scarcely possible to contest their incomparable value on the level of physical and mental hygiene. In the spirit of Judaism, the observance of the divine laws constitutes the most effective preventive medicine against disease.

Prophylactic hygiene raised to the level of a legal, national and collective institution, has been the object of a great many specialized studies.[3] These have analyzed the effect of the laws of circumcision and of abstinence and purification on the occasion of the menses on sexual hygiene; the effect of the laws of ritual slaughter, of forbidden foods and mixtures, of the preparation of meat, of the rules for meals, on sanitary hygiene; the effect of the laws dealing with the Sabbath, their consequences and extensions, on social hygiene; the effect of the laws concerning the divine services, soberness, religious studies, etc. on mental hygiene; the effect of the laws on married life and sexual relations on eugenics.

An extremely powerful effect is thus accomplished for the preservation of our physical beings. The same tight network of rules which serves to sanctify our life, serves at the same time as the shield of our health. Considered in this perspective, the prevention of disease becomes the major preoccupation of Hebrew medicine, for which an imposing discipline of restrictive measures, extending to all spheres of human activity, is erected. Disease itself appears, consequently, as being only an exception to the rule. The hypothesis that therapeutics, relegated to a secondary position, has suffered in its development as a result of this conception, and that anatomical dissection was scarcely practised for the same reason, cannot be dismissed.[4]

This system of prophylactic hygiene on the widest social scale has brilliantly proved itself in its application to the Jewish people. In spite of the fact that the reasons for many prohibitions are beyond the capacities of human logic, the historical fact remains that the so-called ritual laws have conferred on Israel, throughout the generations, an extraordinary vigour and power of physical resistance. In the midst of living conditions often characterized by the most intense misery and the extremes of privation, these laws have sufficed, because of their real sanitary and hygienic value, to form a chain of generations perfectly healthy in mind and body and secure against disease and death to a remarkable degree.

2. Another basic principle, no less important, is Jewish medicine's concept of unity, which possesses a double aspect. On the one hand, there is the identity of religion, morality and hygiene which form an indivisible whole, and on the other hand, there is the unity of the human being, wherein body and mind form an inseparable whole. These two axioms are the direct consequence of the doctrine of absolute monotheism. In effect, we find in the Bible and the Talmud many medical notions tightly bound up with strictly religious and moral prescriptions. "What is particularly

notable," writes A. Castiglioni in his *History of Medicine,* "and what makes the history of Jewish medicine more interesting, perhaps, than that of the other peoples of antiquity, is that one can often observe that traditions and concepts have been absorbed and, so to speak, filtered through the moral and legislative system of Judaism, and what a decisive role has been exercised in this process of assimilation by the concept of monotheism which gives the divinity the power of healing. As a result of this concept, Hebrew medicine differs from that of all the other peoples of antiquity. . . . It is in this same manner that many centuries later, Christianity turns away from empirical medicine to return to the pure virtue of the healing power of faith, which, in the eyes of the early Christians, was to eradicate and make the people forget their faith in magic and occult practices, thus returning to the initial Jewish concept according to which there is no salvation outside the faith, nor medication without prayer." [5]

It would, however, be as false to conclude that Hebrew monotheism has an exclusively spiritualistic aspect, as it would to attribute to it an exclusive materialism. It is both at once. The laws of the body are not only recognized but profoundly studied in the same way as those of the spirit. The sanitary regulations are placed on the same plane as those of morality, of the love of one's neighbour and of justice. Mortifying one's body is as bad as committing a social wrong. It is a religious duty to preserve one's health, and Maimonides, at the beginning of his detailed presentation of the rules of physical hygiene, insists upon the fact that every man has the duty to take care of his health in order to be able to serve God with all the vigour of his body and the lucidity of his mind.[6]

This intertwining of the ethico-religious and hygienic domains corresponds to the intertwining of body and mind in the human being.[7] Man is a microcosm whose multiple components of both, a spiritual and physical nature, harmo-

nize together in a perfect balance, established by an act of
extreme precision. The slightest deviation from this pre-
established balance, the least dissonance, immediately pro-
vokes repercussions which are that much more formidable in
that, once set in motion, they have the distinct tendency to
accentuate themselves.

The interdependence of the soul and the body leads to
the consequence that affections of the body can have causes
whose origins are to be found in the sector of the soul and
vice versa. It follows necessarily that medical therapy must
take into account this empirical fact. The famous physiologist, Claude Bernard (who died in 1878) expresses the
Hebrew theories when he affirms that "physiologists and
doctors must never forget that the living being forms one
organism and a single individuality".

The Bible and the Talmud are impregnated with this
spirit. For them, the plagues of leprosy, of which the Torah
gives us detailed descriptions, have moral causes.[8] This case
serves as the classical example for many other diseases which
are mentioned in Scripture in relation to defective moral and
religious conduct.[9] While Jewish doctrine has developed
this notion to its extreme consequences, it has not, however,
remained alone in its profession. Professor W. Riese writes
in this respect in his book cited above[10]: "The idea of sin as
the cause of disease appears already in primitive medicine.
It reappears in its Christian form in Paracelsus in the 16th
century and is at its apogee in Heinroth at the beginning of
the 19th century. Amongst the contemporary authors,[11] C.
von Monakow maintains the thesis that one can fall ill for
having betrayed the interests of the community and of humanity. From the earliest times, man has incriminated the
passions as causes of disease and inasmuch as the former form
a part of ethics, a distinctly moral problem is raised by the
diagnosis of sickness caused by the passions. It is not sur-
prising to find the passions ranged in the foreground of the
etiologic factors admitted by the school to which the moral

treatment of madness is dear (Pinel, Esquirol). But there are other factors in the etiology of disease which reflect even more eloquently the relation of man to man and, therefore, their moral nature. La Rochefoucauld, in a small chapter of his *Reflexions Diverses*, entitled 'On the Origin of Disease', prepared a list of these, there being as many vices as there are causes of disease. The early periods of humanity were exempt from diseases which, he affirms, only make their appearance as a result of the moral corruption of mankind, a product of more recent centuries. Ambition produced acute and frenetic fevers; envy produced jaundice and insomnia; out of laziness came the lethargies, paralysis and languish; avarice made the tinea and scabies; sadness made scurvy; calumny and false report have spread the measles, smallpox and purpura, and to jealousy we owe gangrene, the pest and rabies, etc. The theory of Rousseau, according to which the misery and disease of civilization are to be attributed to man's untiring search for satisfactions beyond his natural needs and to his avidity which knows no limits, is well known. Disease in this theory figures as the first stage in the destruction of a world destined to collapse under the disastrous effect of the rapacity of man consuming everything and remaining, finally, alone on earth."

Furthermore, the action of psycho-physiological elements in the phenomena of the faculties of sensation has been recognized many times by eminent psychologists as well as by the Sages of the Talmud.[12] It is, therefore, natural that these tendencies, towards which the Bible itself orientates us, should have largely influenced the therapeutic principles of Jewish medical science.[13] Maimonides, especially, repeats in various forms the principle that the acquisition of the moral virtues constitutes the best of all medication. He brands the vices, the bad habits contracted in the domain of manners, moral and social depravity, as being the profound causes of physical degeneration.[14] Parallel to this, he establishes a veritable regimen of the soul, giving precise indications as to its nature and constitution and as to the laws of moral health, to which he consecrates several special treatises.[15] He insists also on the importance which every doctor should attach to the psychological factor in the treatment of disease.[16] Other Jewish doctors have followed in the footsteps of the rationalistic school of Maimonides, while the mystical movements of Jewish thought have reached entirely identical conclusions.[17]

This directing idea of reciprocal relations in the inseparable union of body and soul is proper to Jewish medicine.[18] It makes it a precursor of psychosomatic medicine whose principle has been defined in the following terms: "Every disease arises at the same time from the mind and the body, and every therapy is, consequently, part of psychosomatic medicine. When everyone will be adequately persuaded of this truth, the term psychosomatic will be discarded, the fundamental idea which it translates being henceforth implied in the term medicine."[19] Actually, the point of view of the unity of the individual and the fact that, in disease, it is the whole man, including his mind, which is involved, is still at its beginning in modern medicine. It rests on the discovery by modern psychology of the moral conscience, on the physiology of the emotions and the psychoanalysis of Freud.

The Americans were the first to raise the dam of psychosomatic medicine against the "dehumanization of world medicine" (Pierre Mauriac). The revolution of mechanical and technical progress; the instrumentation in surgery, the fragmentation of medicine into a foliation of specialties have led to abolishing the personal relation between doctor and patient and to reducing the latter to the rank of an object, with neither soul nor personality, to be treated.

The merit and originality of Jewish medical science has been to proclaim, from its earliest days, that the patient can only be healed if his being is considered as a body endowed with a soul and as an entity in which the reactions of body and soul mutually condition each other.

3. Certain attitudes of Jewish medical ethics may seem paradoxical to those who are not familiar with the spirit of Judaism; some explanation is necessary. It appears, in effect, that Jewish law, whose severity and moral discipline generally surpass those of other religious systems, reveals itself on many occasions much more supple and tolerant than other systems, although it is not always possible, on a first appreciation, to discern the criterion applied by the Law. The reader will find several examples in the chapters of this book dealing with the treatment of the dying (Chapter XI), eugenics (Chapter XIII), abortion (Chapter XIV) and elsewhere. The cases which confront the legislator in these different domains and which involve the ineluctable choice in the conflict between a religious principle and a vital necessity are frequently resolved by canon law in a purely dogmatic fashion; whereas Mosaic law reveals itself more inclined to take into account these vital necessities and to admit certain exceptions within well-defined limits. Thus, it tolerates, in exceptional circumstances, dissection,[20] sterilization[21] and the destruction of the embryo.[22] Its attitude in other domains, such as divorce legislation or birth control[23] is similar in spirit. Jewish ethics prefers treating the problems raised by health considerations and vital necessity as individual cases and regarding these, after conscientious examination, as exceptions, justified by reason of *force majeure*, rather than incurring the risks of serious reactions of a moral, physical and social nature.[24]

Judaism considers that the great moral principles are profoundly enough rooted in the religious conscience of the nation to make it possible to tolerate exceptional cases without, for that matter, doing the least violence to the principle involved or undermining its authority. It acts thus in conformity with its general spirit which is to be strict in its principles, but human and clement in its application as it concerns the individual person.

This rule of procedure confirms that, in the field of medicine, it is the human factor of the ethical code which will complete the lacunae of the Law, as is equally the case in the field of civil and criminal law. B. Pascal (who died in 1662) said that the least application of charity, which is on a plane infinitely higher than all human science, is often alone capable of surmounting the highest summits of pain. But ethics itself also has its laws and its criteria. In the medical realm, however, they have never been analyzed in a systematic and exhaustive manner, and it is the merit of the present work to offer us a veritable code of Jewish medical ethics. It thus renders an eminent service to all those who desire to know and to find inspiration in the immortal principles of the tradition of Israel in the exercise of one of the noblest arts which man was given to practise.

JEWISH MEDICAL ETHICS
INTRODUCTION

INTRODUCTION

Religion and medicine have been in alliance with each other in every land, among all peoples, and almost throughout the entire course of recorded human history. The Egyptian god-physician IMHOTEP at the head of medical history, the biblical "I am the Lord, thy physician"[1] (*Ex. xv.* 26), the Greek temples and priests of AESCULAPIUS — who had "the most successful run" of all gods made with hands,[2] the rise of Christianity as "a healing faith",[3] the ascription of sainthood to HIPPOCRATES in Jewish writings[4] and Christian churches,[5] COSMAS and DAMIAN as the patron-saints of medicine and surgery,[6] "monastic medicine" and the rabbi-physician in the Middle Ages, the "Ministry of Healing" and the consecration of bishops "to heal the sick"[7]—these are but some of the forms in which this association has found expression among different creeds and civilizations. SIGERIST[8] attributes the close relationship between religion and medicine to "the helplessness of the sick man, the limitations of medical science and the proximity of death"; SINGER[9] asserts that "nearly all the ancients—and especially the ancient physicians—considered that there were at least some bodies and forces . . . that could not be treated on the merely phenomenal level", and "that 'nature' must be conceived as permeated in some way or another by God"; and OSLER[10] recognises that both systems "arose out of the same protoplasm".

The partnership of religion and medicine has not been always either holy or healthy. By its association with physical healing, religion often tended to become utilitarian in outlook, spurious in appeal, and amoral in aims. Yet, generally speaking, it was medicine that paid the higher price.

The alliance frequently diverted man's attention from the true causes of disease, shrouded medicine in a cloak of mystery and superstition, opposed the alleviation of suffering as an unwarranted intervention in divine Providence, and hampered medical practice by irrational doctrines. The religio-medical association did, however, also yield substantial profits to both partners. Religion was ennobled by its special solicitude for the sick, enriched by its concern with the moral problems raised in medical practice, and strengthened through man's discovery of his own frailty and his dependence on a Higher Being. Medicine, for its part, is indebted to religion for its hospitals, its emphasis on the supreme value of human life and health, its control of the conscientious physician, and its spiritual assistance in the mitigation of pain and distress.

Our present study on Jewish medical ethics is limited to the examination of only one aspect in this mutual relationship: the impact of religion, and of Jewish law in particular, upon the attitude to medicine and its practice. In this connection, we use the term "religious medical ethics" in its widest sense and in preference to "pastoral medicine" which, though perhaps more accurate, is not quite so expressive of some of the broader ramifications of the subjects under consideration. "Medical ethics" is not, therefore, here used in the more technical, narrow meaning of professional propriety, but rather in the sense in which it is understood in Roman Catholic moral philosophy.

SCOPE OF JEWISH MEDICAL ETHICS

The fields of medical ethics covered by Jewish law are considerably wider and more numerous than the comparative material provided by the Christian and Moslem faiths. All three religions, of course, are concerned, to a greater or lesser extent, with such issues as affect the legality of human acts of healing, the recourse to prayer and irrational cures, the moral responsibilities of physicians and in particular the arbitrary termination of life (whether before or after birth). But the great bulk of the medico-religious regulations in Jewish law deal with the problems raised whenever the interests of life and law would seem to be in conflict. While, in Christianity, health considerations affect only (or mainly) three church laws—church-going, fasting and abstinence[11] —in Judaism they have a bearing on the observance of laws relating to the Sabbath, the various festivals and fasts, the dietary prescriptions, prayer, mourning, circumcision and other fields of legislation. The rights and obligations of the physician, too, feature prominently in Jewish medical ethics. In common with the theologians of other denominations, the rabbis included in their legislation certain provisions regarding medical fees, licenses, and liabilities for injuries sustained by patients in the course of their treatment. The legal systems of the various religions also concern themselves with the attendance of male practitioners on women. But these items apart, the special interests of the different creeds in the physician vary considerably. The masters of the Church have, for many centuries, dealt with the right of her clerics to engage in medicine and particularly surgery—for which there is only an insignificant and remote parallel in Jewish law. Jewish sources, on the other hand, devote much attention to the "physician's trustworthiness" in matters affecting religious decisions. Another unique sphere in which Jewish law operates is the surgical treatment of one's parents.

For the solutions of some more distinctly spiritual problems in medical practice the physician may also seek religious guidance. In advising his patient, particularly in sexual matters, he may have to decide whether or not he is morally justified in recommending a procedure which, while physically beneficial, conflicts with the dictates of his faith. When the patient nears death, further problems may confront the physician. Should he, for instance, inform the patient of his condition, or continue treatment if he refuses to call a priest for confession? Again, under what conditions would one be entitled to ignore the respect due to the dead in order to promote the health of the living? The directives of the various religions on how to solve such conflicts between humanitarian and theological considerations may show some superficial similarities, but on closer examination the views of the different creeds will be found to vary substantially. Considerable divergencies also exist in the attitude to certain eugenic regulations and to the establishment of death. All these medico-religious questions are among the main subjects treated in the present work.

Although the general relationship between religion and medicine has been discussed in several scholarly works,[12] there exists no comprehensive historical study on the effect of religious teachings on medical practice in respect to any period or any religion. There are only a number of monographs illustrating the history of this relationship in the light of specific subjects, such as the healing power of nature, [13] medical licensure, [14] sterilisation,[15] contraception,[16] abortion,[17] dissection,[18] and, above all, magic and irrational beliefs as an element of pseudo-medicine.[19] The historical treatment of these and many other kindred subjects provides the mosaics that form the multicolored picture of the impact of religious thought and legislation on medicine.

The Jewish literary material in this field is especially scant, and our compilation of the relevant sources from the principal works of Jewish law will be the first attempt at a comprehensive presentation of the Jewish medical legislation. A series of articles in a Hebrew periodical published a few years ago[20] dealt exhaustively with a limited number of medico-religious subjects, but the sources used were drawn almost entirely from the rabbinical responsa literature only. These sources also formed the chief basis of ZIMMELS's recent work[21] which, however, referred only briefly and occasionally to religio-legal problems in the practice of medicine. PREUSS, too, touches on our field in his unsurpassed work on medicine in the Bible and Talmud,[22] but as a rule only incidentally and merely in so far as it relates to the earliest sources of Jewish law. Otherwise, the medical content of post-Talmudic rabbinic literature has never been collected, classified or studied. Nor are there any "manuals" for doctors setting forth the Jewish religious directives governing the practice of their profession. For guidance, they and their patients must resort to rabbis or halachic works (appearing almost invariably in Hebrew). Yet, the absence of popular writings on these subjects has never been seriously felt in practice, due to the generally liberal attitude of Jewish law itself, no less than to the liberal outlook of most Jewish physicians. On the whole, Jewish law clashes with medical opinion very rarely indeed.

The paucity of Jewish works on medical ethics contrasts sharply with the profusion of Roman Catholic literary material in this field. Treatises on the religious administration of medicine from the Catholic point of view date from the 16th century.[23] Further religio-medical compendia appeared in the 17th,[24] and particularly the 18th,[25] centuries. Among these, F. E. CANGIAMILA's *Embryologia sacra* (first published in Venice in 1763) long enjoyed exceptional popularity. Since then an entire library of this class of literature has grown up in various modern languages, comprising many learned studies,[26] numerous popular handbooks,[27] some periodicals[28] innumerable articles in theological magazines, a "hospital code",[29] and even a nine-page manual of *Ethical and Religious Directives for Catholic Hospitals* published in the United States in 1949.[30] These regulations are widely used by Catholic physicians and in institutions under Catholic control.

Between the relevant Jewish and Catholic sources there is, moreover, one characteristic difference: The rabbis in their responsa—by far the greatest store of material on

Jewish medical ethics—normally deal with the perplexities of individual questioners, not with general rules for impersonal application. In most cases, the rabbinic formulation of the law is addressed to *patients* requesting personal guidance. The directives of the Church, on the other hand, are usually given to *doctors* working in a Catholic society and in Catholic hospitals.

RECOGNITION OF MEDICAL ADVANCES IN JEWISH LAW

To introduce our study of the Jewish sources, we may here also consider the position of the main rabbinic authorities cited in the present work in relation to the advances of medical knowledge and practice. To appreciate the historical significance of our principal sources, the important fact must be emphasised that the great medieval codes of Jewish law are fundamentally codifications of talmudic law and practice, with relatively very few amendments. [31] In their contents and largely in the illustration of their legal principles, therefore, they mirror the conditions of Jewish life and law at the time of the Talmud rather than those prevailing in their own days. This consideration applies in particular to the medical data contained in these codes. Even in the *Shulhan Arukh*, the last and most authoritative of them, most of the diseases,[32] treatments,[33] and medicaments[34] mentioned had their origin in the Talmud over a thousand years earlier. Little or no account is taken of medical facts observed in the intervening millenium, relatively insignificant as these may have been. This does not imply that the codifiers of Jewish law ignored the changes around them or that they accepted the medical authority of the ancients as infallible. They simply limited the deposition and classification of their rulings to laws treated in the Talmud and some later masters, leaving the study of new precedents mainly to their many collections of responsa.

In some cases, however, the codes themselves (and particularly their commentaries), while still recording certain talmudic health rules and medico-religious laws, indicate that these were no longer operative in post-talmudic times. The rabbis, to justify such modification or invalidation of the original laws, argued that they had lost their validity owing to changes in time, local conditions or even nature since their enactment—a device also used by some 16th century physicians to explain discrepancies between the anatomical teachings of the ancients and the discoveries of later times.[35]

This reasoning is already found in the Talmud itself. Thus, the School of HILLEL opposed reducing the legal minimum age at which males could beget children from nine to eight years—although such cases had (according to tradition) occurred in biblical times[36] — because (they argued) "we do not make analogies with earlier generations".[37] RAV likewise desired to cut from ten to two and a half years the period of childlessness (after marriage) which renders a divorce obligatory, since "the earlier generations lived long, whereas the years of the latter generations are short".[38] But as a recognised legal principle this proposition was employed only by TOSAPHOTH and some subsequent masters of Jewish law. In this way, "changes in nature" were said to account for the ineffectiveness of talmudic medicaments,[39] for the decrease in the minimum gestation period of a viable offspring from seven or nine complete months to seven or nine incomplete months in the case of human beings,[40] and from three years to two in the case of cows,[41] and for the abrogation of laws directed against the supposed danger of uncovered liquids,[42] even numbers[43] and evil spirits.[44] Other authorities in the 15th and 16th centuries had recourse to the same principle to explain why, contrary to the Talmud, cows could produce milk before calving,[45] and why fasts during a plague increased the danger to those afflicted.[46] In the last century, the argument that nature had changed was also put forward to vindicate the omission of certain talmudic health regulations in the code of MAIMONIDES.[47] Sometimes, again, the law would change, not with nature, but with local variations (climate?), a point mentioned by TOSAPHOTH[48] and SOLOMON LURIA[49] in connection with the safety "in our lands" from the hazards of even numbers and dangerous spirits, and by KARO in regard to the talmudic restrictions on blood-letting[50] "which applied only in Babylonia".[51]

The general limitations in the efficacy of remedies mentioned or recommended in the Talmud were already recognised at an earlier date. SHERIRA Gaon, in the 10th century, commenting on the popular cures listed in the seventh chapter of the tractate *Gittin*, gave the lead. "We must tell you", he wrote, "that our sages were no physicians; they only recommended that which experience had proved helpful. Their counsels in this field are by no means laws. You must not, therefore, rely on medicines mentioned in the Talmud. Only he may use them who has had them examined and confirmed by experienced physicians, and who has the assurance that at least they can do no harm. Thus our forefathers also teach us that one may employ only those remedies of which one is certain they produce no injurious effects".[52]

This advice is very similar to the attitude adopted, centuries later, by Arab teachers to "the Prophet's Medicine" —a systematic collection of the scanty medical material furnished by the *Koran* and other Mohammedan traditions. Thus the great Arab writer IBN KHALDUN (*c.* 1400)— referring to MOHAMMED's own withdrawal of his ban on the artificial fecundation of the date palm, in view of its disastrous effects on the fruit crop ("You know better than I what concerns your worldly interests")—asserts that the Prophet's medical rules need not be followed, because his "mission was to make known to us the prescriptions of the

Divine Law, and not to instruct us in medicine and in the common practices of ordinary life".[53]

SHERIRA's views paved the way for even more radical opinions by later Jewish teachers. Accordingly, it was not only unnecessary or unwise, but positively wrong to rely on the medical prescriptions in the Talmud. Several sources mention that it was, in fact, forbidden to put the application of talmudic remedies and medicines to the test, since their failure might be attributed, not to the changed conditions of time and place, but (possibly without justification) to the limted or erroneous knowledge of the talmudic sages.[54] This consideration, it was suggested, explains the exclusion of these recommendations by MAIMONIDES and in the later codes; for the operation of such cures and treatments might lead people "to disparage our rabbis, of blessed memory".[55] Some authorities, including SOLOMON LURIA,[56] even refer to the imposition of a formal "ban by the ancient masters" on those who try out the remedies mentioned in the Talmud—other than certain specific cures.[57] But others, confirming the prohibition as such, appear to have no knowledge of such a ban.[58] Its origin, too, cannot be traced.

We may now list the relatively few instances in which such reservations regarding the validity of medical statements in the Talmud have found their way into some of the codes of Jewish law. According to the Talmud,[59] water may be heated on the Sabbath to bathe an infant before and after its circumcision, because the absence of such warm baths may endanger its life.[60] MAIMONIDES[61] and JACOB BEN ASHER[62] still codified this law almost in its original formulation. But KARO omitted it from his code, since the supposed danger no longer existed.[63] Again, the Talmud[64] mentions a rabbinic enactment prohibiting the consumption of liquids that were left uncovered, lest a snake had injected some poison into them. MAIMONIDES[65] recorded this law without qualification; but

JACOB BEN ASHER[66] and KARO, while including it in their codes, added (following TOSAPHOTH[67]): "Now-a-days, however, since snakes are no longer found in our midst, it is permitted [to consume such liquids]" (*Y.D., cxvi*.1). Similarly, ISSERLES questioned the claim in the Talmud[68] that a viable child could only be born following a pregnancy lasting for nine *full* months (unless it was a seven-months' baby)—a claim which (he asserted) "is contradicted by our senses" and refuted by practical experience[69] (*E.H., clvi*.4, gloss).

Far more frequently the modification or suspension of the Talmud's medical rules is found in the commentaries. Thus, ABRAHAM GUMBINER ruled that there was no longer any danger to health in consuming food without salt or liquids without water,[70] in neglecting the washing of hands between eating fish and meat dishes,[71] as well as in several other practices regarded as harmful by the Talmud;[72] he also prohibited all fasting in times of pestilence.[73] Other relaxations of talmudic law in these matters include the abolition of the rules against talking during meals,[74] against blood-letting on certain days,[75] and against the performance of circumcisions on cloudy days.[76] Some of these modifications are justified by the common phrase: "Since people have become accustomed not to mind—'the Lord preserveth the simple' (Psalms *cxvi*.6)"[77] i.e. He will protect from harm those who, by popular custom, ignore such rabbinic enactments intended to safeguard health. The Talmud itself uses this phrase in similar contexts on several occasions.[78] But these modifications, it is often emphasised, are all strictly confined to purely rabbinic regulations based on medical considerations; the validity of laws enjoying biblical status remains unaffected even if the advance in medical knowledge and experience seems to nullify the supposed motive for their enactment.[79]

An important element in the reference to "changes in nature", which guided the attitude of the rabbis to medical progress, was no doubt a general belief that the natural faculties of man were gradually declining with the passage of time.[80] We have already referred to the reduction in human longevity mentioned in the Talmud. NACHMA-NIDES[81] gave legal expression to the same principle when he recorded that women in his day had testified that the physiological symptoms leading to ritual impurity, as given in Talmud,[82] could no longer be observed. Later authorities explained this change as due "to the weakening of the senses and the mind in our times".[83] CHAYIM J.D. AZULAY,[84] in the 18th century, resorted to the same argument to defend the departure from the talmudic ideal[85] and practice of marrying at the age of thirteen years.

It may well be this belief in the decline of man which, on the intellectual plane, motivated the second important principle—viz., "we are no longer competent experts"—in the application of medico-religious rulings. Though of earlier origin,[86] this principle was introduced as codified law mainly by ISSERLES. He uses it frequently in relation to data or diagnoses which, according to the Talmud, could be established by certain prescribed experiments or by observation, and regarding which (he rules) our tests are no longer reliable.[87] In such cases the benefit of the doubt, which thus remains unresolved, goes to the stricter interpretation of the law. The following instances of this principle are of medical interest: KARO, as well as the earlier codes[88] still accepted the talmudic directive[89] that, if a woman died on the Sabbath "whilst she was seated in the travailing chair", a knife should be brought even through a public thoroughfare (which normally constitutes prohibited work) for opening her abdomen to remove the child in case it be found alive (*O.H.*, *cccxxx.5*). But ISSERLES adds that this is no longer done, even on weekdays, because "we are no more competent" to recognise the moment of the mother's death with sufficient accuracy to enable the child to live (*ib.*, gloss) and to prevent hastening the mother's death by a premature incision.[90] KARO, though he retained the law in its talmudic form, obviously knew of its practice no more than his glossator did.[91] Both believed that medical knowledge (or daring?) had declined so much since the times of the Talmud that the operation could no longer be carried out with safety.[92] Elsewhere ISSERLES states that "we are no longer competent" to ascertain the exact cause of death, and that we cannot, therefore, rely on a physician's opinion in this matter if it will determine the validity of a bill of divorce whose terms provided that it should become effective only if death ensued from the particular illness afflicting the husband at the time of its commission (*E.H. cxlv*.9, gloss). In a further passage ISSERLES claims that the symptoms of sterility given in the Talmud[93] can no longer be relied upon for legal purposes (*E.H., clxxii*.6, gloss). The same principle is occasionally also applied in later sources; GUMBINER,[94] for example, uses it to challenge our competence to determine whether a new-born child "has completed the months [of its gestation]".

Sufficient evidence has now been submitted to show that Jewish medical ethics, though commanding no literature of its own, is a subject of broad dimensions, built on an abundance of literary material, that the sources we shall utilise do not necessarily reflect the outlook of the time of their composition, and that the medico-religious views recorded in them are, in certain respects, flexible enough to allow for continuous revision and adjustment. The following chapters will endeavour to indicate how the leading masters of Jewish law integrated the needs of man's body with those of his soul, and point to the contribution Judaism can make to the solution of some of the most crucial moral and social problems of our own day. They may thus also bear witness to the many pilots of religious thought who, if they did not perhaps make medical history, certainly contributed massively to its record.

CHAPTER ONE

THE ATTITUDE TO MEDICINE.

HUMAN HEALING v. DIVINE PROVIDENCE
THE RIGHT TO HEAL AND THE EFFICACY OF
FAITH AND PRAYER

Sickness has not always or universally been considered an unmitigated evil to be shunned by man. SIGERIST,[1] in an analysis of the evolution which the attitude to the physical sufferer has undergone in the three chief constituents of the Western heritage, classifies the following distinct phases: Among the Semitic civilisations of the ancient orient, the sick man found himself burdened with a certain odium, since disease was believed to be the consequence of unrighteousness and to atone for it. In Greece, again, illness was looked upon as a great curse, destroying the ideal of perfect harmony (health); the sick were regarded as inferior. Finally, Christianity introduced a "revolutionary change" in the outlook on disease by addressing itself, as "the religion of healing", especially to the weak and the sick. Suffering assumed the character of purification and became grace; it was the friend of the soul and ennobled the afflicted. Thus, the sick man occupied a "preferential position" in society.

The attitude of Jewish law to disease and healing combines elements of all three approaches. On the one hand, it strongly encourages and facilitates man's struggle against, and escape from, the grip of illness, which is considered a profound misfortune.[2] On the other hand, it implicitly subscribes to the belief in the atoning power of physical suffering and in its moral motivation.[3] But, at the same time, it also affirms the view that disease forges an especially close link between God and man; the Divine Presence Itself, as it were, "rests on the head of the sickbed"[4] (*Y.D.*, *cccxxxv*.3). In this attempt to blend concepts of human suffering originally quite incongruous into a single system, Judaism could not evade the crux of the theological problem created by man's surrender to the physician's "interference" with the deliberate designs of Providence.

Every religious system has recognised this inner conflict between the essentially divine (and therefore providential) character of disease and the human efforts, through medical treatment, to mitigate or, if possible, to frustrate its effect. For the monotheistic faiths this problem was particularly acute. The solutions offered, which varied widely and significantly, materially affected the entire course of medical history, often in its most decisive aspects.

Basically, the difficulty could be, and was, resolved by three completely divergent approaches. The most radical, and perhaps logical, was to reject medical aid altogether, making suffering something to be borne, if not welcomed, as a fated visitation from God; any effort to escape from it would be tantamount to an unwarranted attack on the divine scheme of life. This fatalistic attitude appealed to the ascetic tendencies of certain small Jewish sects[5] and of considerably larger and more authoritative groups in early and medieval Christianity.[6] The second approach was simply to ask whether there was any less moral justification for curing illness, especially where it was caused by human negligence, than for the application of water to the thirsty throat or of the plough to the virgin soil. On the contrary, it was the prerogative and duty of man to harness his intellect and the resources of nature in his conquest of disease as in his striving for prosperity. This solution was favoured by some talmudic savants.[7] MAIMONIDES[8] also would seem to adopt it. As we shall observe, LUTHER solved the problem on similar lines. Finally, there was the view which, while it retained the concept of disease as a divine visitation, still affirmed the legality of human intervention. Its advocates resolved the conflict by resorting to the "divine sanction"; God expressly granted man the right to cure disease in the Bible, and it was on the strength of such scriptural sanction that the physician was permitted to practise his art.

This opinion, already found in the Talmud,[9] ultimately prevailed in the codes of JACOB BEN ASHER[10] and KARO: "The *Torah* gave permission to the physician to heal; moreover, this is a religious precept, and it is included in the category of saving life" (*Y.D.*, *cccxxxvi*.1). The reference here is to R. YISHMAEL's interpretation of the phrase: " . . . he shall cause him to be thoroughly healed" (*Ex. xxi*.19). The context deals with one's responsibility for the treatment of wounds or injuries inflicted on another. From this passage the rabbis quite logically deduced that the Bible explicitly warranted the employment of physicians and medical cures.

Christian schoolmen in the Middle Ages resorted to the same theological device in quoting the verse "The Most High created medicines from the earth" (*Ecclus. xxxviii*.4) as evidence of divine sanction for human healing; this argument was used specifically to prove that such action was "not contrary to the Catholic faith".[11] MOHAMMED likewise encouraged the medical care of the body by claiming that "God has not inflicted diseases upon us without at the same time giving us the remedy".[12]

In Jewish sources, the reasons underlying this sanction and the need for it have been variously explained. RASHI simply states that such permission is required "lest it be said that God smites and man heals".[13] TOSAPHOTH[14] and ADRETH[15] similarly point out that, without such sanction, "he who heals might appear as if he invalidated a divine decree". But NACHMANIDES,[16] followed by JACOB BEN ASHER,[17] regards the warrant as essential because doctors might otherwise hesitate to treat patients for fear of fatal consequences—"seeing there is an element of danger in every medical intervention: that which heals one, may kill another". The 18th century commentator DAVID PARDO[18] follows the same trend when he argues that the biblical reference presupposes the existence of physicians; there would be none, were they liable to penalties for injuries arising from erroneous treatment.

As has been rightly observed,[19] no code ever existed among Jews which imposed a prohibition on healing. Yet, the classic codes of ALFASI, MAIMONIDES and ASHERI omit the talmudic reference to the biblical sanction. This omission, particularly in the case of MAIMONIDES, has surprised some scholars.[20] Others have justified it by explaining that the sanction merely *permits* the practice of medicine, whereas the healing of the sick is, in fact, *obligatory*.[21] This obligation, as MAIMONIDES expressly asserts in his *Mishnah Commentary*,[22] is derived from the biblical commandment "thou shalt restore it to him" (*Deut. xxii.*2) which, according to the Talmud,[23] includes "the restoration of one's fellow-man's body" (i.e. his health) as well as his (lost) property. NACHMANIDES, again, in addition to the warrant for medical practice on the basis of the phrase " . . . he shall cause him to be thoroughly healed" already noted, also considers the injunction to love one's neighbour as oneself (*Lev. xix.*18) as a mandate for the infliction of wounds by surgical treatment.[24] Finally, there is the view of the 15th century commentator and philosopher ISAAC ARAMA,[25] who proves from the Pentateuch narratives (e.g., the Patriarchs' efforts to save themselves when in danger) and legislation (e.g., the duty to construct parapets around roofs for the prevention of accidents[26]) that man must not rely on miracles or Providence only, but must himself do whatever he can to maintain his life and health.

While these authorities evidently saw some necessity for "proving" that the Bible did not object to medical inter-

vention, it should be remembered that this method of exegesis also stemmed from the general outlook of rabbinic
Judaism. In their endeavours to subordinate life in all its
phases to the service of God, they aimed at finding some
scriptural authority for every possible sphere of activity.[27]
Contrary to the assumption of some scholars,[28] therefore, the
efforts to find biblical support in defence of medical treatment need not be construed as evidence for the existence
of schools of thought which opposed human healing. In
isolated cases such schools did exist, particularly among the
Karaites who strongly objected to the use of physicians and
medicines;[29] but it is quite improbable that the rabbis' recourse to these biblical passages arose from a practical consideration of such opposition.

To some Jewish scholars the sanction did, however, suggest certain limitations. The chief biblical reference to the
legality of healing deals, as we have seen, with the treatment of injuries resulting from an assault. Hence, the scope
of the mandate might be regarded as covering only injuries
caused by man, especially since their treatment does not, in
any event, raise the same theological difficulty as the cure
of "divinely-inflicted" ills.[30] While, according to TOSA-
PHOTH,[31] the mandate's validity is expressly extended to
"diseases that come through Heaven", ABRAHAM IBN
EZRA,[32] in fact, restricts the sanction to the healing of
"wounds and injuries which appear externally", whereas
internal diseases are in the hands of God only. The same
distinction is made by the early 14th century Cabbalist and
exegete BACHYAH.[33] In the second half of the 18th century we meet a similar distinction in the halachic commentary of JONATHAN EYBESCHUETZ;[34] he does not,
however, mention the earlier protagonists of this view.
NACHMANIDES,[35] while not accepting this distinction,
applies the sanction only to the physician's right to heal,
but not to the patient's right to engage his services. This
reservation was already attacked by ARAMA[36] as illogical,

since it would be contradictory to permit the doctor to heal whilst forbidding the patient to be healed. Various attempts have been made to explain this apparent anomaly.[37] These mainly academic distinctions of IBN EZRA and NACH-MANIDES—both said to have been practising physicians[38]—can be understood only in the context of their cosmological outlook in which the perfect man, not being subject to the natural law, is not in need of doctors or medicines.[39] Not to seek medical help is, therefore, to be taken as a blessing rather than as a religious law.

Among the teachers of traditional Judaism the rejection of medicine as a legitimate art is virtually unknown. Even the East European mystical movement of Hassidism (though, as we shall see, it occasionally tolerated a form of faith-healing) possessed only one great leader who was radically opposed to the application of medical aid; this was R. NACHMAN of Brazlav, the great-grandson of the movement's founder, R. ISRAEL BAAL SHEM TOV.[40] R. NACHMAN's bitterness, his cynical hatred of physicians, may have been due to the unhappy personal experiences which led to his death from tuberculosis in 1811.[41] But apart from this isolated instance, Jewish thought and practice invariably concurred with the views expressed by BAAL SHEM TOV's younger contemporary, CHAYIM J.D. AZULAY, in the 18th century: "Nowadays one must not rely on miracles, and the sick man is in duty bound to conduct himself in accordance with the natural order by calling on a physician to heal him. In fact, to depart from the general practice by claiming greater merit than the many saints [in previous] generations, who were cured by physicians, is almost sinful on account of both the implied arrogance and the reliance on miracles when there is danger to life. . . . Hence, one should adopt the ways of all men and be healed by physicians . . . ".[42]

Indeed, none of the aforementioned reservations, academic or otherwise, found their way into any code of Jewish law. The reference to the biblical sanction is combined with the unqualified statement that the physician's right to heal is a religious duty and that he who shirks this responsibility is regarded as shedding blood (*Y.D.*, *cccxxxvi*.1). The law also rules emphatically: "It is forbidden to rely on miracles or to endanger one's life" (*Y.D.*, *cxvi*.5, gloss), and the codes list several detailed injunctions for the protection of one's life and limb (*Y.D.*, 1*x*.2; *cxvi*.1-7; *H.M.*, *cdxxvii*.7-10; and *O.H.*, *clxx*.16). In fact, regulations concerning health must be observed more stringently than ritual laws (*O.H.*, *clxxiii*.2; and *Y.D.*, *cxvi*.5, gloss).

We may now make a comparative survey of the attitude of Islam and Christianity before examining some practical implications of the teachings of all three faiths. MO-HAMMED, as already mentioned, gave every encouragement to the care of the body and its health. Moslem rulers generally promoted medical science and practice. Islam, like Judaism, also codified the precepts of health and hygiene and made these religiously binding on all.[43] Arab physicians thus shared with their Jewish colleagues an almost complete absence of religious restrictions on the practice of their art.[44] But this held true only in the earlier stages of Moslem medicine. Later, this tolerant outlook gave way to an increasingly inhibiting attitude. From the time of the 11th century religious teacher, AL-GHAZALI, there was a tendency to oppose scientific enquiries "because they lead to the loss of belief in the origin of the world and in the Creator".[45] Consequently, in the later phases of medieval medicine, the relative freedom of Jewish physicians from the religious restraints which restricted Arab doctors tended to increase the former's preponderance.[46] The growing divergence of views is well illustrated by their respective attitude to AVERROES who "opposed the combination of religion and science";[47] while Islam, and the Church, hated him on that score, Jews developed "Averroism" with enthusiasm up to the 16th century.[48] Thus ended eventually the long and significant Arab-Jewish partnership which sprang from a remarkable community of outlook and contributed so illustriously to the finest chapter of medical history in the Middle Ages. ·

Medieval Christianity had inherited rather different, and in some respects more contradictory, traditions of the relationship between religion and medicine. A medical historian has warned with some justice against blaming theology for all the aberrations of medieval folk-medicine showing a religious colouring. The diversity of the literary material used to testify to the Christian attitude to medicine is enormous. But reliable investigations should be limited, in the same scholar's judgment, to "authoritative theology", as expressed in papal decretals, Council decrees and similar sources.[49] A number of these documents give evidence of an uncompromisingly favourable outlook on physical healing. The *Gratian Decretals*, for instance, show that the medical treatment of disease was regarded as a Christian duty in that one must not rely on miracles[50]—in fact, this duty bore the character at least of *"exhortatio"*;[51] that a wilful refusal leading to injury or illness was considered as suicide;[52] and that there was no conflict between Providence and medical treatment.[53] Some of these principles were also confirmed by THOMAS AQUINAS[54] and ANTONINUS.[55] It will be noted that the references to "duty", "miracles", "suicide" and "Providence" are strikingly similar to the corresponding concepts taught by Jewish law.

But the anti-medical elements of Christian teachings possessed roots no less deep and authentic. We have the authority of as dispassionate a scholar as ALLBUTT for the assertion that already " . . . the Church Fathers, or most of them, . . . indignantly rejected material means of healing; for to make use of such means was to deify earthly things".[56] The leading historians of medieval medicine are almost unanimous in ascribing its stagnation largely to the influence of the Christian views of life. PUSCHMANN speaks of the direct opposition to science of " . . . Christian dogma when it [i.e. science] made the manifestations of nature, as e.g. the human body—which the Christian faith held as impure and worthless, if not despicable—the subject matter of its study".[57] OSLER,[58] too, attributes the "desolation" of medieval medicine, among other factors, to the disregard of science by Christianity, which looked upon the "vile body" as the one barrier between man and his redemption. SINGER[59] likewise assigns the cause for the "Dark Ages" of medicine partly to the negative Christian attitude to life and the human body, regarded as contemptible and unimportant. As evidence of this outlook, he refers to the figures of skeletons and decaying corpses often found on tombs, finger-rings, house-ornaments and in manuscript illuminations. At times the aversion to the physical care of the body was particularly pronounced. In the 4th century, St. JEROME had said that "the purity of the body and its garments meant the impurity of the soul", and, a thousand years later, the expression "odour of sanctity" symbolised the relationship between filth and holiness in the lives of many saints, monks and nuns.[60] In LUTHER's time, Dr. CARLSTADT still preached against calling on physicians, and in 1656 DES MARETS had to prove in detailed argument that "a Christian who is ill may solicit the physician's help".[61] Traces of this attitude outlived the Middle Ages. Whether certain prophylactic measures conflicted with the decrees of God still formed the subject of a French parliamentary enquiry to the theological faculty at the Sorbonne in 1763 and of a question addressed to the philosopher IMMANUEL KANT.[62]

The one-sided emphasis on the hereafter was not the only factor in the retarding effect of Christianity on medical progress. Christian theology used only speculative means, involving sophism and casuistry, to develop its own dogmas; hence observation and experiment disappeared also from other branches of knowledge, with authority enthroned as the sole guide to intellectual endeavour.[63] Consequently, the doctor's task was not to observe and examine his patient, but to explain the teachings of HIPPOCRATES and GALEN[64]—an approach often embodied in the medical syllabuses laid down in papal bulls.[65] In this way, Christianity promoted the dogmatic-compilatory direction of medicine well into the 16th century.[66] This factor may also account for the Christian tendency to oppose the application of doubtful cures[67] and experimental operations.[68] Naturally, such handicaps gravely hampered the development of medical science.[69]

These varied religious teachings assume particular significance when we study their impact on some practical aspects of medicine in more limited spheres. In the long conflict between religious and medical claims for prior consideration, there are probably no criteria by which its outcome can be more reliably assessed than the attitude to flight from deadly epidemics and the extent to which prayer and faith were resorted to as the sole therapeutic agents in the fight against disease.[70]

ATTITUDE TO FLIGHT FROM PLAGUES

No form of physical affliction lent itself more convincingly to a theurgical interpretation of illness as a divine visitation than the fearful ravages wrought by outbreaks of the plague. As LECKY poignantly observed, "if men are employed in some profession which compels them to inhale steel filings or noxious vapours, or if they live in a pestilential marsh, the diseases that result from these conditions are not regarded as a judgment or a discipline, for the natural cause is obvious and decisive. But if the conditions that produced the disease are very subtle and complicated, . . . if, above all, it assumes the character of an epidemic, it is continually treated as a divine judgment".[71] Indeed, the terrible effects of the many devastating epidemics, which decimated the population during the first centuries of the Common Era, may be regarded as an indispensable leaven in the rise of Christianity as a healing faith.[72] Already in the Bible, plagues were among the principal instruments of divine retribution.[73] It is, therefore, only natural that, when such calamities occurred, man's faith in his right to frustrate, and to flee from, the "providential scourge" was severely put to the test. Fatalism is always the child of desperation and anguish, never of hope or prosperity.

Jewish religious leaders in all ages have consistently urged those threatened by pestilence to put to flight without hesitation. This verdict was unanimous; there is no record of a dissenting opinion anywhere in Jewish literature. The authentic ruling on the subject is: "It is proper to flee from a town in which the plague has broken out; and it is right to evacuate the place at the commencement of the outbreak and not at its end" (*Y.D.*, *cxvi.5*, gloss). ISSERLES bases this decision on a responsum by JACOB MOLIN[74] in the first half of the 15th century, but the advice to escape rests on much earlier sources. Indeed, JEREMIAH already warned his stricken and besieged fellow-citizens in Jerusalem: "He that abideth in this city shall die by the sword, and by the famine, and by the pestilence; but he that goeth out, . . . he shall live" (*Jer. xxi.*9). The Talmud, too, counseled people: "When the plague is in town, gather your legs!"[75] Following these instructions, the Jewish spiritual guides of the 16th and 17th centuries time and again emphasised that it was proper, indeed imperative, to flee from the epidemics which raged so disastrously at that period. SOLOMON LURIA endorsed the ruling of his contemporary, ISSERLES, in a special chapter devoted to the subject. The duty to escape by flight from the plague, he maintains, devolves on all except two categories of people: those who were regarded as immune to the disease because they had once been afflicted and cured; and those who could be useful to the community by personal service. LURIA adds that "after the pestilence, however, has definitely spread one should remain in one's own house, particularly as fleeing in such a case constitutes a greater danger to those who flee among the Gentiles than the plague itself".[76] The last remark sheds a revealing light on the motive underlying the same qualification (*viz.*, not to flee "at the end" of the epidemic) by ISSERLES. Early in the 17th century, ISAIAH HOROWITZ[77] likewise confirmed that flight from the plague was the accepted Jewish practice, and he expressed surprise at the criminal negligence of parents who failed to evacuate their children from a district smitten by an outbreak of smallpox. These strictures were also repeated by YECHIEL M. EPSTEIN in his abridgement of HOROWITZ's *Shenei Luhoth Haberith*,[78] first published in 1683. GUMBINER,[79] too, refers to this complaint against parents.

While the position in favour of evading the plague was, therefore, undisputed in law and practice, the moral and religious problems created by the need to seek safety through flight did engage the attention of some scholars. BACH-YAH,[80] commenting on the directive given to MOSES and AARON: "Separate yourselves from among this congregation" (*Nu. xvi.21*), asks: What need was there for this physical separation from those about to be stricken? Was it not in God's power to smite and to save as He wished? The commentator solved the difficulty along two lines. He cites earlier authority for the view that there is no discrimination between the righteous and the wicked when the divine judgment is turned on man. Moreover, the separation of the survivors was necessary, "so that the evil air of the pestilential plague should not infect them, in the same way as it is written in regard to LOT's wife: 'But she looked back from behind him . . . ' (*Gen. xix.26*)". This is a reference to the belief, already recorded by NACH-MANIDES[81] in his commentary on the passage, that infection of plagues and other contagious diseases was spread by looking at those stricken with them.[82] Another facet of the same problem is discussed by SOLOMON DURAN[83] in the 15th century. He enquires into the *usefulness* of fleeing from the outbreak, not into the *need* for it, as BACH-YAH had done a hundred years earlier. Since the duration of a man's life is predetermined by divine judgment every New Year (he reasons), what harm could befall a person fated to survive if he stayed in the infected area, and what benefit could accrue to him who is destined to die if he escaped? After a lengthy argument, DURAN is forced to the conclusion that there are people whose length of life is not determined on New Year and that, for such, flight from pestilence is efficacious. These entirely academic speculations again show that no philosophical or theological doubts were allowed to affect the practical requirements of human life and health.

Among Christian teachers the problem already caused a good deal of embarrassment to the Church Fathers.[84] Sometimes doubts concerning the right to flee from the plague did not lead to purely academic conclusions only, nor were they confined to any one Christian denomination. Even in the 19th century, such doubts were still quite prevalent. When, for instance, a virulent outbreak of smallpox occurred in Montreal in 1885, it was soon controlled among the Protestant population through vaccination, but Catholics suffered incredible losses of life as their clergy opposed compulsory vaccination on theological grounds.[85] On the other hand, when Scotland was hit by the dreaded cholera thirty-two years earlier, it was the Presbytery of Edinburgh who caused the Moderator to address a petition to the English Home Secretary for the proclamation of a national fast by royal edict. This was regarded "as a dignified rebuke addressed to the irreligious habits of the English people who, seeing the cholera at their doors, merely occupied themselves with sanitary measures, and carnal devices to improve public health . . . ".[86] The violent controversy aroused by JENNER's discovery of vaccination—hailed with enthusiasm by ISRAEL LIPSCHUETZ and other leading rabbis[87]—has been surveyed in a special monograph.[88] Much additional material on medical practices which, in France, England and America during the 18th century, were regarded as "flying in the face of Providence" has been collected in another work.[89] Churchmen in all ages, including the present, often recoiled from the idea of defeating Providence or thwarting the divine vengeance for sin. This outlook caused the ecclesiastical condemnation of the pioneering efforts in plastic surgery by GASPARE TAGLIACOZZI in the 16th century;[90] it induced Pope LEO XII to ban the employment of the condom against syphilis in 1826;[91] it prompted the opposition to SIMPSON's use of chloroform to ease the pains of childbirth later in the same century;[92] and it animated those "who were deeply disturbed" by EHRLICH's discovery of salvarsan for the treatment of syphilis in the present century.[93]

During the 16th century, our test-case (the attitude to epidemics) engaged the special attention of LUTHER. He was asked whether it was proper for a Christian to flee when the plague broke out in Breslau in 1525. His answer is significant, and characteristic of the perplexities weighing on him and his age. On the one hand, he could not altogether conceal his admiration for those who maintain that fleeing was not permissible and who, therefore, submitted passively, but with fortitude, to death as a punishment for their sins. On the other hand, he vindicated the majority who could not be expected to demonstrate the same placid resignation to a cruel fate.[94] In arguments reminiscent of those used before him by MAIMONIDES[95] and ARAMA[96] in similar circumstances, LUTHER justified the flight from the plague by asking rhetorically whether a man might not alleviate his hunger by taking food, and by recalling the biblical heroes who promptly fled from the sword or famine to save their lives. But while LURIA (as we have seen[97]) *exempted from the duty to flee* people who could be of service to the community, LUTHER *denied the right to leave* the infected area to men holding public office or who might be needed by their relatives or neighbours.[98]

There are apparently only few Mohammedan sources on the subject. But it is recorded that, among the Turks, the Ulema declared in 1837 that every precaution against a pestilential outbreak was sinful. A little later, however, a Mufti found it expedient to state that a Moslem did not commit a religious offence if he escaped from a plague-stricken town, provided he called on the mercy of Allah.[99]

HEALING BY FAITH AND PRAYER

We can now turn to our second criterion for the religious attitude to medicine in practice: the substitution of faith and prayer for rational healing. We shall here be concerned only with religious faith-healing; the resort to other irrational cures will be discussed in the next chapter.

Recourse to religion in the face of pain or danger is not, of course, necessarily an indication of despair in the efficacy of rational means of relief. Nor need such appeal to supernatural intervention betray a tendency to reject, as either wrong or futile, the benefits of medical experience. Some of the most outstanding protagonists of rational medicine have not hesitated to confess that the success of their work depended on divine assistance, from the Hippocratic writer who taught: «ὁ ἰατρὸς τῆς φύσεως ὑπηρέτης» to the great surgeon PARE, over two millenia later, who often concluded the description of his operations with the words: *"Je le pansay, et Dieu le guarist"*.[101]

The theurgical bias of medicine did not necessarily decline with the passage of the Middle Ages. In the 14th century, the celebrated Christian physician GUY DE

CHAULIAC ridiculed " . . . the sect of women and many idiots who place patients with any disease in the hands of the saints, doing this because 'the Lord has given me what it pleases Him' "; yet, three hundred years later, another famous doctor, GUY PATIN, wrote: "What saved the king were three good blood lettings and the prayers of good people like ourselves".[102] But it was left to the medical revolutionary, PARACELSUS, to define the relationship between God and medicine in terms which approximate most closely the Jewish attitude. "All health and all diseases", he stated,[103] "come from God, and in God is the cure. Some diseases, however, do not directly come from God, but are natural (although they, too, come from God indirectly, because Nature is a manifestation of the power of God), but other diseases are sent directly from God as a punishment for our sins . . . The physician is only a servant of God who works to accomplish His will . . . The physician may cure the sick by using remedies, but it is God who makes the physician and the remedy. God does not perform miracles without man; He acts through the instrumentality of man, and restores the sick to health through the instrumentality of the physician. Therefore, the physician should be in possession of faith (in harmony with God) . . . ".

Similar sentiments have inspired many Jewish physicians in the Middle Ages to compose and recite special prayers for the success of their work, without compromising their reliance on rational cures. FRIEDENWALD[104] has collected a number of these stirring supplications for divine help. Some of them may be mentioned here as a background to the legal affirmations in the Jewish codes. Thus, the great poet-physician, JUDAH HALEVY, sang:—
"My medicines are of Thee, whether good or evil, whether strong or weak,
  It is Thou who shalt choose, not I,
  Of Thy knowledge is the evil and the fair.
  Not upon my power of healing I rely;

Only for Thine healing do I watch".[105]
The renowned physician, ABRAHAM ZACUTUS (Lusitanus) opened the first volume of his *Opera Omnia*, first published in the middle of the 17th century, with *Precept I*: "The physician should be a faithful worshipper of Divine Majesty"; yet, in discussing a medical problem elsewhere, he remarked: " . . . for we are physicians, not theologians". His second volume concluded with "a deeply pious and moving prayer of gratitude for Divine help".[106] A little later, JACOB ZAHALON, the rabbi-physician who was regarded as "one of the three most learned men of his generation", wrote a long and beautiful prayer in which he declared: "I am minded to busy myself with the practice of medicine in Thy Holy Name and through Thy assistance . . . I do not rely upon my wisdom, nor do I place my trust in the drugs and herbs and medicaments which Thou hast created, for they are but the means to fulfil Thy will and to proclaim Thy greatness and Thy providence . . . ".[107] At the beginning of the 18th century, we find an anonymous doctor's prayer to be recited every morning; this was republished in a *Book of Devotion* in 1867.[108] In 1863, there appeared a German translation of a "Daily Prayer of a Physician before Visiting His Patients". This "very lofty and beautiful prayer" gained much fame and wide currency as the "Prayer of MAIMONIDES" to whom it was often ascribed, but it is probably the work of MOSES MENDELSOHN's physician, MARCUS HERZ.[109] All these fine compositions emphasise the ethical and moral responsibilities of the physician as a divine agent in the alleviation of human suffering. While they all recognise God as the ultimate Healer of disease, they also assert the indispensable part played by the physician, his art and his medicines in the "harmonious preservation in all its beauty of the body, which is the envelope of the immortal soul"—to quote from the "Prayer of MAIMONIDES".

We here interrupt the pursuit of Jewish sources in order

to give some parallels of the Christian approach to faith and prayer in medicine. Faith-cures were a dominant factor in the acts of healing wrought by JESUS[110] and also in the Apostolic age.[111] The most vivid example of faith-healing in the Patristic Church is given by St. AUGUSTINE.[112] He tells the story of a man at Carthage who was only partially cured by an operation for fistula, but totally restored by prayer. He also relates how a Carthaginian lady was relieved of an incurable cancer of the breast by the sign of a cross made over her. Towards the end of the 13th century, the Christian ARNOLD of Villanova—claimed as "the best known physician" of the period and "one of the most interesting figures of the Middle Ages"[113]—prescribed many prayers to certain saints as the best means of healing the particular diseases with which they were associated as patrons.[114] Comparing the "dream oracles in Christian shrines" with the pagan cult of incubation in the temples of AESCULAPIUS, a modern scholar finds the "chief difference" in "that the saints are represented as indignant at any suggestion that their cures are not miraculous throughout, and inflict severe punishment on a rash physician who declared that some of their prescriptions might be found in GALEN and HIPPOCRATES".[115] For most of the Common Era, the Virgin MARY in particular was worshipped as the intercessor for the sick. In France alone about forty churches were dedicated to her in her healing capacity, bearing such names as *Notre-Dame des Malades, N.-D. des Infirmes, N.-D. du Remède, N.-D. de Santé,* etc.[116] To this day, the promise of miraculous cures has remained an important element in the propagation of the Catholic faith.[117] Indeed, in most Christian denominations faith-healing in one form or another is now once more gaining tremendously in popularity and official support.[118]

But there are only few periods in which the blind belief in the sole efficacy of faith and prayer obscured rational medicine altogether. There is much logic in the argument:

"If the popes had been interested only in the miraculous healing of disease . . . , they would have had no physicians in regular attendance on them".[119] Numerous faithful devotees of the Church, including some of her most illustrious dignitaries,[120] were themselves medical practitioners of no mean standing. There are also no indications that recourse to natural means of healing ever came under any formal ban. But the authentic account of the Roman Catholic attitude to cures by prayer and faith is sufficiently at variance with Jewish teachings to show that, in this respect, a considerable gulf separates the views of the two faiths. "The Church's teaching", it is stated authoritatively,[121] "is not that all the ailing are to go to such places [as, e.g., Lourdes] to be cured, nor that all those who go there will be sure of a cure, but that some of them for special reasons will be granted the favour of a cure as a demonstration that the arm of the Lord is not shortened and that wonders of healing are being worked in our day. The Church has been very careful to insist that there should be proper investigation of the patient's history and the proper diagnosis of their actual condition made by physicians. Only when there is assurance of a cure of physical and not merely psychoneurotic disease is any question raised of a miraculous cure".

The belief in the curative powers of religious shrines and saintly relics is unknown among the Jews. To be sure, it is reported that to this day sick people are carried to the synagogue in Cairo bearing the name of MAIMONIDES to sleep there hoping to obtain healing through the spirit of the great physician,[122] but our information is that these pilgrims are mainly Arabs. A similar custom is known among Moslems who visit the tomb of AVICENNA at Hammadan where "cures are said to be not uncommon".[123] The nearest Jewish parallel to this outlook is to be found among the Hassidic "wonder-rabbis" in modern times. Some of these occasionally resorted to faith-healing, but— as a leading medical historian has testified—"their cures were generally limited to moral or hygienic prescriptions and to the use of certain prayers, formulae or cryptograms . . . Their medical system was of only the mildest sort; its suggestive therapy was often educational, always fantastic, but certainly not dangerous".[124]

The relevant references to prayer in the codes of Jewish law are few but significant. A prayer for the sick, based on the wording of Jeremiah *xvii*.14, is to be recited three times every weekday among the *Nineteen Benedictions* (*O.H., cxvi*); this is included in the statutory Jewish prayer-book.[125] Provision is also made for the insertion of a special intercession for the recovery of a sick relative or other specified individual[126] (*O.H., cxix*.1). The purpose of these petitions is to "seek mercy" from God. That is also the principal object of the obligation to visit the sick; "and whoever visits the sick without pleading for mercy has not fulfilled the precept" (*Y.D., cccxxxv*.4, gloss). The law also lays down a formula for the success of medical treatment about to be administered: "May it be Thy will, o Lord our God, that this treatment shall be a healing unto me, for Thou art a gratuitous Healer"[127] (*O.H., ccxxx*.4). Upon the safe deliverance from any illness it is obligatory to recite a special benediction of thanksgiving in public[128] (*O.H., ccxix*.1 and 8); but ISSERLES limits this to the restoration from dangerous diseases (*ib.*, gloss).

Detailed regulations governed the proclamation of special fasts,[129] accompanied by the blowing of the *Shofar* horn,[130] whenever a city was struck by an outbreak of the plague or other diseases in epidemic proportions, such as diphtheria, delirious fever and certain types of skin infection[131] (*O.H., dlxxvi*.2-5). We have already noted[132] that the obligation to fast in times of pestilence was subsequently revoked. There are also records of special prayers against the pestilential scourge, such as the plague-prayer written by R. SOLOMON BEN R. MORDECAI of Meseritz (printed in 1602 with the approbation of MOR-

DECAI JAFFE and other rabbis). Another rabbi composed a liturgical poem against the threat of smallpox among children; published thirteen years later, it was included in the penitential liturgy of the Polish rite.[133]

Apart from these public appeals for divine intervention to stave off disease and to secure relief, Jewish law also provides for the resort to more mystical media. Following the ancient Jewish belief that the prayers of the righteous are especially efficacious,[134] ISSERLES records the view of some medieval authorities advising people who have a patient in their house to repair to the "scholar of the town", so that he shall "seek mercy" for the sufferer (*Y.D., cccxxxv.* 10, gloss). The *New Testament* offers similar counsel: "Is there any sick among you? let him call for the elders of the church; and let them pray over him, anointing him with oil in the name of the Lord. And the prayer of faith shall save the sick . . . " (Epistle of James, *v.*14 and 15). Some scholars assume that these verses betoken a belief in the sufficiency of prayer and the rejection of all but theurgical cures,[135] but we would scarcely be justified in inferring that ISSERLES's advice was meant to take the place of rational means of healing. He further adds: "It was also a custom to recite a blessing for the sick in the synagogue and to give them a new name therein; for a change of name tears up the [evil] decree against one"[136] (*ib*).

At the same time, the law severely limited the legitimate recourse to supernatural agencies. "He who whispers an incantation over a wound or over a sick person and expectorates and then recites a verse from the *Pentateuch* has no share in the world to come; if he does not expectorate, he still commits an offence;[137] but in cases of danger to life, all is permitted" (*Y.D., clxxix.*8), because, "although such charms are of no avail, the rabbis have allowed them when life is in danger, so as to prevent the distraction of the patient's mind"[138] (*ib.*, 6). To substitute faith-cures by prayer for rational healing is even more emphatically condemned in the following ruling: "If a child is stricken, one must not read a scriptural verse, nor place a scroll of the Law, over it" (*ib.*, 9). For "the words of the *Torah*", explains MAIMONIDES,[139] "are given not to heal the body, but to heal the soul". Scriptural passages may, however, always be recited for the protection of healthy persons from affliction and injury (*ib.*, 10). In this case, such readings serve merely a prophylactic, not therapeutic, purpose, and one is not tempted to trust their efficacy.[140]

These laws indicate unmistakably that, while every encouragement was given for the sick to exploit their adversity for moral and religious ends and to strengthen their faith in recovery by prayer, confidence in the healing powers of God was never allowed to usurp the essential functions of the physician and of medical science. Judaism repudiates, therefore, as altogether incompatible with its religious teachings, the doctrine of "Christian Science" and similar movements, even when they are completely divorced from their Christological associations.[141]

The frequency with which Jewish law consistently subscribes to medical measures to combat disease, and the long history of the rabbis' resort to medicine as their favourite profession, shows how wrong it is to speak with some historians[142] of "the theurgical character of Jewish medicine", unless indeed the constant reminder of the physician's dependence on the "Healer of all flesh" can be construed to bear out such a claim. The wholly positive attitude to medicine evidenced in these pages must, moreover, decisively qualify the critical verdict on the rabbinic approach to science which finds that " . . . it is a special feature of talmudic preoccupation that it tends to occupy the whole area of thought as do few other studies; for the Talmud is not only a subject of study, it is a habit of thought, a cast of mind, a way of life. The practical test lies in the historical record. Very few if any talmudists have made contributions to science. Why should this be? The answer must be in terms of Jewish sociology or psychology . . . ".[143] This thoughtful statement is substantially correct and yet incomplete. In the sphere of medicine, it is true, Jews have scarcely been noted for any outstanding discoveries or pioneering theories outside the modern period. But this lack of scientific creativeness was by no means restricted to students of the Talmud, and it cannot be ascribed exclusively to the effect of such studies.[144] Moreover, this deficiency may well be more than offset by what is, perhaps, a far more momentous contribution to medical progress: the maintenance and uncompromising encouragement, throughout the Middle Ages, of an eminently sound approach to disease and its cure. It was in such soil, freed from its weeds of quackery and superstition, and fertilised in great measure by talmudic traditions, that the seeds of enquiry and experiment eventually, in the period following the 16th century, bore such rewarding fruit.

CHAPTER TWO

IRRATIONAL MEDICAL BELIEFS.

SUPERSTITIOUS, OCCULT and SCATOLOGICAL CURES

The evolution of medicine from a primitive fight against evil spirits, demons, witches and astrological omens into a rational science was a long and tedious process. The modern outlook on disease and healing as the manifestation and treatment of purely natural phenomena only dates from the 17th century. Popular beliefs in the grossest superstitions even among civilised peoples to the present day show how difficult it is to dislodge the deeply-rooted faith in supernatural and occult forces. Throughout almost the length of human history, the disposition of the stars was considered a more potent cause of illness than indifference to cleanliness. Amulets and magic formulae ranked equally with herbs and minerals among the main *materia medica*, while impostors skilled in sorcery and witchcraft competed successfully with the scholastically proficient alumni of the medical schools as advisers of the sick.

There were, of course, periods when some gleams of reason penetrated the clouds of obscurantism. The medical systems of classic Egypt and Greece, in particular, had been remarkably free from the aberrations of sophistry and intellectual blindness. Yet, among the often quite rational prescriptions in the Egyptian *papyri* we also find references to magic and exorcism.[1] In the opinion of one scholar, "there cannot be the slightest doubt that Egyptian medicine is the direct offspring of Egyptian magic, and that it never became really emancipated from its parent".[2] In Greece, again, Hippocratic medicine flourished side by side with the cult of AESCULAPIUS whose popularity among the masses remained virtually unaffected by the early progress of medical science.[3] GALEN himself is said to have sought healing in a temple of AESCULAPIUS[4] and to have recommended amulets and other charms for various diseases.[5] The Greek assault on human credulity and superstition met with a notable, even relatively lasting, success; but eventually, with the decay of the civilisation born a thousand years earlier, rational medicine also retreated before the wave of unreason and mysticism in the first few centuries of the Current Era. The introduction of magical elements into classical medicine was due mainly to the two Greek writers, ALEXANDER of Tralles and AETIUS of Amida, both of the 6th century;[6] thereafter the essential characteristics of European medicine, with comparatively few exceptions, differed little from what they had been for more than a millenium before the emergence of Hellenistic thought and culture.

To appreciate the historical background to the relevant Jewish literature, a further consideration is necessary. Due to a variety of factors, historical and especially perhaps religio-cultural, neither Egypt nor Greece—the two homes of rational medicine in ancient times—appears to have exerted any material influence on the scientific outlook of the Talmud. The foremost historian of talmudic medicine, PREUSS, regards it as significant that there is no trace in the Talmud of the three chief factors in the Egyptian system of dietetics and prophylactics: the use of enemas, sneezing-stimulants and emetics.[7] Again, although scores of Greek names occur in the Talmud, none (as has been observed[8]) is of a man of science. It is perhaps also not without significance that even the *Zohar*, in discussing the religious attitude to healing, of all classical physicians mentions only KRITO.[9] It is, therefore, apparent that whatever foreign influences were brought to bear on the development of talmudic thought came from the East rather than the West, particularly when it is remembered that it was the Babylonian Talmud, and not its Palestinian counterpart, which became the accepted guide to Jewish religious life.

The countries in and near Mesopotamia were not merely the cradle of human civilisation; they also represented the original home of astrology and the occult virtues. As a specialised study[10] has shown, on the basis of numerous sources, it was particularly in Babylonia and Assyria that the widespread *"Volksmedizin"* still practised today had its origin. Their ancient medical systems were, almost entirely, of an irrational character. Among the Parsees, "those who cured diseases by prayer alone were looked upon as the most excellent doctors; they were, so to speak, 'doctors of doctors'. Then came those who ordered medicinal herbs, and the lowest place was assigned to those who handled the knife".[11] The very word "Chaldean" (Babylonian) is used as a synonym with "soothsayer".[12] Babylonia possessed no medical schools as Egypt did, and its system of medicine was mainly of a supernatural order[13] in which it was "the task of the priest-physician to discover and interpret the intention of the gods in order to placate them".[14] Such, then, was the cultural background in which the foundations of rabbinic law were laid; it was in this climate of magic and superstition that the medical concepts of the Jewish people and its leaders first took shape.

In the middle ages, too, Jews found themselves mostly in an environment where the popular form of medical thought and practice was of the crudest order. As an example of the widespread belief in supernatural forces, reference might be made to the extraordinary part played by astrology in medieval medicine. As late as 1699, the Paris Faculty discussed the thesis: "Whether comets were harbingers of disease".[15] At Bologna University astrology was one of the regular studies in the medical department.[16] No less a scholar than ROGER BACON had stated: "If a doctor is ignorant of 'astronomy' [i.e. astrology], his medical treatment will be dependent upon chance and fortune", while another doctor had asserted early in the 14th century: "Those doctors who are ignorant of astronomy kill many patients".[17] The common belief in the effect of heavenly bodies on illness is well illustrated by the term "influenza", short for "*influenza coelestia*".[18] To this day, the long-lived association between medicine and astrology is still symbolically indicated by the ℞-sign at the head of doctors' prescriptions—probably a remnant of Jupiter's zodiac sign ♃, used on medical prescriptions since shortly after the beginning of the Common Era.[19] The irrational outlook on medicine, therefore, was not peculiar to ignorant laymen alone; its universality was virtually unchallenged in medieval times.

Whether the human addiction to unreasoned beliefs has, in fact, produced only negative effects in the wider sphere of social relations is open to some doubt. In his learned "defence of superstition", the leading authority in this field, FRAZER, has put forward a convincing claim that "among certain races and at certain times, superstition has strengthened the respect for government . . . , private property . . . , marriage . . . , and human life . . . ".[20] In any case, it is not, of course, the task of theology or religious leadership to correct all human illusions and errors of scientific judgment, and it would be illogical to hold the teachings of religion responsible for the persistence of such fallacious beliefs as are strictly outside its province. There is, therefore, nothing intrinsically irreligious in the approbation of medical teachings which do not correspond with the more enlightened outlook of our age, except in so far as these teachings may involve idolatrous practices[21] or resort to remedies causing greater spiritual damage than physical benefits.

The reality of demons, magic and other occult virtues has been acknowledged by religious guides of all faiths. In

Christianity, the tradition of exorcising people "possessed of devils" goes back to the New Testament, where such cases are quite frequently found,[22] though there is no mention of them in the Hebrew Bible.[23] In the 5th century, St. AUGUSTINE declared: "All diseases of Christians are to be ascribed to demons",[24] and this belief was shared by ORIGEN, TERTULLIAN and GREGORY of Nazianzus.[25] Pope INNOCENT VIII issued a bull to provide the faithful with an efficacious formula for exorcising incubuses who assailed the chastity of women.[26] His bull *"Summis Desiderantis"* of 1484, which regarded witches as a factor in disease, storms and various human misfortunes, paved the way for what has been called "one of the most fearful monuments of theological reasoning and human folly"[27]—the massacre of witches, involving 100,000 victims in Germany alone, between the years 1550 and 1650.

Much of early Arabian practice, too, was based on amulets with a distinctly religious flavour. Often they would consist, for example, of a phrase from the *Koran* which had to be written by a priest on a Friday, shortly before sunset, with ink containing certain drugs.[28]

From time to time we also hear more enlightened voices raised against the prevailing superstitions in the name of theology. Already in the 7th century, St. ELIGIUS, or ELOY, Bishop of Noyon, declared in a sermon: " . . . you shall observe none of the impious customs of the pagans, neither sorcerers, nor diviners, nor soothsayers, nor enchanters; nor must you presume for any cause, or for any sickness, to consult or enquire of them, for he who commits this sin loses unavoidably the grace of baptism . . . Let none presume to hang amulets on the neck of man or beast; even though they be made by clergy, and called holy things, and contain the words of Scripture . . . , for they are fraught . . . with the poison of the Devil. . . . Moreover, as often as any sickness occurs, do not seek enchanters . . . or make devilish amulets . . . , but let him who is sick trust only in the mercy of God . . . and faithfully seek consecrated oil from the church . . . ".[29] In general, the Church offered strong opposition to witchcraft and astrology, even though the latter in particular was widely tolerated and taught everywhere.[30] But, on the whole, neither Christianity nor Islam regulated the employment of occult remedies in precise terms showing the border-line between lawful and unlawful cures involving magic and the like, as was done by the masters of Jewish law.

Jewish sources, and more especially the Talmud,[31] abound with references to the occult virtues both in legend and law. Those mentioned in the Talmud are almost all of Babylonian or Persian origin. Already HAI Gaon, the head of the Pumpaditha Academy, wrote at the end of the 10th century: "Sorcery and amulets sprang from the Sura Academy, because that lies near to Babylonia and to the house of NEBUCHADNEZZAR".[32] But in general the Talmud largely retained the biblical hostility to superstition. The next great influx of demonological and magical ideas into Jewish writings occurred mainly in the 13th century. GUEDEMANN, who has subjected the superstitious practices among Jews at that period to a very thorough comparative study, has adduced various parallels from non-Jewish sources for every such practice found in Jewish literature.[33] He has shown that the intrusion of these beliefs into Jewish works on such a large scale was an entirely new phenomenon for which no precedent could be found either in the Talmud or in rabbinic writings before the 13th century.[34] He regards the exclusive use of Latin, French or German expressions— or their crude translation into an artificial Hebrew—to describe the different categories of demons in Hebrew sources as conclusive proof that "we are not dealing here with originally Jewish superstitions".[35] It is also significant that the "epidemic of superstition" affected predominantly the Jewish communities in the Franco-German regions of the Rhineland, where the general level of enlightenment was very low, whereas the Jews of Spain and Southern France[36]—and, to a lesser degree, of Northern France, too[37] —were protected from the crudest excesses of such irrational beliefs by the superior standard of culture around them. The essentially foreign character of occult usages is again revealed by the fact that Jews evidently repaired to monks for the exorcising of evil spirits, as suggested by the refusal of AMATUS LUSITANUS to treat a Jewish boy in such circumstances.[38]

Among medieval Jewish authors, there were especially two who distinguished themselves by their enlightened attitude in this sphere.[39] ABRAHAM IBN EZRA denied in set terms the very existence of demons.[40] This was indeed "a remarkable feat for the 12th century",[41] making IBN EZRA "one of the first medieval theologians of church or synagogue to denounce the popular belief in the ubiquity of minor representations of the supernatural".[42] The second, and in many ways even more radical, protagonist of this view was MAIMONIDES[43] who even modified some halachic rulings through the re-interpretation of talmudic laws based on the existence of demons.[44]

The chief medieval codes, in their outlook on superstitious practices, contain some elements of all these diverse currents. In the main, they faithfully and uncritically reflect the approach of the talmudic savants. The great majority of the irrational beliefs these codes recorded are drawn directly from the Talmud; so is their strong opposition to sorcery and the generally sober discretion with which they repeatedly sift the true from the dubious. While incorporating some of the occult usages which had intruded into Jewish life in the earlier Middle Ages, they also assimilated important features of the enlightened attitude of MAIMONIDES, particularly his belief in the futility of magic charms and incantations[45] (*Y.D.*, *clxxix*.6). Significant, too, is their complete silence on the many folkloristic prescriptions for strengthening one's memory and the warning against acts thought to impair it—based on popular beliefs found in the Talmud[46] and medieval rabbinic writings,[47] often strikingly similar to the views on aids and impediments to memory given in Mohammedan sources.[48] There is, therefore, no complete uniformity in the general outlook on irrational practices in the classic formulations of Jewish law.

The codes naturally reveal but few clues to the rabbinic theories of aetiology. But such hints as there are betray a decidedly rational tendency and a pronounced aversion to assigning the cause of all diseases to fortuitous chance or divine punishment. Thus the law distinguishes between "accidents" and "negligence" as factors leading to illness; a person is "negligent" if he falls ill through walking in the snow in the winter or in the heat in the summer[49] (*H.M.*, *clxxvii*.2). Similarly, it was recognised that a man's reproductive faculties could be impaired by persistent immersion in water or snow (*E.H.*, *v*.13) and that disease could be aggravated by disobeying the doctor's orders (*H.M.*, *cdxx*. 20). The limitation of fate and other adventitious causes is also indicated by the assumption that superior medical skill is likely to result in more effective cures (*ib.*, 22-24). Again, the widespread mystical fear that dispositions made during life, and especially on the sickbed, for the eventuality of death may portend evil is boldly challenged as unfounded; one should advise a gravely sick person to settle his affairs in time, "and he should not be afraid of death on this account" (*Y.D.*, *cccxxxv*.7)—for "words cause neither life nor death".[50] In the same way, the dying should be encouraged to recite the confessional prayer with the assurance that "many have confessed and did not die, and many who did not confess died" (*Y.D.*, *cccxxxviii*.1).

HEALING BY WITCHCRAFT

The most important factor determining the attitude of Jewish law to superstition is, of course, its prohibition of sorcery and allied practices. The biblical interdict under this heading expressly includes, apart from sorcery and witchcraft, the practices of divination, soothsaying, the consulting of auguries, magic spells and necromancy (*Deut. xviii.*10 and 11). Moreover, the closely attached command "Thou shalt be perfect with the Lord thy God" (*ib.*, 13) is rabbinically interpreted to extend the ban to prognostication by horoscope or the casting of lots (*Y.D., clxxix.*1, and gloss).

Among the various superstitions, sorcery and witchcraft are the most severely condemned. The reality or possible efficacy of the sorcerer's powers was not in question; even the *Shulhan 'Arukh* on two occasions still objects to certain practices in the exercise of bodily functions "on account of sorcery" (*O.H., iii.*3 and 11). On the other hand, the rabbis went so far as to make some religious concessions in order to remove from Jews even the suspicion of sorcery among their Gentile neighbors. Thus the talmudic law to lower the couch as a sign of mourning[51] was no longer observed, "lest the non-Jews will say they practise witchcraft" (*Y.D., ccclxxxvii.*2). Several more concessions for this purpose can be cited from various rabbinic works.[52] It has been shown that this fear of arousing the suspicion of Gentiles originated mainly in the 15th century, when the dreaded resort to witchcraft by the "heretics" was popularly attributed to Jews, too.[53]

Whether the use of sorcery for medical ends was exempted from the prohibition was a moot and much debated question raised by various medieval authorities.[54] According to some views, the appropriate usages in the Middle Ages were no longer of the idolatrous type banned in the Bible as sorcery proper; hence, the consideration of the precept to "be perfect with the Lord" could be waived if such measures were adopted to effect cures.[55] But others held that the original ban continued to stand, and that it could be overridden only in cases of grave danger to life; all agree that sorcery may then be resorted to.[56] According to yet another view, such cures may be used only to heal conditions believed to have been likewise caused by witchcraft.[57] Rabbinic literature, in fact, mentions several instances of Jewish patients invoking the aid of sorcerers.[58] But it is significant that the practitioners consulted were nearly always non-Jews.[59]

Closely akin to sorcery are the idolatrous customs termed in rabbinic writings "the ways of the Emorites"—the nearest rabbinic equivalent to "superstitious practices" in general.[60] Their identification with the cult of another specified nation illustrates once again the Jewish consciousness that such practices were essentially foreign in origin and character,[60a] and banned because of their heathen, if not idolatrous, nature. A very long list of acts falling within this category is given in the Talmud, particularly in the *Tosephta*.[61] But the Talmud expressly excludes from this category "anything done for the sake of healing".[62] The codes, too, accept this ruling (*O.H.*, *ccci*.27); hence, it is permitted (even on Sabbaths) to carry as amulets the egg of a certain species of locust (against ear-ache), the tooth of a fox (against insomnia or drowsiness), or a nail from the gallows (against swelling)[63] (*ib.*).

MEDICAL CHARMS AND INCANTATIONS

The rabbis often discussed the question whether incantations and amulets were, in principle, included among the general provisions regarding "the ways of the Emorites".[64] ADRETH,[65] who dealt with this issue at great length, inclines to the view that the ban extends only to the practices expressly enumerated in the Talmud. ASHERI[66] also rules that charms used for the promotion of health are covered by the exemption of "anything done for the sake of healing". But RASHI[67] holds that the exemption does not include charms, although even he appears to restrict the prohibition of magic therapy only to acts not performed on the patient himself.[68] KARO decides that all magic measures are permitted, so long as their futility has not been conclusively exposed by trial;[69] but he adds that there are some who object to any "untested" amulet as belonging to "the ways of the Emorites"[70] (*ib.*). In this latter view he follows MAIMONIDES, who permits only such supernatural cures as have been found efficacious on the evidence of physicians, particularly when their employment would violate any religious law.[71] KARO also agrees with MAIMONIDES that such charms as whispering an incantation over a scorpion's bite "are of no avail whatever"; they are permitted only in cases of grave danger, "so as not to distract the patient's mind" (*Y.D., clxxix.*6)—that is, to calm him by suggestive treatment.[72] As with sorcery, the practices listed as belonging to "the ways of the Emorites" are likewise, in the opinion of various authorities, to be treated as heathen beliefs only "in the former times" when idolatry was rampant.[73] The 13th century *Sepher Hasidim*, for instance, mentions with approval several practices which had been prohibited in the Talmud as "Emorite" customs, because— as a commentator[74] explains—they were no longer peculiar to the pagan cult of the "Emorites" who had long ceased to be identified with them.

Sharply differentiated from sorcery are some supernatural aids to therapy, especially incantations and amulets to which reference is made most frequently in the codes. The general attitude to their employment, as far as they border on sorcery or idolatry, has already been considered. It now remains to collect and classify these distinct beliefs and customs, largely on the basis of the many quite incidental references to them in the codifications of Jewish law.

The medical effectiveness of incantations was, as we have seen, never in doubt. But that such procedures were regarded as quite harmless is shown by the permission to resort to heathens for cures by the whispering of charms, notwithstanding the general ban on accepting medical treatment or drugs from them "because we are afraid of bloodshed" (*Y.D.*, *clv*.1), there being no danger to the patient's life in this case.[75] Incantations to heal a scorpion's bite are permitted even on the Sabbath (*Y.D.*, *clxxix*.6), despite the rabbinic objection to indulgences normally incompatible with the spirit of that holy day.[76] Similarly, it is allowed to charm snakes or scorpions to prevent injury by them (*ib.*, 7), and such acts are not deemed to violate the Sabbath law against hunting or capturing animals (*O.H.*, *cccxxviii*.45). But there are restrictions—detailed in the preceding chapter[77] —on the incantatory recitation of scriptural verses over wounds or stricken children, unless life is in danger.

The amulets mentioned in our sources usually were pendants containing some written text—presumably a mystical formula or biblical verses. These were generally worn by the user at all times to cure, or more often to prevent, certain ailments.[78] Various other objects, too, are mentioned as efficacious against specific complaints. We have already referred to some talismans and their purpose.[79] To prevent or heal bruises, a coin tied to the sole of the foot was worn (*O.H.*, *ccci*.28); it was suggested that the healing properties of this talmudic remedy[80] were derived "from the moisture exuded by the silver of the coin and also from the imprint stamped upon it".[81] Finally, mention is made of a "preserving stone" (*O.H.*, *ccciii*.24) which, as was widely believed in ancient times, was supposed to guard the wearer against the danger of miscarriage.[82]

Regarding the use of amulets in general, a distinction is made between their prophylactic and therapeutic employment in the following ruling: "It is permitted to make medical use of amulets, even if they contain [divine] names; similarly, it is allowed to wear amulets containing scriptural verses, provided they serve to protect the wearer from falling ill and not to heal him when afflicted with a wound or a disease. But it is forbidden to write scriptural verses on amulets" (*Y.D.*, *clxxix*.12).[82a] Most references to amulets, as to many other subjects of medical interest, occur among the extensive Sabbath laws. The issue is whether, and on what terms, it is permitted to carry them outside private property, seeing that the removal of anything not strictly part of one's wearing apparel constitutes a desecration of the Sabbath (*O.H.*, *ccci*.7). In the case of the above-listed charms and talismans, sanction for their wear on the Sabbath is invariably given if medically indicated, but there are reservations in regard to ordinary amulets. Only those may be worn in public places on the Sabbath as are "tested by experience". What constitutes such "experience" is defined in very great detail (*ib.*, 25). Briefly stated, amulets are considered "approved" if either the script or its writer has proved efficacious in three separate cases where the same magic formula was used. A like "test" is also applied to amulets consisting of roots. All such "approved" charms may be taken out on the Sabbath by persons who suffer from, or are genetically disposed to, any ailment, however mild (*ib.*). Domestic animals, too, may carry amulets on the Sabbath, but again only if they are "tested"; at the same time, those "approved" for human beings are not necessarily efficacious, and thus sanctioned, for animals[83] (*O.H.*, *cccv*.17, gloss). But the mere handling of any kind of amulet is permitted on the Sabbath, even if it is "untested" (*O.H.*, *cccviii*. 33). Whether amulets containing biblical verses may be rescued from the flames on the Sabbath is the subject of a rabbinic controversy[84] (*O.H.*, *cccxxxiv*.14). Amulets, if they bear sacred inscriptions, may not be taken into a privy unless they are enclosed in leather (*Y.D.*, *cclxxxii*.6).

EXORCISM OF DEMONS

In contrast to amulets and incantations, demons and their exorcism are only very rarely mentioned in Jewish law, although they constituted (as we have seen) an important element in the medical theories of ancient and medieval times. While the codes (apart from that of MAIMONIDES[85]), following the Talmud, clearly affirm the belief in the existence of demons, references to them occur almost exclusively in entirely non-medical contexts. The marriage laws, for instance, twice accept the possibility that certain unauthenticated statements heard to come from a field, or a pit, or a ruin may have been made by a demon, thus invalidating the alleged evidence (*E.H.*, *xvii*.10; and *cxli*.19). In the 16th century, faith in the power of these supernatural beings was so strong that a leading rabbi seriously discussed the question whether a certain woman, alleged to have had intercourse with "a spirit or demon called '*Tracht*' ", should be separated from her husband as an adulteress.[86] It is all the more remarkable that the codes make no mention of demons as a cause of illness. The only two relevant references to them are (i) the rather cautious statement that "in regard to the consultation of demons, whatever is permitted on weekdays is also permitted on Sabbaths" (*O.H.*, *cccvii*.18), and (ii) the warning, first found in the *Zohar*,[87] that "most people who engage in this [employment of demons, even for the sake of the sick[88]] will not escape in peace from them; hence, he who wishes to guard himself should keep away from them" (*Y.D.*, *clxxix*.16, gloss). But outside the codes, some rabbis deal at length with the legal relationship between demons and sorcery.[89] KARO[90] holds that the recourse to demons for healing purposes need not generally be regarded as sorcery.

Apart from common demons, some other supernatural beings and forces also appear occasionally. A species of incubuses termed "destroyers" is mentioned twice in connection with the laws of prayer (*O.H.*, *xc*.6; and *cdlxxxi*.2, gloss). Another spirit, known as "bitter destruction",[91] was believed to rule at certain hours during the three weeks of national mourning ending on the Ninth of Av; hence, one should not walk alone during those hours or chastise pupils on these days (*O.H.*, *dli.*18 and gloss). The anxiety to put "the spirits of defilement" to flight, so that they shall not enter into the grave with the dead, accounts for the custom recorded by ISSERLES of setting down the bier every four cubits as it passes through the cemetery[92] (*Y.D.*, *ccclviii.*3, gloss).

THE "EVIL SPIRIT" AND THE "EVIL EYE"

Reference is made somewhat more frequently to "the evil spirit". It finds its way into Jewish law in two entirely distinct forms. Firstly it is to be found on one's hands or food. Thus, one should be careful to pour water on one's hands three times every morning "in order to remove the evil spirit resting on them"[93] (*O.H.*, *iv.*2, *et pass.*; *cf.* *dcxiii.*2, gloss). A similar spirit attaches to food or drinks under a bed[94] (*Y.D.*, *cxvi.*5) and to water used for the washing of hands after meals[95] (*O.H.*, *clxxxi.*2). The second manifestation of "the evil spirit" may well be of a more rational type. In these cases "the evil spirit", by possessing or "pursuing" human beings, causes a condition which, as the context suggests and as MAIMONIDES[96] and others[97] assume, corresponds to any, or possibly some specific, form of mental disease.[98] The matrimonial regulations refer to a husband, wishing to divorce his wife, who "is seized by the evil spirit and turned insane" (*E.H.*, *cxxi.*1). Again, "an individual pursued by the evil spirit" is regarded as being in immediate danger[99] (*O.H.*, *cclxxxviii.*10), and one may cry for him even on the Sabbath when expressions of grief should normally be avoided (*ib.*, 9; and *dlxxvi.*13). Such a person should also refrain from fasting "so as not to break his strength" (*O.H.*, *dlxxi.*3). It was popularly believed that a person "in whom the evil spirit had breathed" could be cured by milk squirted on him by a nursing mother;[100] but in the absence of danger this procedure must not be carried out on the Sabbath (*O.H.*, *cccxxviii*.35, gloss).

Among other examples of folklore and superstition which have crept into the codes, the following should be mentioned. The "evil eye" has haunted men since immemorial times,[101] and Jewish law refers to two remedies against its harmful effects. For humans there was a special charm,[102] which might be worn even on the Sabbath (*O.H.*, *ccciii*.15), whilst horses could be protected against the "evil eye" by a fox-tail suspended between their eyes—a charm with which they must not go out on the Sabbath (*O.H.*, *cccv*.11). Following an old talmudic belief,[103] for which the New Testament[104] and TACITUS[105] also furnish parallels, the saliva of a man's first-born son served to heal eye-diseases; in fact, the efficacy of such a cure could legally be relied upon to support the claim for a double portion of inheritance which is due only to a first-born son on the father's side (*H.M.*, *cclxxvii*.13). Other irrational remedies included the measuring of a sick person's girdle to restore his health —an act also permitted on the Sabbath[106] (*O.H.*, *cccvi*.7) —and the preservation, or perhaps interment, of the placenta to keep a new-born child warm—an ancient practice which, again, does not contravene the Sabbath laws[107] (*O.H.*, *cccxxx*.7). ISSERLES records the advice of some authorities to draw water every Saturday night, "since the well of MIRIAM travels around all wells every Saturday night, and he who strikes upon it and drinks from it is healed of all his ills"[108] (*O.H.*, *ccxcix*.10, gloss).

Among the few bad omens mentioned is a "tradition that there is a certain hour during the months of Teveth and Shevat, and that a slaughterer will die if he kills a goose at that hour without eating of the bird"[109] (*Y.D.*, *xi*.4, gloss). Into a similar category belongs the law that distant visitors should not call on the sick before the lapse of three days (*Y.D.*, *cccxxxv*.1), because a premature visit may "shake his luck" by attaching the name of "patient" to him too soon.[110] Another portent of ill-fate was to submit to blood-letting on the eve of festivals, particularly of Pentecost[111] (*O.H.*, *cdlxviii.*10, gloss). The custom to respond "health!" to a sneeze—derived from popular fears which survived for very long—also finds legal expression[112] (*O.H.*, *clxx.*1). In the only codified reference to spiritualism, KARO permits one "to abjure a sick person to return to the petitioner after death and to tell whatever asked" (*Y.D.*, *clxxix.*14); ISSERLES adds that this request may be made even after the death of the medium, "so long as one abjures not his corpse, but his spirit[113] (*ib.*, gloss).

The old belief—evidently also supported by modern scientific evidence[114]—that the cries of a foetus could be heard in the mother's womb appears in the codes, although the Talmud did not consider this feasible except if the head of the child had actually emerged from the birth-canal.[115] Such *"vagitus uterinus"* determines a child's birth-day for fixing, eight days later, the date for the circumcision, even if the birth was delayed by several days (*Y.D.*, *cclxii.*4), unless the mother testified that the position of the foetus was entirely normal and that she felt no labour pains at the time[116] (*ib.*, gloss). As already noted, Jewish law also accepted the popular notion — which infiltrated into the Talmud from non-Jewish sources, lasted among the medical profession until the 18th century and still persists as a common belief[117]—that a child born in the eighth month of gestation is not likely to survive and is to be treated as a non-viable birth (*Y.D.*, *cclxvi.*11); if such child nevertheless showed no signs of prematurity (i.e. the absence of hair and nails), it is to be regarded as a seven-months' baby which had "tarried" in the womb for another month.[118]

We may conclude this list of folkloristic beliefs scattered in the codes of Jewish law by two examples indicating that concessions to superstitious fears were not always tolerated. It is forbidden to say: "Slaughter the cock that crows like a raven, or this hen that crows like a cock"[119] (*Y.D.*, *clxxix.*3);

but others permit this, provided one did not state why one wished the bird to be killed (*ib.*, gloss). Again, an animal "slaughtered in the name of mountains . . . or heavenly bodies" is ritually unfit for consumption, "even if the intention was not to perform an idolatrous act, but to serve medical ends . . . on heathen advice" (*Y.D., iv.5*).

THE "DRECKAPOTHEKE"

Finally, we have to consider a closely related group of beliefs which enjoyed a curiously widespread popularity. So universal was the faith in the healing powers of repugnant substances that this strange department of pharmacology was given the special name *"Dreckapotheke"*. The prescription of drugs compounded of various offensive human and animal excretions was as popular in the *Ebers Papyrus* of ancient Egypt as it still was in 1862 when Dr. JOHN HASTINGS wrote the pamphlet entitled: *"Value of the Excreta of Reptiles in Phthisis and some other Diseases"*.[120] Trust in such odd concoctions was not limited to quacks and wonder-healers. GALEN, who had averred that he would "not mention the abominable and detestable as XENO-CRATES and others had done",[121] himself later included in his *materia medica* such items as dung of dogs, goats and doves, and burnt human bones in drink.[122] PARACELSUS used human excrements for his drug *"Zebethum Occidentale"*[123] and other repulsive medicines.[124] A hundred years later, MOSES CHARRAS's *The Royal Pharmacopoeia* (published in London in 1678)—claimed as "the most scientific work of the day"[125]—was again full of scatological directions.

On the whole, Jewish sources are surprisingly free from this evident desire to repel the carriers of disease with the most nauseous weapons. We have the evidence of a Christian scholar that "the *'Dreckapotheke'* which could be assembled from the talmudic literature is greatly surpassed in unsavouriness by what is to be read in the *Ebers Papyrus*, PLINY and GALEN".[126] PREUSS, too, collecting all the relevant talmudic passages in a few lines, regards this group as "strikingly small in comparison with the Greek and Roman '*Dreckapotheke*' ".[127] But his judgment that "this is manifestly connected with the general disgust of oriental people for anything unclean and vile" is open to doubt if one consults the Index to BUDGE's edition of the Syrian *Book of Medicines* under such entries as "dung", "excrements" and "urine".[128] One will discover that an important medical work of an oriental country situated between Palestine and Babylonia—where the two parts of the Talmud were produced a little later—was not at all averse to recommending a wide variety of obnoxious compounds. The reason for the paucity of such repulsive elements in Jewish sources must rather be sought in a different direction.

Judaism may well be the only religion which invested the abhorrence of filthy food with the authority of a legal enactment or which, indeed, offered any direct opposition to the consumption of coprolitic substances: "It is prohibited to consume food or drink containing an admixture of dirt or excrements . . . Similarly, it is unlawful to eat or drink from filthy vessels for which the human soul feels an aversion, such as vessels of a privy or glass-receptacles used for blood-letting and the like; nor may one eat with soiled hands . . . , for all this is included in the law: 'You shall not make yourselves abominable' (*Lev. xx.*25)" (*Y.D., cxvi.*6). For the same reason, it is forbidden to eat fish and edible locust in a live state (*Y.D., xiii.*1, gloss).

The codes refer only twice to specific scatological foods. While the authorities differ on the permissibility of the urine from unclean animals, they agree that human urine[129] is not forbidden (*Y.D., lxxxi.*1). But this ruling is concerned only with the ritual aspect of the question—that is, to indicate whether the biblical ban on consuming certain animals covers their urinary excretions; moreover, such sanction as is given can be utilised for sick people only.[130] The second reference permits the consumption of "a burnt unclean reptile" (including probably the carbonised remains of any ritually impure substance) for medical purposes, but only "because it is like mere dust" (*Y.D., lxxxiv.*17). ISSERLES adds that the sanction extends even to mildly ill persons, but in all such cases the drug must be "known or prescribed by an approved physician"[131] (*Y.D., clv.*3, gloss). MORDECAI JAFFE[132] and others[133] generally exempt articles taken for medical reasons from the law "You shall not make yourselves abominable". In some rabbinical responsa[134] we find further references to some offensive preparations, items such as snake broth, mummies' flesh and the pulverised ashes of human skulls. But the refining influence of Judaism must have been strong indeed to explain the absence from any code of Jewish law of references to the medicinal use of human bones, menstrual blood,[135] animal *faeces* or other "nasty recipes" which featured so prominently in the pharmaceutical armoury of the medieval practitioner.

The small segment of the cultural history of man surveyed in this chapter may not be very edifying, nor can it be said that the role played by religion in freeing the human mind from its mystical encumbrances has been particularly conspicuous. Theology and superstition were only too often more in league than in conflict with each other. But the deeper causes for this strange alliance lay, perhaps, not so much in the fallibility of ecclesiastical leadership as in man's innate psychology. Fear of the unknown, especially when accentuated by acute physical or mental suffering, has always encouraged human recourse to the supposed forces beyond man's limited comprehension. The hiatus created by lack of knowledge must be filled by some belief. Creed and credulity, though at opposite poles, spring largely from the same human quest for security. Their relationship is, therefore, essentially natural. But religion and superstition meet only at their lowest level where the element of fear is their common denominator; their association grows more tenuous in proportion to the degree to which the worship of God is sublimated and divested of its primitive urges and emotional origins.

Judged by this standard, there can be little doubt as to the place occupied by Judaism right up to the end of the Middle Ages. Many of the above illustrations make it clear that, by and large, Jewish law, where it did not altogether proscribe superstitious practices, at best tolerated them as a concession to human addiction.[136] It found very little space for the faith-healer and none at all for the professional quack — the favourite character in the medical legislation of the past millenium and more. It knew nothing of healing shrines or relics, and next to nothing of the exorcism of demons. On the other hand, Jewish law treasured the protection of human life so intensely that it was prepared, as a general rule, to give the accepted claims of magic and the occult virtues, however questionable, the benefit of the doubt, often even at the expense of its own religious injunctions. For, whenever law and life are in conflict, Judaism usually shows a strong bias in favour of life. The problems created by such clashes, and their solution, will engage our attention in the following chapters.

CHAPTER THREE

LAW AND LIFE — 1.

GENERAL PRINCIPLES

The Jewish view on the supreme value of human life is well expressed in the stern warning which, according to the Talmud, must be given to witnesses in a capital indictment. Admonishing them that they are "answerable for the blood of him [that is wrongfully condemned] and the blood of his posterity to the end of the world", the court solemnly declared: "Therefore but a single man was [originally] created in the world, to teach that if any man has caused a single soul to perish (from Israel[1]) Scripture imputes it to him as if he caused a whole world to perish; and if any man saves alive a single soul (from Israel[1]) Scripture imputes it to him as if he saved alive a whole world".[2] The Talmud thus anticipated by over half a millenium the similar thought of the *Koran*: "He who has restored life to a man shall be accounted as if he had restored life to humanity".[3]

The preservation of human life takes precedence even over acts of reverence for the dead. "For a one-day-old child [that is dangerously ill] the Sabbath may be profaned . . . ; for DAVID, King of Israel, once he is dead, the Sabbath must not be violated", says the Talmud.[4] More than a thousand years later, the *Sepher Hasidim*[5] ruled that one must rescue from the flames any living infant rather than the dead body of one's own father. The same idea is reflected in the ruling: "If a funeral *cortège* meets a bridal procession, the former must give way to the latter" (*Y.D.*, *ccclx*.1), because "religious duties concerning life always have priority over those connected with death".[6]

Among Jewish teachers, only the sectarian Sadduces[7] and Karaites[8] were in doubt whether it was lawful to ignore the Sabbath and other religious precepts in order to save life. In the Talmud and all subsequent rabbinical works this was taken for granted. They are unanimous on extending this important principle even to cases in which the success of the operation involving the suspension of the Sabbath laws[9] is in doubt; such operations must be continued "however remote the likelihood of rescuing life may be" (*O.H.*, *cccxxix*.3). Moreover, it makes no difference whether the life of the person so saved on the Sabbath is likely to be extended by many years or merely seconds; efforts to free a victim buried in a collapsed building must be maintained "even if found crushed in such a manner that he cannot survive except for a short while" (*ib.*, 4). For, as a contemporary scholar[10] has pointed out, the value of human life is infinite and beyond measure, so that a hundred years and a single second are equally precious. He illustrated this principle by suggesting, on the basis of a discussion in the Talmud,[11] that a person who killed a child falling from a roof would be guilty of a capital offence like any ordinary murderer, even though he expedited the child's certain death by only a few moments.

While the operation of this vital principle was never in dispute, the Talmud[12] records a variety of answers to the question: "Whence do we derive scriptural support for the rule that the saving of life supersedes the Sabbath laws?" Of the seven answers, three may here be given. According to one teacher, the rule is based on the verse: "For it [i.e. the Sabbath] is holy *unto you*" (*Ex. xxxi*.14)—"it is surrendered unto you, but not you unto the Sabbath".[13] Another sage derived the principle from the verse: "Wherefore the children of Israel shall keep the Sabbath . . . " (*ib.*, 16)— "[it is right to] profane one Sabbath for a person, so that

he may [be able to] fulfil many Sabbaths [afterwards]".[14]
The prevailing view[15] held that the concession was implied
by the verse: "Ye shall therefore keep My statutes . . . ,
which if a man do, *he shall live by them*" (*Lev. xviii.5*)—
"that 'he shall live by them', and not that he shall die by
them".

These variations of exegesis are significant and may
indicate important divergencies of outlook and, possibly,
law. Thus, the early 18th century mystic and exegete,
HAYIM ATAR,[16] argued that the second reasoning may
not apply when the duration of the life to be saved will
certainly be less than a week, since the profanation of "one
Sabbath" would then not render possible the observance of
"many Sabbaths [afterwards]". Following this view, it has
been suggested, in fact, that in such cases the saving of "temporary life" can override only rabbinic laws (such as the
removal of debris on the Sabbath), but not biblical commandments (such as lighting a fire).[17] Consequently, the
justification for the suspension of any divine law would lie
solely in the net gain resulting from weighing the moral
damage of violating a single law once against the expected
benefit of fulfilling many laws later on. But this is a minority opinion. The various teachings of the other six sages
agree, whatever the scriptural derivation, that the Sabbath
is superseded by the absolute and supreme value of human
life itself, and not by the superior virtue accumulating
through the performance of numerous laws.[18] MAIMO-
NIDES, who accepts the derivation from " . . . he shall
live by them", expounds this view in clear terms: " . . . this
teaches that the judgments of the *Torah* are not meant to
bring vengeance into the world, but [are intended to secure]
compassion, kindness and peace in the world".[19] The first
argument (that the Sabbath is subordinate and not superior
to man), like the other talmudic expositions not mentioned
here, similarly emphasises the view that the overriding consideration in suspending religious laws is the intrinsic value

of life, which transcends the moral worth of religious observance.[20]

A rather different reasoning altogether is introduced by MENAHEM ME'IRI, a leading talmudist of the 13th century. He holds that the profanation of the Sabbath is justified to gain even a short extension of life, because this may enable the person so saved to win sufficient time for repentance and atonement.[21] This view evidently again measures the value of life primarily in terms of the moral perfection achieved. But, in practice, it may be assumed that ME'IRI agrees that it is imperative to desecrate the Sabbath even when the circumstances clearly rule out any possibility of repentance during the limited respite afforded by the attempt.[22]

The exact nature of the suspension principle is further illustrated in the following controversy: If meat required on the Sabbath for a dangerously sick person can be obtained either by specially slaughtering a beast or by taking meat from an animal which was not ritually killed, which alternative is to be preferred? Some authorities favour the latter course, since it involves only the transgression of an ordinary "negative commandment" (normally carrying corporal punishment) on the part of the sick person (*viz.*, by consuming ritually forbidden meat), whereas the first alternative would necessitate the commission of a capital offence (*viz.*, by killing a beast on the Sabbath) on the part of someone else.[23] Most authorities, however, recommend the adoption of the first course, unless the food is immediately required and none but ritually unfit meat is available (*O.H., cccxxviii.*14). They argue that the consumption of ritually unfit meat may be repugnant to the patient.[24] Moreover, the slaughtering of a beast on the Sabbath constitutes merely a single breach of the law, while the second alternative means that a precept is ignored every time the patient takes a bite of the forbidden food.[25] According to ADRETH,[26] the solution of the problem depends on whether the law, when it clashes with the interests of life, is rendered altogether nugatory or simply superseded without thereby ceasing to exist. ADRETH, who himself opts in favour of the latter interpretation, explains that if the law becomes completely inoperative, the special killing of an animal is to be preferred; for the *degree* of the offence committed to save life then becomes entirely irrelevant. But in the contrary view, the consideration of life merely overrides the law to the minimum extent necessary; hence, it is better that the patient himself commit a relatively minor offence than that he should cause others to transgress a capital law.[27]

These practical arguments no doubt also express, in characteristically rabbinic fashion, fundamental differences of moral reasoning. It appears that the controversy again revolves around the motivation for the suspension principle. The view that, in relation to whatever is required for the saving of life, the Sabbath laws simply cease to exist may be assumed to correspond with the line of thought which regards the preservation of life as man's supreme duty transcending every other consideration. The validity of all laws would thus be contingent on the proviso that man "shall live by them and not die by them", or that he "shall not be surrendered unto [them]". The opposing schools of thought, again, would hold that the operation of biblical laws was never intended to be conditional, and that it is the observance of the divine law, and not the intrinsic value of life, which constitutes the absolute factor. The sanctity of "one Sabbath" is merely suppressed, not eliminated (as emphasised by the significant term "desecrate"), by the greater weight of "many Sabbaths", because the law itself invariably remains intact.[28]

OVERRIDING DUTY TO SAVE LIFE

In this controversy the broadly humanitarian definition of the suspension rule is generally accepted in the codes with little or no reservation. This outlook is reflected in a number of regulations indicating, in practical terms, (i) that the duty to promote life and health, and any acts performed to that end, enjoy a specifically religious character; (ii) that it is obligatory to disregard laws conflicting with the immediate claims of life, and that such action is hallowed and not in need of atonement for the "offence" committed; and (iii) that it is sinful to observe laws which are in suspense on account of the danger to life or health.

We have already referred to the general religious obligation to heal the sick and to protect human health.[29] In order to amplify the first item (i) listed above, we may here add some details. A beast which had eaten some man-killing poison or been bitten by a snake, though ritually fit, must not be used for human consumption (*Y.D., lx.*2). "Because of the danger", it is prohibited to place a vessel containing hot water on the abdomen (*O.H., cccxxvi.*6). Particular caution is urged in the performance of circumcisions,[30] "because danger to life overrides everything; for it is possible to perform a circumcision after its proper date, but it is impossible to restore a [lost] life" (*Y.D., cclxiii.*1). That services rendered to the sick are regarded as purely religious acts is shown by several laws. If a person vowed to forswear the benefit of his services to another, he may still render him medical assistance (*Y.D., ccxxi.*4), because such service constitutes not a favour but a religious duty.[31] A light kindled for a sick person legally has the same religious character as lights burning in a synagogue or lit on festive occasions at home (*O.H., dclxxiv.*2, gloss), and acts required by the sick are generally placed into the category of religious requirements (e.g., *O.H., dli.*9, gloss).

The following rulings illustrate the second point mentioned above (ii) and indicate that it is not merely permitted but imperative to disregard laws in conflict with life or health. "It is a religious precept to desecrate the Sabbath for any person afflicted with an illness that may prove dangerous; he who is zealous is praiseworthy, whilst he who

asks [questions] sheds blood"[32] (*O.H., cccxxviii.*2). The
emphasis on the praiseworthiness of such zeal is repeated in
identical terms in two further clauses (*ib.,* 13; and *cccxxix.*1).
The duty to ignore the law, if necessary, for health reasons,
is particularly stressed in connection with the fasting of
children on the Day of Atonement (*O.H., dcxvi.*2 and gloss)
and of expectant and nursing mothers on ordinary fast days,
especially if they are in considerable pain (*O.H., dl.*1, gloss;
and *dlxxv.*5, gloss). For reasons of health it is also wrong
to observe two consecutive Days of Atonement[33] (*O.H.,
dcxxiv.*5, gloss).

Any dispensation granted to the sick and the weak, as
specified by law, is complete and unqualified. Hence, although it is normally forbidden to derive any advantage
from acts unlawfully performed, even healthy people may
benefit from work done on the Sabbath for the sake of sick
persons, such as the killing of a beast to provide meat (*O.H.,
cccxviii.*2) or the kindling of a light for them (*O.H.,
cclxxvi.*1), because these acts have been carried out "in a
legitimate way" (*O.H., dcxxiv.*5). For the same reason,
vessels used to cook food for patients on the Sabbath are
not affected by the ban on utensils thus used unlawfully in
the ordinary way.[34] Still more striking is the ruling that the
statutory benedictions should be said before and after the
consumption of forbidden foods when required by considerations of health (*O.H., cxcvi.*2; and *cciv.*9), despite the general rule that the recitation of blessings over prohibited articles is strongly condemned as contempt of God (*O.H.,
cxcvi.*1). But in this case the patient "performs a religious
act" by eating such food,[35] and it thus loses its forbidden
character. By the same token, several codes rule that a
gravely sick person, eating on the Day of Atonement, shall
insert in the Grace after Meals the special formula otherwise recited only on the other festivals (*O.H., dcxviii.*10);
for, as MAIMONIDES[36] put it, "to him the Day of Atonement is as ordinary festivals are to us, seeing that he is not

only free, but religiously obliged to break the fast". Indeed, neither the patient nor his assistants need have any qualms of conscience, or require any atonement, when compelled to carry out acts forbidden under normal circumstances.[37]   Even if a number of people, in an attempt to rush aid to a patient, violated the law, they are all free from sin; in fact, "they will receive a good reward from the Lord, even if the patient had recovered [before the aid reached him]"[38] (*O.H., cccxxviii.*15).

There is, therefore, absolutely no virtue in observing laws at the risk of life. Such conduct, rather, is branded as both sinful and foolish. Anyone who is not sufficiently strong or healthy and yet indulges in regular fasts is "called a sinner" (*O.H., dlxxi.*1). According to many authorities,[39] a seriously sick person who refuses a cure because it would involve a breach of the law should be forced to submit to it, since such a refusal amounts to a "piety of madness".[40]

THE JEWISH OBJECTION TO MARTYRDOM AND SELF-SACRIFICE

The attitude represented by these regulations does not spring merely from theological principles; it is deeply rooted in the moral approach of Judaism to life and its sanctity. In the Jewish field of virtue and saintliness, the ideal of martyrdom occupies a strictly confined place. The cult of self-sacrifice to the point of death never appealed to the Jew. He generally preferred living in misery to dying in glory. To him survival mattered more than the heroics eventually recorded on imposing monuments. Of course, there were important exceptions—they will be considered presently in some detail. But, on the whole, Jewish law stemmed from, and strongly encouraged, this life-affirming attitude. Indeed, the *Midrash* regarded the profanation of the Sabbath for the saving of life as no less natural than the avoidance of a "martyr's death" at the hands of robbers by fleeing from them when in jeopardy of one's life.[41] In another midrashic passage, two rabbinic disciples excused their disguise as heathens in order to escape detection and consequent death during a wave of religious persecution, by arguing that "it was not the way of man to commit suicide".[42]

Hence, according to MAIMONIDES,[43] anyone who sacrifices his life for the fulfilment of a religious precept when this is not required by law is guilty of a deadly sin, a view evidently shared by KARO (*Y.D.*, *clvii*.1), though disputed by some other authorities.[44] But even the dissentients agree that the right of an individual to choose death rather than to violate the law applies only to transgressions exacted by external compulsion; in cases of illness, all admit that such voluntary martyrdom must be opposed, if necessary by force.[45] The same outlook is revealed in an entirely different context: "Whoever cannot subsist except by taking charity—such as old, sick or ailing persons—and who yet arrogantly refuses to accept such [aid] is shedding blood and guilty of a mortal offence; to his distress he only adds iniquities and sins" (*Y.D.*, *cclv*.2). It was, therefore, inconceivable that a conscientious Jew would endanger his life in contravention of this principle, and referring to ISAAC HALEVI, of the 12th century, who died after fasting on the Day of Atonement against his physician's orders, the 16th century halachist DAVID IBN ZIMRA[46] explained the action as due to the conviction that he would die in any case.

EXCEPTIONS REQUIRING DEATH RATHER THAN BREACH OF LAW

The supreme sacrifice was demanded, and sanctioned, only in certain clearly defined cases. By a rule "voted and passed . . . in Lydda" at the time of the Hadrian persecution in 135 *C.E.*,[47] death—whether at the hands of an oppressor or as a consequence of disease—must be chosen if life could be purchased only by committing any of the three cardinal crimes against God, one's fellow-man or oneself, *viz.*, idolatry, murder or incest.[48] There are, however, two distinctions between the threat of physical violence and the affliction of disease as the compelling *force majeure.* For the purpose of healing, any act save the three cardinal sins is legitimate. But an oppressor's challenge to "break the law or die!" must in certain circumstances be resisted to death to maintain the integrity even of minor laws; for instance, when the challenge is specifically aimed at breaking down the Jew's loyalty to his faith (*Y.D., clvii.*1). The second difference concerns the *refusal* to obey the three cardinal laws in the face of mortal danger. If the threat of violence caused a person to succumb to these offences, he is free from all legal liability as the victim of superior pressure, unless he was in a position to flee but failed to do so (*ib.*, gloss). But if medical considerations prompted him to save his life by resorting to idolatry, bloodshed or incest, he is—as MAIMONIDES[49] explicitly states—subject to the appropriate penalty; in this case the circumstances do not militate against the culpability of the offence, since it was committed freely and deliberately.

The ban on being healed by recourse to idolatry includes the medical use of any object dedicated to, or associated with, idol-worship. But some authorities prohibit such cures only if the heathen offering them expressly stated that they were of idolatrous origin (*Y.D., clv.*2). It is also forbidden to put one's mouth to the sculptures of human faces ejecting water in front of an idol, since it may appear as if one kisses the idol (*Y.D., cl.*3); but others permit this in cases of danger to life, holding that life need not be sacrificed to avoid an act condemned only for appearance sake (*ib.*, gloss).

Homicide for medical purposes is considered in Jewish law merely in connection with abortion, a subject to be considered at length in another chapter.[50] To appreciate the significance of this limitation, it must be remembered that, in ancient and medieval times, murders committed in the name of medicine were not rare. The belief in the medical efficacy of human blood, in particular, often led to the most gruesome massacres in which children were especially favoured victims. There are many reports of these brutal practices in history,[51] but no-one could have anticipated the large-scale murder for medical experimentation officially sanctioned and practised during the 20th century in the heart of Central Europe.[52] It is significant that the Jewish moral consciousness recoiled from the horror of legalising murder in any circumstances even more instinctively than from the thought of justifying idolatry or immorality under similar conditions. For, while the unconditional prohibition of the latter crimes required the support of biblical evidence, the rejection of homicide as a means to save life was, in the words of the Talmud,[53] based simply on the "obvious argument: What right have you to assume that your blood is redder than your neighbour's?", or—as MAIMONIDES[54] has it—on "the reasoned consideration that one does not destroy one life for [the sake of] another."

The unconditional proscription of incest covers all incestuous, adulterous or other carnal relationships which are biblically forbidden,[55] whether under pain of death or not, with the exception of a union between a non-Jew and a Jewess (*Y.D.*, *clvii*.1, gloss). But the offence must be of an active nature; hence, a woman forced to submit to illicit intercourse need not expose herself to martyrdom (*ib.*).[56] On the other hand, the Talmud[57] widely extends the scope of the prohibition by ruling that a person, who is seized by a "vehement passion" and medically advised that his life can be saved only by some surrender to his lust, must die rather than commit any immoral act, even to the extent of refusing to gratify his voluptuousness by conversing with a maiden from behind a screen. This ruling is expressly endorsed by MAIMONIDES,[58] who — in common with

KARO (*E.H.*, *xx.*1)—regards every lascivious physical contact between forbidden relations as a violation of biblical law.[59]

The practical meaning of these laws can be understood only in the context of the popular faith in the therapeutic value of illicit relationships. Several scholars[60] have shown how common was the ancient belief in the medical efficacy of such relations against certain (mainly venereal) diseases, especially with virgins and children.[61] The notion that some sensual gratification could promote health was, in principle, also shared by MAIMONIDES in his rules on conjugal propriety when he included "medical reasons" among the legitimate grounds for intercourse between married partners.[62]

These regulations also affect the relations between a husband and his wife during the *tempus menstruationis*.[63] If she is ill in that state, the husband—according to some authorities[64]—must not attend her by rendering services involving physical contact (*Y.D.*, *cxcv.*16), nor may he feel her pulse if he is a doctor (*ib.*, 17); this applies even when no other attendants or physicians are available to serve the sick woman, because all such actions may be included in the unqualified prohibition as "appurtenances of incest".[65] But other authorities, recognising the absolute ban only when such acts are motivated by voluptuousness,[66] permit the usual suspension rule to operate in favour of lifting the ban if urgently required and if the husband's services cannot be replaced by anyone else (*ib.*, glosses). But in the reverse case of the husband being ill, all agree that his wife may attend to his needs, avoiding any direct contact as far as possible, provided there is no-one else to do so[67] (*ib.*, 15).

These exceptions to the suspension rule make it clear that the duty to uphold the law at all costs supersedes the claims of human life only in the rarest (and often hypothetical) cases. When, therefore, an 8th century Gaon asserted that "indeed not one commandment whose performance is dangerous has God enjoined upon Israel",[68] he expressed a truism which can be accepted for practical purposes with very little reservation. If Jewish physicians or rabbis still sometimes insisted on limiting the means of healing to prescriptions which would not invoke the right to suspend religious laws, they did so only when convinced that the application of wholly permitted cures would be equally effective to ward off any danger to life. Thus, we learn that R. JOSEPH BARUCH CAZES of Mantua, on taking up the medical profession in 1716, "entered a covenant" that he would not prescribe any remedies containing substances forbidden in Jewish law, since (as is recorded) "he was certain that such medicines were not indispensable for any disease, for he found in all medical books that numerous alternative treatments and drugs existed for every illness".[69] This statement may well be compared, as significantly similar and yet in contrast, with the gloss invariably added by many Arab copyists to prescriptions in which wine occurred: "Allah proscribed wine for us; if the patient is destined to recover, he will recover without wine, too".[70]

The principle of suspending religious injunctions for the purpose of safeguarding life is, of coures, also recognised in the moral philosophy of the Church. But the Christian attitude to conflicts between law and life is, on the whole, less clearly defined, and occasions for the emergence of such problems can arise only comparatively seldom.[71] Generally, even the strictest demands of religious practice may be set aside for urgent medical considerations. Thus, CAPELL-MANN,[72] a leading expert on Catholic pastoral medicine, while refusing to allow a pregnant woman to gratify a "morbid desire" for meat during a period of abstinence, relaxes this rule if she experiences an insurmountable horror of eating any substitute. On the other hand, the Church often carries her opposition to concessions in favour of life much farther into the realm of pure theology than does Judaism. According to Christian doctrine in the Middle Ages, man's spiritual salvation was more important than physical heal-ing.[73] This crucial tenet found practical expression, too. In 1236 the Council of Canterbury charged that "no physician may give a patient advice which is harmful to his soul",[74] and GALEN's teachings were opposed by the saying of AMBROSIUS: *"Contraria sunt divine conditioni precepta medicine"*.[75] The fulfilment of the obligation to confess before death, in particular, was counted among the cardinal duties surpassing the intrinsic value of human life, as we shall observe in another chapter.[76]

CHAPTER FOUR

LAW AND LIFE — 2.

DETERMINING THE DANGER TO LIFE

When the interests of life conflict with the demands of religious law, vital decisions must be made quickly and, perhaps, irrevocably. Any delay may result in fatal consequences; on the other hand, misjudgments as to the nature of the disease may lead to unnecessary breaches of important laws. Doctors cannot always be available at once to ascertain whether a patient is in a serious state, and action may be required before their advice can be sought. While observant Jews, or their spiritual guides, could hardly be expected to familiarise themselves with the professional knowledge conveyed in medical text-books, they could be assumed to have some reliable acquaintance with the great religious codes governing their conduct. Jewish law itself, therefore, comes to the assistance of those whose lives it controls, by offering them a practical set of rules on the medical conditions justifying the suspension of religious laws.

These rough-and-ready rules, to be found in all rabbinic codes and extensively supplemented in the responsa literature, stem mostly from the Talmud.[1] But they are framed in sufficiently general and flexible terms to serve as a competent laymen's guide in all ages.[2] On the principle that "where a doubt exists involving danger to life, the more lenient view prevails" (*O.H.*, *cccxxviii*.10), there are numerous safeguards to ensure that all uncertainties are invariably resolved in the patient's favour. Provision is also made for such variations between talmudic and contemporary medicine as may be discovered with the advance of scientific research. The rabbis agree on accepting claims by medical experts that a disease may be mortal even when the Talmud and the codes explicitly regard it as not dangerous.[3] In the reverse case, however, conditions should be treated as dangerous if so defined in the Talmud even against medical evidence.[4] The benefit of the doubt is once again given to life rather than to the law.

DEFINITION OF DANGEROUS DISEASES

For legal purposes, all diseases are broadly divided into internal and external sores.[5] The former category is defined as ailments manifesting themselves "from the teeth inwards, the teeth themselves being included . . . , provided one of the internal organs is damaged through a wound or an abscess or a similar cause; but mere pains are not called sores" (*O.H., cccxxviii.*3). In such cases, "no medical assessment is necessary; even in the absence of experts and if the patient himself says nothing, one does for him [on the Sabbath] whatever is normally done for him on weekdays. But if one knows and identifies a particular illness as one not requiring any immediate desecration of the Sabbath, one must not profane it for his sake, even though he suffers from an internal affliction" (*ib.,* 4).

Apart from this generalisation, the following maladies are specifically listed as dangerous and as justifying the immediate suspension of biblical laws: "A 'seizure of blood',[6] even if [the patient] walks on his feet and even on the first day [of the attack]" (*ib.,* 8); anal inflammations[7] (*ib.,* 7); carbuncles[8] (*ib.*); fevers accompanied by high temperature or tremor[9] (*ib.*); aching eyes showing secretions (blennorrhoea?[10]) or discharge of blood or tears (through pain),[11] including incipiency of eye cancer[12] (*ib.,* 9); "*bulimus,* that is a disease caused by hunger; its symptom is a [temporary] dimness of the patient's eyes, so that he cannot see" until he is given food[13] (*O.H., dcxviii*.9); and a morbid desire for food, attended by a change in facial colour[14] (*O.H., dcxvii*.3), especially in pregnant women[15] (*ib.*, 2). Among fatal epidemics, mention is made—à propos the proclamation of special fasts—of the (bubonic) plague (*O.H., dlxxvi*. 2), diphtheria, delirious fever, and certain skin diseases[16] (*ib.*, 5).

Other conditions which warrant the immediate profanation of the Sabbath are: Sores on the palm of the hand or the sole of the foot[17] (*O.H., cccxxviii*.6) and any wound caused by an iron instrument[18] (*ib.*, 7); a bite by a mad dog[19] or a poisonous snake[20] (*ib.*, 6); the swallowing of a leech[21] (*ib.*); chills following blood-letting[22] (*ib.*, 18); and the pursuit by "evil spirits"[23] (*O.H., cclxxxviii*.10), though there are cases when this does not presage any danger to life[24] (*O.H., cccxxviii*.35, gloss). Fatal consequences may also ensue from interrupting the seven-day course in taking a solution of *assa-foetida* in warm or cold water[25] (*O.H., cccxxi*.18); from failing to attend adequately to the needs of a new-born child, including its washing,[26] its salting (to strengthen the skin[27]) and the severance of the umbilical cord[28] (*O.H., cccxxx*.7); and from the failure to suck the circumcision wound[29] (*Y.D., cclxiv*.3) and to treat it with medicinal powder[30] (*Y.D., cclxvi*.4). A woman in confinement is always regarded as being in danger (*O.H., cccxxx*.1). The Sabbath may be violated for her from the moment when "she is seated on the birth-stool", or when she begins to discharge blood, or when she has no longer the strength to walk unaided (*ib.*, 3). She retains this status for three days following the birth, and thenceforth to the seventh day if she requests assistance involving the breach of the Sabbath laws; thereafter, until the thirtieth day, she is considered like any patient not in danger[31] (*ib.*, 4), except in regard to making a fire for her even in the summer (*ib.*, 6) to prevent her catching a cold.[32]

In several cases, however, unlike those already listed, there are various doubts on whether, and to what extent, the desecration of the Sabbath may be justified. Thus, the element of the danger to life in epileptics[33] and in persons threatened with the loss of an organ or a limb[34] (*O.H., cccxxviii*.17) was the subject of many rabbinic controversies. Opinions also differed on the right to disregard religious laws for saving the lives of deaf-and-dumb or insane persons,[35] of people in a dying condition[36] and of capital convicts.[37] A similar dispute concerns the claims of unborn children;[38] although the Sabbath may be desecrated by a post-mortem operation on the mother to save her fruit (*O.H., cccxxx*.5), it is doubtful whether this implies a general permission to violate the Sabbath laws for the protection of the life of a foetus.[39] But it is agreed that the suspension rule must not be applied to infants, within the first thirty days of their life, who were born after an eight months' gestation, unless their hair and nails showed signs of maturity[40] (*ib.*, 7).

Of far-reaching practical importance to Jewish physicians was the problem of how far they were justified in ignoring the Sabbath laws and other religious precepts when attending to non-Jewish patients. According to the Talmud,[41] the positive duty to maintain life—over and above the obligation not to destroy it—is incumbent on Jews in respect of the "stranger"[42] as well as of their fellow-Jews. Indeed, MAIMONIDES[43] and others[44] plainly held that it was obligatory to heal non-Jews as well as Jews once they accepted the basic laws of humanity. But the special sanction to disregard religious laws in the face of danger to life originally operated only in regard to Jewish lives,[45] an attitude still upheld, in theory at least, by the *Shulhan 'Arukh* (*O.H., cccxxix*.2; *cccxxx*.2; and *E.H., iv*.34). But already in the 13th century MENACHEM ME'IRI[46] had suggested that the prohibition to desecrate the Sabbath for the sake of Gentiles was applicable only to "the ancient heathens

. . . because they professed no religion at all, nor did they acknowledge their duty to the human society". Evidently the problem was not very acute until the 17th century, when many responsa began to be devoted to it.[47] In principle the more rigorous view of the Talmud and the codes was generally maintained, but in practice it was admitted that Jewish doctors and midwives—even the most religious among them—often violated the Sabbath in their attendance on non-Jews, however legally indefensible their action might be.[48] Some doctors avoided forbidden work on the Sabbath by telling their patients to do what was necessary themselves.[49] The rabbis naturally advised Jewish practitioners to reduce any breaches of the Sabbath laws to a minimum[50] and, wherever possible, to seek a legitimate excuse for avoiding professional calls on the Sabbath altogether, if these would involve forbidden acts.[51] But they were not required to withhold their services, even at the risk of violating major Sabbath laws, in defiance of government regulations[52] or if threatened by other grave consequences.[53] These restrictions may equally apply to the treatment of nonconforming Jews.[54]

So far we have treated only with symptoms and conditions which are declared dangerous by the law itself and which invoke the suspension rule irrespective of any competent medical verdict as to the nature and prognosis of the illness. But over and above these specified cases, the violation of the Sabbath is justified for any sickness (even when it manifests itself externally), if either the physician or the patient believes that such action is required to avoid a risk of life (*O.H.*, *cccxxviii.5*). It is not necessary for the doctor to state that the patient may die if the law is not set aside; he need merely assert that the refusal to break the law may aggravate the illness (*O.H.*, *dcxviii.1*). Some authorities even hold that such evidence need not be given by a professional doctor, "since everybody is deemed partly competent"—at least to raise sufficient doubt on the gravity of the disease to sanction a breach of the Sabbath laws (*O.H.*, *cccxxviii*.10). Others stipulate that this concession applies only to Jews and that non-Jewish laymen are not legally presumed to be experts in this matter (*ib.*, gloss).

DISPUTES AMONG PHYSICIANS

Detailed rules are also given to determine whether religious laws may be suspended if differences of opinion arise among the attending physicians, or between them and the patient himself. These regulations are probably unique in religious and medical legislation. They set out with great precision the course to be adopted when doctors fail to agree with each other, or with the patient, on the seriousness of his condition. For safety's sake, the more critical verdict on the state of his health is generally accepted without reservation, even when it conflicts with the view of the majority, unless the majority is challenged by only a single opinion. Once the patient himself asks for a cure which contravenes the law, his own estimate of his needs is invariably approved, however many doctors express a contrary view; for it is assumed that "the heart knoweth its own bitterness" (*Prov. xiv*.10) better than anyone else.[55] But in the reverse case, the patient's view is ignored even if only one physician regards a breach of the law as essential, unless another competent opinion supports the patient's claim that such a breach is not required. However, the recommendation of two or more medical men to violate the law cannot be challenged by any combination of views to the contrary.

The following list tabulates these regulations in detail, mainly on the basis of the laws regarding fasting on the Day of Atonement:—

Table Showing Decisions in Cases of Conflicting Views among Physicians and Patients on the Need to Violate Religious Precepts

If illness is such that breach of law is deemed necessary by	unnecessary by	and	the law should be	Source O. H. dcxviii.	Comments
one doctor	the patient	even if doctor is non-Jewish	set aside	1.	"Because we say the patient is distracted" (TaZ, a.l., 2).[56]
the patient	even 100 doctors		set aside	1.	"Because 'the heart knoweth its own bitterness' " (TaZ, a.l., 3).
one doctor	one doctor		set aside	2.	So also cccxxviii. 10.
two doctors	two doctors	even if the latter more competent	set aside	2, gloss	Some authorities dispute this ruling.[57]
one doctor	the patient & one doctor		upheld	3.	
one doctor	two doctors	if the patient has no views	upheld	3.	Unless the first doctor is more competent (M.A., a.l., 5).
two doctors	even 100 doctors	even if patient objects	set aside	4.	
the patient and one doctor	even 100 doctors		set aside	4, gloss	"And we do not suspect that patient merely relies on first doctor" (Isserless, ib.).
	the patient	if the doctor is in doubt	set aside	5.	"i. e. he knows the disease but doubts if it is still in dangerous state" (TaZ, a.l., 7).
	the doctor	if the patient says he does not know	upheld	5.	"Since most patients are not familiar with their diseases" (BETH YOSEPH, a.l.).
If the doctor says he is not familiar with the disease			unaffected by his words	6.	"Because the doctor is then merely like any layman" (Karo, ib.)
If the patient is so weak that most people around him deem him in danger			set aside	6, gloss	

The extent to which medical evidence by physicians is admissible in ritual issues is a much debated question in rabbinic literature, to be discussed in another chapter.[58] But the problem regarding the "trustworthiness of doctors", particularly if they do not themselves confess the Jewish faith, arises only when their claims are of religio-legal consequence without affecting human life; for instance, when a medical diagnosis purports to find whether an abnormal vaginal discharge is menstrual or ulcerous—to determine the application of the purity laws in particular cases. However, when professional experts are consulted to establish the urgency of a patient's requirements to save his life, the admission of their testimony is not in question, for any doctor's assertion that a danger to life exists is enough to produce at least a state of doubt which, in turn, is sufficient to warrant the disregard of religious laws.[59]

CHAPTER FIVE

LAW AND LIFE — 3.

RELIGIOUS CONCESSIONS
FOR PATIENTS IN DANGER

The two foregoing chapters have dealt with the conditions under which it is lawful to disregard religious laws in the interest of human life. We shall now consider in some detail *what* contraventions of the law are sanctioned under those circumstances. The rabbis are unanimous in permitting any act (whatever breach of the law it involves, apart from the three cardinal offences) directly required to relieve any threat to life,[1] but they differ materially on the interpretation of this rule. These differences concern in particular the extent of the sanction in cases where it is possible to limit the violation of the law without increasing the risk of life.

Some authorities[2] hold that, in the face of grave illness, it is permitted to profane the Sabbath even by acts not directly conducive to the mitigation of the danger, as long as they are of some benefit to the patient. KARO, by ruling simply that for a dangerously sick person "one may do whatever one usually does for him on weekdays" (*O.H.*, *cccxxviii*.4), evidently shares this view.[3] But in the opinion of the majority, including RASHI[4] and ADRETH,[5] the suspension rule permits only such acts as are calculated to ward off the danger to the patient's life.[6] This opinion, it has been suggested,[7] is also supported by ISSERLES when he states, in another context, that "one must not violate any law for the sake of a sick person if he can be cured with equal effect by recourse to whatever is permitted, even if this will involve a little delay, provided there is no danger in the matter" (*Y.D.*, *clv*.3, gloss). The argument is no doubt related to the dispute (treated in an earlier chapter[8]) on whether the consideration of life cancels the Sabbath laws altogether or merely overrides them to the minimum extent necessary for its preservation.

A similar difference of views on fundamental principles may account for a further dispute between KARO and his glossator. The former accepts the talmudic ruling[9] that, when compelled to profane the Sabbath for a patient in danger, "one should endeavour to do so, not through [invoking the aid of] non-Jews, children or women, but through adult and responsible Jews" (*O.H.*, *cccxxviii*.12). According to ISSERLES, however, the necessary work should rather be done either "in an uncommon manner"[10] or by a non-Jew, unless this may lead to delays or negligence (*ib.*, gloss). The motive for the talmudic decision has been variously explained. NISSIM[11] and ASHERI[12] attribute the preference for adult Jews to the fear lest in other cases (when non-Jews may not be available) one will be reluctant to call on Jews and thus perhaps endanger life, thinking that the rabbis granted the sanction only with demur. In the view of TOSAPHOTH,[13] it is suspected that non-Jews may not be zealous enough in the prompt performance of the required work. MAIMONIDES,[14] on the other hand, insists that the essential services shall be rendered preferably by prominent and learned Jews, because ordinary people, violating the Sabbath in such cases, may come to treat it lightly on other occasions, too. It is also suggested that the example of such scholars will impress other Jews with the urgency and absolute legality of breaking the law for the maintenance of life.[15] In view of these considerations, DAVID HALEVI[16] and others[17] find it difficult to reconcile the amendment of ISSERLES with the Talmud; hence, they contest his decision as not based "on the usage of the ancients". ISSERLES himself, however, is perfectly consistent; his view follows logically from his principle that no law may be broken if the necessary aid to the sick can be rendered in a lawful manner[18] (*Y.D., clv.*3, gloss).

In regard to the Day of Atonement, all authorities are agreed that any essential break of the fast should be reduced to a minimum. In some cases, as we have seen,[19] a "morbid desire" for food, if not satisfied, may endanger the lives of those so afflicted; yet, one must first "whisper into their ears[20] that it is the Day of Atonement", in case this reminder will pacify them, and only if this proves unsuccessful may they be given food until their mind is at ease (*O.H., dcxvii.*2). Moreover, whenever sick people are obliged to break the fast, the amount of food or drink to be consumed should not constitute the volume whose consumption normally carries the penalty of "extermination"[21] (*O.H., dcxviii.*7), unless it is estimated that this measure is insufficient to overcome the danger (*ib.*, 8). The thus forbidden volume amounts to the size of a large date (a little less than an egg) in the case of food (*O.H., dcxii.*1), and to the fill of one's cheek in the case of drinks[22] (*ib.*, 9). Any smaller amounts combine to make up the legal size if the aggregate consumed reaches the prohibited volume within approximately nine minutes[23] (*ib.*, 3, 4 and 10). Hence, whenever possible, the amount of food or drink taken by the sick should not exceed these limits (*O.H., dcxviii.*7 and 8). Again, permitted articles are to be preferred to forbidden foods when feeding a patient on the Day of Atonement; if the former cannot be procured, items involving lesser offenses should be given priority over more gravely prohibited substances[24] (*ib.*, 9).

Similar considerations apply to minimising, as far as possible, the gravity of other breaches of the law for the sake of the severely sick. For instance, if a patient is estimated to require two figs on the Sabbath, and none could be found but two growing on two separate peduncles or three on one, the latter should be plucked (*O.H.*, *cccxxviii*.16) to reduce the offence to a single act;[25] likewise, it is better to remove a stalk bearing two figs than one with three fruits[26] (*ib.*). "But", adds ISSERLES, "if the matter is pressing, one should not be particular, so as not to risk any delay" (*ib.*, gloss).

The sanction to violate the law extends only to whatever is actually required by the patient. Hence, after slaughtering an animal on the Sabbath to provide meat urgently required,[27] the statutory "covering of the blood" with earth[28] should be omitted—or delayed until after the termination of the Sabbath if a trace of the blood can still be found[29] (*Y.D.*, *xxviii*.16). On the other hand, zeal in the desecration of the Sabbath for the sick is commendable "even if one thereby also accomplishes another [normally prohibited] purpose; for example, if one spread out a net to rescue a child that had fallen into a river, and one thereby also caught some fish" (*O.H.*, *cccxxviii*.13). For a similar reason, one need not await the termination of the Sabbath before commencing an urgent course of medical treatment lasting eight days in order to obviate the necessity for violating two Sabbaths (*ib.*, 11).

FORESTALLING DANGER TO LIFE

The law is in suspense not only to overcome but to forestall any danger to life. Thus, flames should be extinguished on the Sabbath before they threaten to engulf properties in which human lives would be unsafe[30] (*O.H.*, *cccxxix*.1), and food may be rescued from a conflagration if required for sick, old or ravenous people (*O.H.*, *cccxxxiv*.5). Likewise, it is permitted to capture snakes, scorpions or other dangerous creatures to prevent being bitten by them[31] (*O.H.*, *cccxvi*.7). Animals whose bite is lethal may be killed unconditionally on the Sabbath; but if the injury they cause is not usually fatal, their destruction is lawful only if one is actually pursued by them, or if one treads them to death without making it obvious that one is intent on killing them (*ib.*, 10).

Although all laws are equally in abeyance when their observance may endanger human life, some instances are singled out for special mention, such as the statement: "It is permitted to extinguish a light [on the Sabbath] in order to enable a dangerously sick person to sleep" (*O.H.*, *cclxxviii*), if there is no other way to protect the patient from the glare.[32] Again, regarding a woman in confinement, the general permission to desecrate the Sabbath for her sake is amplified to include the right to "summon for her a midwife from one place to another,[33] to deliver her child, and to kindle a light for her even if she is blind" (*O.H.*, *cccxxx*.1) because the mere knowledge that her assistants can see properly is likely to ease her mind.[34] In a further reference to a specific law, KARO permits the payment of interest on a loan required for the saving of life[35] (*Y.D.*, *clx*.22).

HEALTHY PERSONS BENEFITING FROM ACTS FOR THE SICK

Finally, we may here record the rulings on how far healthy people may lawfully benefit from breaches of the law in the service of the sick. We have already referred to the right of anyone to utilise lights kindled, vessels used, or meat of animals slaughtered on the Sabbath for the sick.[36] But such meat may be consumed by healthy persons only in a raw state;[37] they must not, however, eat of food specially cooked on the Sabbath for a patient, as it is to be feared that the amount cooked may be increased for their sake[38] (*O.H.*, *cccxxviii*.2). Again, none but gravely ill patients may eat fruit plucked for their benefit on the Sabbath, because such fruit—if not quite ripe when removed from the tree[39]—continues to grow until plucked and is thus rendered unfit for handling on the Sabbath[40] (*O.H.*, *cccxviii*.2, gloss). But some authorities contest this ruling, since the effect of such maturing on the Sabbath is too negligible to be considered.[41]

CHAPTER SIX

LAW AND HEALTH.

CONCESSIONS AND RESTRICTIONS
FOR PATIENTS NOT IN DANGER

In the preceding chapters we have examined the attitude of Jewish law to people on "the danger list". The rules governing these cases are relatively simple and general, because virtually every law must give way to the claims of life. But when the law is likely to clash with the interests of health rather than life, the possibilities of accommodation are far more limited—and, therefore, also more complex and varied. Here it is necessary to assess the relative importance of a law and set it against the degree of sickness or discomfort arising from the indisposition, before a ruling in favour of, or against, a particular concession can be given.[1] The most voluminous part of the Jewish medico-religious legislation is concerned, accordingly, with listing the conditions in which modifications of the law are justified for health reasons.

Physical complaints involving no risk of life are classified as "diseases in which there is no danger". This category includes all indispositions, especially if they confine the sufferer to bed (*O.H.*, *cccxxviii*.17), and mere pains if they affect the entire body, even though the person so afflicted walks about (*ib.*, gloss). For the benefit of small children, even when healthy, it is also usually permitted to do anything normally sanctioned for the sick in this group (*ib.*; and *cclxxvi*.1, gloss). In addition, these provisions extend to healthy adults if they may otherwise suffer from feeling cold; for "all are [deemed] sick in respect of the cold"[2] (*ib.*, 5). Women from the seventh to the thirtieth day after childbirth, as already noted,[3] invariably count as "not dangerously sick persons" (*O.H.*, *cccxxx*.4).

In general, it is lawful in all these cases to request non-Jews to render any necessary services on the Sabbath (*O.H.*, *cccxxxviii*.17). Some hold that, for the sake of people in this class, even Jews may disregard such laws as are of rabbinic status (*ib.*) on the assumption that the rabbis "did not institute their decrees in cases of illness".[4] But no Jew may violate any biblical law to relieve such afflictions, though the patient himself may render some assistance to his non-Jewish attendant in the administration of any necessary medical treatment or service (*ib.*, gloss). In the case of lesser complaints (that is, such as do not affect the whole body), the opinion prevails that even a non-Jew must not be called on except for acts only rabbinically prohibited (*O.H.*, *cccvii*. 5). But this ruling (which is not unanimous) cannot be applied indiscriminately, since rabbinic enactments often vary in importance.[5]

These general regulations are supplemented by numerous detailed laws, the great majority of them again connected with the observance of the Sabbath. Of these, one group derives from the rabbinic ban on the general use of medicines on the Sabbath, and the other concerns the modifications, on account of ill-health or wounds, of the rules based on the thirty-nine principal acts which define work prohibited on the Sabbath, together with their derivatives and rabbinic extensions.[6]

SABBATH BAN ON MEDICINES

The sabbatical ban on medicines, introduced to guard against the possibility of pounding spices on the Sabbath[7] (*O.H.*, *cccxxxviii*.1), is of talmudic origin.[8] The decree is directed against the employment of all medicinal drugs, potions, ointments, lotions or other medicaments, whether taken orally or applied externally, including any food or drink not normally consumed by healthy people (*ib.*, 37). But one may eat or drink anything which can serve as ordinary food, even if it is hard for some healthy people and is, in fact, consumed for obvious remedial purposes (*ib.*). Under this ban—which does not apply to people who either have no pain at all (*ib.*) or whose pain is so acute as to confine them to bed (*ib.*, gloss) or to affect the whole body[9]—it is also prohibited on the Sabbath to chew gum-mastich and rub it on the teeth as a cure, unless this is done against bad oral odours[10] (*ib.*, 36); to quaff vinegar through the teeth and then spit it out against toothache[11] (*ib.*, 32); to take oil to lubricate a painful throat,[12] unless the oil is properly consumed (*ib.*); to employ wine as an ophthalmic agent if applied to the eye itself,[13] though it may be put on the lid without opening and closing the eye at the time[14] (*ib.*, 20); to apply insipid saliva[15] (*ib.*) or a turpid paste to the eye[16] (*O.H., cclii.*5); and to bathe the eye in collyrium[17] dissolved on Friday, if its application is accompanied by opening and shutting the eye (*O.H., cccxxviii.*21). A person suffering from a pain in his loins[18] must not apply a mixture of oil and vinegar; he may use oil alone, provided it is not rose-oil[19] save in a place where this is employed also as a general ointment (*O.H., cccxxvii.*1). But where ordinary oil, too, is applied to the body solely for medical pusposes, no oil may be so used (*ib.*, gloss).

The ban also imposes some restrictions on the treatment of wounds and injuries on the Sabbath. Old wool or pieces of clothing must not be applied, because they are believed to have medicinal properties; but if they had been used on a wound before, or if they are dry and new, they may be used to prevent one's clothes being soiled[20] (*O.H., cccxxviii.* 23). A medicinal plaster may be placed only on a wound already healed, to protect the sore (*ib.*, 27). On an open wound, a plaster may be replaced if it accidentally fell off and rested on a vessel[21] (*ib.*, 25). A non-Jew, however, may always be asked to prepare and affix a plaster[22] (*ib.* and gloss). Calcined ashes, too, since they have healing properties,[23] may be applied to sores only by a non-Jew (*ib.*, gloss). Leaves may be placed on a wound to protect it, so long as they have no curative powers; this excludes the leaves of the vine (*ib.*, 24) and the bulrush (*ib.*, gloss). Bruises may be contracted by the application of wine, so as to check the blood; but vinegar must not be so used, since its action is so strong that it actually heals the injury[24] (*ib.*, 29). Scabs of a wound may be removed and treated with oil, but not with fat which is thereby dissolved[25] (*ib.*, 22). If the emollient consists of a mixture of oil and warm water, it must not be placed on a wound or the wool covering it;[26] but it may be applied outside the wound so as to percolate into it[27] (*ib.*). While a dislocated bone may be reset[28] (*ib.*, 47), it must not be rubbed much in cold water, since that is the usual cure;[29] but it may be bathed in the ordinary way, even if the procedure will effect a remedy (*ib.*, 30).

The use of hot water for bathing or douching the entire body is forbidden,[30] unless the water comes from natural hot springs and is not contained in artificial tanks (*O.H.*, *cccxxvi.*1). Health baths, too, are permitted in natural waters, whether hot like the Palestinian springs or saline like the Mediterranean;[31] for it is usual to bathe in them and there is no obvious indication of the medical motive (*O.H.*, *cccxxviii.*44). But such baths are not permitted in waters normally used only for health reasons, such as in the bad parts of the Mediterranean or in loathsome ponds,[32] unless one merely immerses in them, so that it appears as if one just wishes to cool oneself (*ib.*).

The decree against medicines also covers the use of emetic and laxative stimulants. Even on weekdays, the gourmand's practice of deliberately inducing vomiting is condemned as an unlawful waste of food[33] (*ib.*, 39). Only in the case of pain due to an excess of food is this permitted, but on the Sabbath the fingers alone should be used to agitate the disgorgement (*ib.*). On the Sabbath it is also forbidden to use suppositories for the relief of constipation, unless done in some unusual manner[34] (*ib.*, 49; and *cccxii*.8); to press against the abdomen of children in order to provoke the movement of their bowels[35] (*O.H.*, *cccxxviii*.42); and to induce perspiration by exhausting physical exercises[36] (*ib.*).

The ban does not generally apply to remedies in which no material substances are used, because the possibility of compounding cannot then arise[37] (*ib.*, 43). Hence, it is permitted to lay a vessel on the eye to cool it[38] (*ib.*, 46); to invert a hot cup on the navel in order to lift it (as a cure against dysentery[39]); to raise the ears (to remedy a luxation of the jaw-bone?[40]) whether by hand or with instruments; and to lift the cartilage at the end of the sternum when this is bent inside (and so presses on the stomach, causing nausea[41]) (*ib.*, 43). Cures by incantation, too, are excluded from the ban (*O.H.*, *cccvi*.7; and *Y.D.*, *clxxix*.11); so are measures to calm drunkards, such as rubbing their soles and palms with oil[42] (*O.H.*, *cccxxviii*.41), and to heal animals[43] (*O.H.*, *cccxxxii*.3 and 4). Nor does the ban cover the consumption of any article not taken for purely curative ends, such as sweet gums or raw eggs to clear the voice[44] (*O.H.*, *cccxxviii*.38).

LAWS OF SABBATH

We now turn to the category of biblically or rabbinically prohibited *work* on the Sabbath, and the exemption from some of these laws granted to ailing people. A number of these concessions concern the interdict on carrying any object, other than the clothing one wears, in or into public property (*O.H.*, *cccxlvi*.1-3; and *ccci*.7 *ff.*). A lame person may use a stick, even if not tied to him, provided he cannot walk otherwise (*O.H.*, *ccci*.17); the same applies to a patient rising from his sick-bed on recovery[45] (*ib.*, gloss). But a stick must not be carried if it is not indispensable to walking, but merely serves as a support to one who limps (*ib.*, 17) or as a guide to a blind person[46] (*ib.*, 18). A similar distinction applies to festivals (*O.H.*, *dcxxii.*1), where the concession is also extended to him "whose femoral tendons are shrunk" (*ib.*, 3). Like provisions govern the carriage of artificial limbs or stumps.[47] These may be worn only to assist in the movement of a cripple, provided they are not likely to slip off (*O.H.*, *ccci.*16), but not as a dummy to simulate a missing limb without facilitating walking[48] (*ib.*, 15). Artificial teeth,[49] too, may be worn so long as there is no likelihood of their removal during a walk out of doors—that is, when their colour is not conspicuously different from that of natural teeth; but in the case of women with gold teeth, it is to be feared that they may be insulted and so remove and carry the offensive object in violation of the Sabbath regulations[50] (*O.H.*, *ccciii.*12).

Bandages affixed to a wound before the Sabbath may be retained on going out, if they possess some healing properties,[51] such as lint, wool, compresses, poultices, plasters and husks of garlic or onion[52] (*O.H.*, *ccci.*22). A cord or a band may not be tied to a wound,[53] except if used merely to prevent the actual plaster from falling off (*ib.*). One may also go out with a sling suspended around the neck to support an injured hand or arm, and with a rag of material wrapped around a wounded hand or finger (*ib.*, 51). Again, while one should not go out with only one shoe,[54] this is permitted if the unshod foot is injured (*ib.*, 7). But a sufferer from gonorrhoea must not go out with a suspensor to protect him from being soiled by his flow,[55] nor a woman with a sanitary towel (except if made in the shape of drawers[56]) to prevent stains on her body, though she may wear such a towel to avert the discomfort resulting from the coagulation of the discharge (*ib.*, 13). For that purpose she may wear a pad of cotton-wool, too (*O.H.*, *ccciii.*15, and gloss). Such wool may also be carried in the ear or shoes (*ib.*).

We have already shown in another chapter[57] that the concession to wear medically required objects on the Sabbath also extends to various charms and "tested" amulets, whether therapeutic or prophylactic in their effect. Special rules are also laid down regarding the carriage of charms[58] and other objects by animals on the Sabbath. For, beasts being expressly included among the beneficiaries of the Sabbath ordinance of rest (*Ex. xx.*10; *xxiii.*12; and *Deut. v.*14), they, too, must be restrained from forbidden work (*O.H.*, *ccxlvi.*3) and, in particular, from carrying any articles other than the ordinary outfit they wear for their protection (*O.H.*, *cccv.*1). Among the list of items with which animals may go out on the Sabbath for health reasons or for the prevention of pain are cushions to protect asses against the cold[59] (*ib.*, 8); fodder-baskets around the neck of calves and foals to relieve their discomfort in picking up their food from the ground[60] (*ib.*, 10); and bandages or coats of splints for wounds or fractures (*ib.*, 11). But they must not wear anything which can easily slip off, such as a sort of shoe to guard the legs against bruises[61] or a bag covering a goat's udder to prevent it from being scratched by thorns (*ib.*).

Under the heading of other forbidden work on the Sabbath, it is an offence to "manipulate an abcess in the manner of the physicians" by dilating the orifice of the wound,[62] except in order to let the pus escape[63] (*O.H.*, *cccxxviii.*28); to place a cloth on a wound discharging blood[64] (*ib.*, 48); and to squeeze it out[65] (*ib.*). Such wounds should be treated by first washing them in water or wine to remove the blood and then spreading a spider-web[66] on the whole area before wrapping a bandage around it (*ib.*). For the removal of a splinter a needle may be used, provided its point or eye is not broken off[67] (*O.H.*, *cccviii.*11). But instruments must not be used to remove partly detached finger nails or skin[68] (*O.H.*, *cccxxviii.*31).

In addition to the general prohibition of compounding medicines,[69] it is forbidden to mash ingredients for a poultice[70] (*ib.*, 26); to dissolve the resin of *assa-foetida* in warm or cold water[71] (*O.H.*, *cccxxi*.18); and to capture snakes, scorpions or other creatures for medicinal preparations[72] (*O.H.*, *cccxvi*.7). But, while there are various restrictions on the pressing of fruit for ordinary drinks,[73] a fruit may be squeezed out for the sake of the juice, if required specifically as a cure (*O.H.*, *cccxx*.1, gloss). A sufferer from an attack of *angina pectoris*[74] may suck milk from an animal[75]—a cure still widely employed in the 16th century[76]—though this concession is not granted to people who merely suffer the pain of hunger (*O.H.*, *cccxxviii*.35).

A number of special concessions are made in respect of new-born children and nursing mothers. We have already mentioned the sanction to perform on the Sabbath such acts immediately after birth as are regarded essential for the preservation of the infant's life.[77] In addition, it is allowed to straighten the child's limbs which may have become deranged in the course of the puerperal labour[78] (*O.H.*, *cccxx*. 9), to swathe it in clothes so that its limbs shall not become crooked[79] (*ib.*, 10), and to place a finger into its mouth in order to "raise its uvular lobula to the right place if it had dropped,[80] even though this sometimes causes vomiting" (*ib.*, 11). When nursing, a mother may not collect the milk from her breasts in a receptacle and then give it to the suckling[81] (*O.H.*, *cccxxviii*.34), but she may squirt her milk into the infant's mouth to induce it to seize the nipple and suck properly[82] (*ib.*, 35). She may also press out by hand any excess milk causing her pain[83] as well as relieve herself by suckling an eight months' baby, though it must not otherwise be handled on the Sabbath[84] (*O.H.*, *cccxx*.8).

Finally, at the other end of life, the usual ban on the administration of divorces on the Sabbath[85] (*O.H.*, *cccxxxix*. 4) is waived for a very sick man who seeks to release his wife from the legal complications of widowhood[86] before his death[87] (*ib.;* and *dxxiv.*2).

On the medical assistance of patients by non-Jews, we may here add some details to the general provisions mentioned earlier in this chapter.[88] It is permitted to ask a non-Jew to extract a painful tooth on the Sabbath[89] (*O.H., cccxxviii.*3, gloss) and to send him beyond the Sabbath limits[90] to call for the relatives of a dying person (*O.H., cccvi.*9). There is a difference of opinion on whether these and similar services may also be rendered by slaves who, despite their bondage to Jewish masters, have not consented to fulfil the "seven Noachidic laws"[91] (*O.H., ccciv.*1). But the restrictions on soliciting medical aid from non-Jews on the Sabbath apply only to acts for the benefit of Jewish patients; to give instructions on the treatment of the non-Jewish sick, as NACHMANIDES already confirmed, "has invariably been the practice of Jewish doctors".[92]

TREATMENT OF ANIMALS ON SABBATH

To conclude our consideration of the Sabbath laws, we will list some further provisions on the treatment of animals.[93] Relaxations of the Sabbath laws for the sake of protecting the health of animals include the permission to capture them[94] (*O.H., cccxvi.*2); to oint their wounds, provided they are fresh and painful[95] (*O.H., cccxxxii.*2); to race them to exhaustion as a remedy for overeating[96] (*ib.,* 3); to place them in water so as to cool them following an attack of congestion[97] (*ib.,* 4); and to ask a non-Jew to bleed them if venesection may save their life (*ib.*) To ease the sufferings of beasts it is also lawful to assist in raising them from water into which they had fallen[98] (*O.H., cccv.*19) and to ask a non-Jew to relieve them of milk causing them distress[99] (*ib.,* 20). While one may not deliver the young of cattle[100] (*O.H., cccxxxii.*1), one may help by holding the young to prevent it from falling to the ground, by blowing into its nostrils, and by placing the dam's teat into its mouth[101] (*O.H., dxxiii.*3) . Of special interest is the following law: "If an animal rejected its young, it is permitted to sprinkle the water of its placenta on the latter and to place some salt into its mother's vaginal orifice so that she shall have compassion on it [through being reminded of her birth-pangs], but one may not do so with an animal of the unclean species [since it will not help to arouse her pity]"[102] (*ib.,* 4).

LAWS OF FESTIVALS

The laws regarding forbidden work on the festivals are, with a few reservations, identical with those affecting the Sabbath, to the exclusion only of acts required for the preparation of food and of work in the categories of "carrying" and "the lighting of fires" (*O.H., cdxcv.*1). With those exceptions, therefore, anything which must not be done on the Sabbath for people not dangerously ill is forbidden on the festivals, too.[103] These rules apply equally to the festival days specified in the Bible and the "second days" of the festivals ordained by the rabbis for the Diaspora, save that on the latter days one may "paint the eye" for medical purposes[104] (*O.H., cdxcvi.*2) and disregard any rabbinical prohibition for the sake of even only moderately sick patients[105] (*ib.,* gloss). But on the "intermediate days" of the Passover and Tabernacles festivals, there are no restrictions at all on performing any medically required acts (*O.H., dxxxii.*2)— even if they constitute work otherwise prohibited on these days.[106] All restrictions on these days are also relaxed for the medical treatment of animals, including venesection (*O.H., dxxxvi.*3). It is even permitted to cut and adjust the hoofs of horses to prevent their discomfort (*ib.,* 1), although it is the accepted practice not to cut human hand- or foot-nails on these days[107] (*O.H., dxxxii.*1, gloss). The removal of flies irritating an animal is allowed even on the main festival days, notwithstanding the small wound thus caused (*O.H.*, *dxxiii.*1).

Occasionally ill-health is also mentioned among the laws relating to specific festivals. On Passover, when no leavened substance may be consumed or used (except, of course, in cases of danger to life[108]), it is forbidden to chew wheat to be used as a poultice on a wound,[109] since the saliva brings about its fermentation (*O.H.*, *cdlxvi.*1). But, despite the practice—codified as law by ISSERLES—not to knead flour in fruit juices[110] lest this accelerate the fermentation of the dough, sick or old people may eat unleavened bread prepared in this way, if necessary[111] (*O.H.*, *cdlxvi.*4, gloss). On the other hand, he who refrains from wine because it harms him (by causing him pain or head-ache) must still drink the obligatory four cups of wine on the first two Passover nights[112] (*O.H.*, *cdlxxii.*10). Although one must not drink anything after these four cups (*O.H.*, *cdlxxxi.*1), an exception is made for people who are delicate or who have an excessive desire for drink (*ib.*, gloss). An epileptic, during an attack, cannot legally discharge any religious obligation;[113] hence, if he ate the statutory unleavened bread whilst in a fit, and he then recovered, he must consume a further morsel to perform his duty (*O.H.*, *cdlxxv.*5).

On Tabernacles, too, the law is relaxed in cases of indisposition. Sick people, together with their attendants,[114] are exempt from the duty of dwelling (that is, especially eating and sleeping) in the festival booth;[115] this concession includes even such as suffer only from some head- or eye ache[116] (*O.H.*, *dcxl.*3). KARO, however, also records a view that attendants are covered by these concessions only at the time their services are actually required by the patient[117] (*ib.*). The exemption is also granted to persons to whom the performance of this law would cause some physical distress, for example through exposure to wind, flies, spiders or evil smells; but the attendants are not included in such cases (*ib.*, 4). On the other hand, people are not free from sleeping in the booth merely because the place is too narrow to stretch out, or if their absence from the booth will not remove the cause of their distress (*ib.*, gloss). The cold, in particular, is a cause of suffering;[118] that explains the usual practice not to sleep in the booth in countries that have a cold climate (*O.H.*, *dcxxxix*.2, gloss).

LAWS OF FASTS

More numerous are the laws affecting the sick and the weak in connection with the Day of Atonement. In addition to all restrictions applicable on the Sabbath (*O.H.*, *dcxi*.2), the day also imposes various duties of mortification, including the complete abstention from eating and drinking, washing and anointing oneself, and the wearing of leather shoes[119] (*ib.*, 1). We have already dealt with the exemption of dangerously ill people from the duty to fast.[120] Further concessions regarding the minor duties of self-denial are made for moderately sick or delicate persons, though such people—including expectant and nursing mothers (*O.H.*, *dcxvii*.1)—are under no circumstances absolved from the fast itself. Washing any part of one's body is forbidden only in so far as it is conducive to pleasure or refreshment; hence, it is allowed to rinse parts which are soiled with dirt and to wash a bleeding nose (*O.H.*, *dcxiii*.1). For the same reason a delicate person may wipe his face with water if his mind cannot be at ease otherwise[121] (*ib.*, 4). But ISSERLES inclines to a stricter view even in regard to the ablution of the eyes,[122] since that may constitute a medical act which is prohibited (*ib.*, gloss). He also forbids rinsing the mouth[123] (*ib.*). But a sick person may wash himself in the ordinary way (*ib.*, 9, gloss). A patient or a person with scurf in his hair is exempt from the ban on unguents, though any anointing is otherwise forbidden even for the removal of one's perspiration (*O.H.*, *dcxiv.*1). The ban on wearing leather shoes is lifted for persons who are ill or suffer from a foot injury, and for women in confinement for thirty days (*ib.*, 3). In the event of rain, a delicate person, too, may wear shoes in the street (*ib.*, 4, gloss).

Less stringent than the Day of Atonement are the other five statutory fasts, since these are only rabbinically ordained.[124] With the exception of the Ninth of Av, they require no abstention from washing, anointing or the wearing of shoes (*O.H.*, *dl.*2), nor does the duty to fast include the preceding night from dusk (*ib.*). On these fasts the general obligation to abstain completely from food or drink (*ib.* 1) is relaxed for women during pregnancy or lactation (*O.H.*, *dliv.*5), if fasting would cause them undue distress (*O.H.*, *dl.*1, gloss), though, when eating, they should do so not for pleasure but only for the health of the children they carry or nurse (*O.H.*, *dliv.*5). On the Fast of Esther, being of a still less binding character than the others,[125] sick people and even such as only complain of aching eyes are excused from fasting (*O.H.*, *dclxxxvi.*1, gloss). The Ninth of Av, on the other hand, shares almost all the stringencies of the Day of Atonement (*O.H.*, *dliii.*2), including the specified acts of self-denial (*O.H.*, *dliv.*1). Even pregnant women must complete the fast (*ib.*, 5); but mothers within thirty days of childbirth and sick people requiring food may be allowed to eat without any medical assessment of their need (*ib.*, 6), though it is the usual practice for all to fast, except in cases of great pain which may lead to a risk of life (*ib.*, gloss). Among the exemptions, for reasons of health, from the special privations[126] is the permission to wash the legs if they feel faint after a journey (*ib.*, 14) and to anoint the head if it is scurfy (*ib.*, 15). The Ninth of Av being a day of extreme mourning, it is also customary to deprive oneself of some comforts one normally enjoys whilst sleeping; yet expectant mothers who cannot bear such discomfort need not do so (*O.H.*, *dlv.*2, gloss). Any patient is also excused from the custom not to eat meat on the nine days terminating on the Ninth of Av (*O.H.*, *dli*.9, gloss).

Further concessions are made for pregnant and nursing mothers on the additional fasts which may be proclaimed as days of intercession in times of national distress or persecution (*O.H.*, *dlxxvi*.14) and of protracted drought in Palestine (*O.H.*, *dlxxv*.5 and gloss). In the case of voluntary, self-imposed fasts by individuals, ill-health, acute pain or weakness are also legitimate grounds for reducing their severity (*O.H.*, *dlxviii*.4, gloss), or for ransoming them by donations to charity (*ib.*, 2, gloss), or for obtaining a formal release from three scholars[127] (*Y.D.*, *ccxiv*.1).

These laws on fasts come closer than other fields of the Jewish ritual legislation to comparative rules in Christian theology. But even here the similarity of conditions is reduced by the fact that the fasts ordained by the Catholic Church are less complete than those in the Jewish calendar in view of the ruling: *"Liquidum non frangit jejunum"*, thus excluding most plain drinks from the ban on alimentary items.[128] According to CAPELLMANN,[129] the numerous exemptions from the duty to fast include, apart from dispensations (for which no parallel exists in Jewish law), any illness or other legitimate hardship, the *tempus gestationis et lactionis*, and possibly the *tempus menstruationis*. He observes that the decision in these matters rests with the doctor and especially the feeling of the person concerned.

LAWS OF PRAYER

The sick are also given special consideration among the Jewish laws on the daily prayers. For medical reasons food or drinks may be consumed before the morning prayer (*O.H.*, *lxxxix*.3), and the recitation of the night prayer[130] may be delayed if prevented from saying it earlier by illness or some other unavoidable cause (*O.H.*, *ccxxxv*.4). The proper posture during the reading of certain prayers may be modified for reasons of sickness (*O.H.*, *lxiii.*1; and *xciv.* 6). If a patient is altogether unfit to recite these prayers, he should meditate on them in his heart (*O.H.*, *lxii.*4; and *xciv.*6, gloss). The laws on the statutory washing of hands before meals are also modified; a person with a wound on his hand need not water the part covered by a plaster (*O.H.*, *clxii.*10). Since phylacteries may be used only in a physically clean state, a sufferer from indigestion is free from the duty to wear them (*O.H.*, *xxxviii.*1); so is any sick person who cannot put his mind at ease (*ib.*, gloss). Leprosy constitutes a complete disability from fulfilling this commandment[131] (*ib.*, 13). Men disposed to head-colds through uncovering their heads may have a thin cap underneath the head phylactery in preference to not wearing it at all (*O.H.*, *xxvii.*5).

LAWS OF MOURNING

The next group of laws to be considered are the extensive mourning regulations and their application to sick people. A patient should not be informed of the death of a close relative "lest his mind will be distracted" (*Y.D.*, *cccxxxvii.*1). Nor should he perform the statutory "tearing of the shirt"[132] (*ib.*), even if he is aware of his bereavement, as that might aggravate his trouble.[133] In his presence it is also improper to weep for or eulogise the dead[134] "so as not to break his heart"; in fact, mourners should be silenced in his vicinity (*ib.*). During the first week of mourning for the loss of a near relative, the law imposes severe limitations on the enjoyment of all pleasures and many comforts, including the restrictions applicable to the Day of Atonement (except fasting), unless their observance may be physically harmful or unduly vexacious. The ban on washing the entire body, and on ablutions in warm water of any part of it, is modified for the removal of dirt (*Y.D.*, *ccclxxxi.*1);

for women in confinement (*ib.*, 3); for people suffering from scabs through uncleanliness (*ib.*); and for delicate persons in general, provided their failure to wash themselves "would cause great hardship and lead to indisposition" (*ib.*). The use of unguents, too, is forbidden only for pleasure or refreshment, not for the removal of the body's perspiration or any medical pupose, such as against dandruff[135] (*ib.*, 2). Within thirty days of childbirth women in mourning need not observe the restrictions on footwear "because the cold is harmful for them"[136] (*Y.D., ccclxxxii*.2). Sick and aged people are not required to sit on the ground while mourning, if they would suffer unduly by observing this custom.[137] According to JACOB MOLIN, the laws of mourning are altogether in abeyance in times of pestilence "on account of the [harm done by] fright";[138] ISSERLES, recording this opinion, adds: "And I have heard of some who have adopted this [view in] practice" (*Y.D., ccclxxiv*. 11, gloss.)

DIETARY LAWS

Among the dietary laws, references to sick people are far less numerous than those found in the Sabbath regulations, possibly due to the relatively infrequent occasions on which rabbinical rulings were sought on problems regarding a patient's diet.[139] In ordinary Jewish households, there would be little difficulty in meeting a sick person's alimentary and medicinal needs compared with the problems arising from his requirements on the Sabbath. The scarcity of medico-dietetic provisions in Jewish law also bears testimony to the overwhelming preponderance of vegetarian over meat substances among the ancient and medieval *materia medica*;[140] for the bulk of the Jewish food laws concerns only meat and its products.[141]

In cases of danger to life, every article may, of course, be employed as a cure, even if used in the normal way (*Y.D.*, *clv*.3), unless there is reason to suspect it was dedicated to an idolatrous purpose (*ib.*, 2). But in the absence of danger, substances banned for use as well as for consumption[141] may be medically utilised only in an uncommon manner,[142] the sole exceptions being a boiled mixture of meat with milk and products of a vineyard growing mixed seeds[143] which must not be used in any form, save to ward off a risk of life (*ib.*, 3). A moderately sick person may, however, even consume any forbidden article once it is transformed into a carbonised state by burning[144] (*ib.*, gloss). Substances rabbinically banned for use may be utilised for the cure of sick people without restriction, provided they are not actually consumed (*ib.*). Any patient is permitted to eat dishes cooked by non-Jews[145] (*O.H.*, *cccxxviii*.19).

While KARO bans the use of wine handled by Gentiles[146] for medicinal baths by sick people[147] (*Y.D.*, *cxxiii*.2), his glossator expressly includes such baths among the permitted cures for patients who are not in danger (*Y.D.*, *clv*.3, gloss). He adds that even healthy people are allowed to inhale the fumes of such wine sprinkled into fire,[148] "since the vapour does not constitute a [forbidden] substance" (*ib.*). The codes do not mention the legality or otherwise of drinking ritually unfit wine as a medicament—a question often treated in rabbinic literature[149]—except to permit the purchase of medicinal pomegranate wine from a non-Jewish dealer without the restrictions normally applicable to the buying of such liquors[150] (*Y.D.*, *cxiv*.5). Historically, it is of interest to observe that, while the Arabs (as previously noted[151]) opposed the inclusion of wine in medical prescriptions, every slaughterer authorised by the Chief Rabbi in England early in the 19th century had to sign a pledge that he would not " . . . drink wine which had not been supervised by Jews, except for medical purposes."[152]

The consumption of human milk — presumably for therapeutic reasons in accordance with the popular belief in its curative value[153]—is sanctioned in Jewish law, provided it is first collected in a vessel (*Y.D., lxxxi.*7) or hand (*ib.,* gloss). An adult sucking from a human breast is to be reprimanded and chastised (*ib.,* 7). Since the boiling of meat in human milk is discountenanced only for appearance sake (*Y.D., lxxxvii.*4), the rabbis raised no objection if this was done for medical reasons.[154] The maximum age up to which a child may be allowed to suck the milk of its mother or wet-nurse is, in common with oriental custom and ancient Jewish practice,[155] fixed at four years for healthy, and five for sick and weak, sucklings, unless the child was previously weaned for a period of seventy-two hours; in that case, breast-feeding must not be restarted after the child's second birthday, except if the interruption was due to illness (*Y.D., lxxxi.*7). A physiologically interesting law first mentioned by ADRETH[156] adds that, though the milk of a non-Jewess is ritually as fit as that of a Jewish mother, a Jewish suckling should not be fed by a Gentile nurse—if a Jewess is available for the purpose—because her milk "obstructs the heart" (*ib.,* gloss). Nor should a child drink the milk of a Jewish woman who, due to illness, consumes forbidden food, "for all that will cause harm in its advanced years" (*ib.*). The antiquity of this belief is attested by JOSEPHUS[157] and the *Midrash*[158] in their almost identical reference to the legend that the infant MOSES refused to be nursed by any Egyptian woman and did not suck until the breast of a Jewess was offered to him.[159]

To our consideration of the dietary laws we may add that herbs and other edible substances grown or produced for exclusively medical ends are not generally regarded as human food in a technical sense. Thus, although food should not be used to cover the festival booth on Tabernacles (*O.H., dcxxix.*9), the herb called "*phinogo*"[160] may be so employed, since it serves only as fodder for animals and as human medicine (*ib.,* 11). Likewise, a plant grown for medical or animal-feeding purposes in a vineyard or field does not render its products liable to condemnation under the laws of mixed wine[161] (*Y.D., ccxcvi*.14) or corn seeds[162] (*Y.D., ccxcvi*.3) respectively. These considerations also affect the benedictions to be recited before eating medicinal herbs[163] (*O.H., cciv*.11, gloss). Yet, a beast ritually slaughtered to provide meat for healing purposes or for animals is still subject to compliance with the law on priestly gifts[164] like ordinary meat (*Y.D., lxi*.6). In the context of medicinal substances, we may also mention the ban on the general use of earth covering a grave; the ban is waived if the earth is required for a medical purpose[165] (*Y.D., ccclxviii*.1, gloss).

The following scattered laws conclude our enumeration of religious concessions for sick people. The biblical ban on "printing marks" upon oneself (*Lev. xix*.28)—"that is, by making an incision into one's flesh and filling the etching with stibium, ink or any other permanent dye" (*Y.D., clxxx*.1)—may be disregarded when treating an open wound with wood-ashes[156] (*ib.*, 3), even if this may leave a permanent mark.[167] The frequency with which a husband must fulfill his marital duties, fixed by law in accordance with his occupational pursuits (*E.H., lxxvi*.1 and 2), may be modified if he is not healthy (*ib.*, 3). Unlike healthy people, the sick and the aged may derive a gainful benefit from their religious learning (*Y.D., ccxlvi*.21, gloss). But the duty to pursue religious education devolves on healthy and ailing persons alike (*ib.*, 1). Any act in the interest of human healing sets aside the laws against cruelty to animals[168] (*E.H., v*.14, gloss). Reference is made elsewhere to the accommodation, in cases of illness, of laws relating to sorcery and other superstitions,[169] to the surgical treatment of one's parents,[170] to contact between a husband and his wife while in a state of impurity,[171] and, in particular detail, to circumcisions.[172]

Finally, we will list some religious acts which, due to wounds or physical disabilities, cannot be fully carried out. The law requires that the ritual waters in which a woman immerses to terminate her period of uncleanliness[173] must be in unbroken contact with every part of her body at the same time (*Y.D.*, *cxcviii*.1). Interpositions which invalidate the immersion include a plaster on a wound (*ib.*, 10 and 43) or hair cleaving to it (*ib.*, 44), a splinter lodged in her flesh if visible from without (*ib.*, 11), blood which is dry (*ib.*, 9) or adheres to the skin (*ib.*, 16), and secretions discharged from an open wound when they become dry[174] (*ib.*, 9). The procedure of the levirate divorce[175] provides for the removal of a special sandal worn on the levir's right foot (*E.H.*, *clxix*.24) by his sister in-law's right hand (*ib.*, 30). If her hands are stumped, she may use her teeth instead (*ib.*, 31); but if the levir's foot is disabled, the rite cannot be carried out (*ib.*, 34). In the absence of the left hand, the performance of the precept of phylacteries is also compromised[176] (*O.H.*, *xxvii*.1, gloss). Various physical abnormalities disqualify priests from "raising the[ir] hands"[177] to recite the "Priestly Benediction"[178] (*O.H.*, *cxxviii*.30) and rabbis from certain judicial functions (*E.H.*, *clxix* [*Seder Halitzah*].1, gloss; and *H.M.*, *vii*.2).

The religious and legal disqualifications of the blind[179] and deaf-mute[180] are too numerous to be detailed here. With the latter category the idiot, too, is generally associated;[181] and both are very often classed together with the minor with whom they share an incompetence to carry out certain religious (*e.g.*, *O.H.*, *dlxxxix*.2) and legal (*e.g.*, *H.M.*, *xxxv*.1, 8 and 11) acts. Epileptics[182] are likewise disqualified for the duration of an attack (*O.H.*, *cdlxxv*.5; and *H.M.*, *xxxv*.9).

CHAPTER SEVEN

ETHICS AND HEALTH.

ETHICAL CONCESSIONS FOR THE SICK
AND MORAL CONSIDERATION IN
THE SAVING OF LIFE

The formal distinction between ethics and ritual is altogether foreign to rabbinic Judaism.[1] The Bible lists laws of social and purely religious concern quite indiscriminately side by side with each other[2]—an arrangement which the rabbis regarded as profoundly significant[3]—and the Talmud adduces evidence from every major part of Holy Writ to prove "that man is obliged to fulfil his duties towards his neighbour in the same way as he must discharge his debt to Heaven".[4] In the traditional Jewish view, every divine precept, whether of a moral or ritual character, derives its validity and binding nature only from the fact that it was revealed to MOSES at Sinai,[5] and MAIMONIDES[6] is at pains to show that this consideration alone justifies the validity of even such laws as were ordained in pre-Sinaitic times. In contrast to the jurisprudence of the Romans, Jewish law does not know of any division between *jus* (legal law) and *fas* (moral law) in its principles or administration.[7] Hence, transgressions against religious injunctions are at the same time regarded as social crimes,[8] while (conversely) the penal system of Judaism extends to both categories of offenders precisely the same juridical norms of trial and punishment.[9]

It follows, therefore, that the rules already established for the suspension or modification of religious laws in the event of illness or other risks of life and health apply equally to the Jewish code of ethics. Accordingly, it is hardly necessary to state that, with a view to saving life, it is permitted, for example, to disregard the law against the payment of interest on a loan[10] (*Y.D.*, *clx*.22); indeed, this decision may be codified for the very purpose of confirming that the setting aside of ethical and religious precepts is governed by identical principles.

Regarding concessions to patients not in danger, separate rulings are required to determine the extent to which health considerations can compromise ethical and social duties, just as in the case of ritual observances.[11] The following is a list of such relaxations on account of sickness. The sick, like mourners, need not rise to honour even the highest dignitary[12] (*Y.D.*, *ccclxxvi*.1, gloss). The rabbis interpreted the injunction "a man shall not put on a woman's garment" (*Deut. xxii.5*) as directed against any activity by men which is peculiar to women,[13] such as the personal use of mirrors (*Y.D.*, *clvi*.2) and the removal of pubic hair in the groin and arm-pits[14] (*Y.D.*, *clxxxii*.1). But an exception is made if these acts serve medical ends;[15] hence, a man may look into a mirror if his eyes trouble him (*Y.D.*, *clvi*.2), and he may cut off any hair causing pain to sores underneath it (*Y.D.*, *clxxxii*.4). On hearing anyone sneeze it was customary to exclaim "health!"; but this social convention should be ignored during meals[16] (*O.H.*, *clxx*.1) as well as in the house of learning[17] (*Y.D.*, *ccxlvi*.17). Again, old and sick people are not required to fulfil the biblical law of assisting in the loading or unloading of beasts of burden in distress (*Ex. xxiii.5*; and *Deut. xxii.4*), even if they themselves own the animals[18] (*H.M.*, *cclxxii*.7). The exemption of the sick from some of Judaism's civil laws will be considered in another chapter.[19]

Into the category of duties towards one's fellow-men belong also vows to abstain from receiving any benefit from another person or from granting any favour to him. In such cases complex rules lay down the exact conditions in which these vows may be disregarded to enable persons thus bound to receive certain paid medical services[20] (*Y.D.*, *ccxxi.*4) and to "wait [on a person so foresworn] with the cup [of hot water, serving as a cure during the use[21]] of the bath-house" (*ib.*, 2). But a vow to abstain from eating another's food includes the chewing of wheat for putting it as a plaster on one's wound[22] (*ib.*, 1). On the other hand, "if a woman swore before her husband, during his illness, that she would not remarry after his death, or *vice versa*, or if one made a vow to the sick on any matter, [it may be regarded] as a vow under duress [requiring no formal absolution], provided it was made on the insistence of the patient, so that his mind should not be distracted"[23] (*Y.D.*, *ccxxxii.* 17, gloss). For the same reason the sick were also exempted from the ban on card-playing pronounced at Bologna in 1415, at Forli in 1418 and at Cremona in 1576 by the communal authorities.[24]

SAVING LIFE WITH NEIGHBOUR'S POSSESSIONS

In all the aforementioned issues, the concessions granted for the protection of life and health are allowed to override the claims of Jewish ethics with no more reservations or scruples than are the ritual demands of Judaism. But one important moral problem created by the clash of the interests of life and ethics has evoked much discussion and some controversy. KARO refers to this problem in the following ruling: "Even if a person is in mortal danger and can save his life only by robbing his neighbour, he must not appropriate [another's possession] except with the intention to repay [him]" (*H.M.*, *ccclix.*4); for "he who saves himself at his neighbour's expense is obliged to compensate him" (*H.M.*, *ccclxxx.*3). The subject is first raised in the Talmud[25] where the question "May one save oneself with one's neighbour's money?" is answered in the negative. KARO's ruling follows the construction of the question by TOSA-PHOTH:[26] "Must one make repayment to one's neighbour if forced to use his money to save one's life?" ASHERI[27] understands the passage in the same sense, since only idolatry, incest and bloodshed are laws overriding life itself.[28] But RASHI[29] appears to imply that it is categorically forbidden to lay hands on one's neighbour's possessions to save one's own life, and NACHMANIDES[30] and others[31] in fact record a minority opinion of a talmudic sage[32] according to whom theft is expressly added to the three inviolable offences. RASHI's attitude has also been explained[33] as motivated by the talmudic dictum: "He who robs his fellow-man of any amount, however minute, is as if he took his life",[34] a dictum later codified as law, too (*H.M., ccclix.*3). But all the later authorities dealing with the problem leave us in no doubt that one has the right, indeed the duty, to safeguard one's life by encroaching on the possessions of another person if necessary, even if one is not at that time in a position to promise compensation.[35]

SAVING ANOTHER'S LIFE AT ONE'S OWN RISK

In practice, therefore, rabbinic opinion is clearly unanimous on sanctioning the violation of property rights in the defence of human life. But there is a wide difference of views on the perplexing question whether one should imperil one's own life and limb in order to rescue one's neighbour. One view recorded by KARO[36] holds that the law "Thou shalt not stand upon the blood of thy neighbour" (*Lev. xix.*16)—from which the rabbis derive the general duty to come to the aid of a person in danger (*H.M., cdxxvi*) —also teaches that one must be prepared to risk a possible threat to one's own life to save that of another; "for the one faces a certain danger, whereas the other [*i.e.* the rescuer] takes only a doubtful risk, and whoever preserves the life of one person in Israel is as if he had preserved an entire world".[37] But in the codes this law is omitted,[38] though various commentators mention it.[39] In this connection, we may also mention that the 17th century Palestinian rabbi MOSES IBN HABIB[40] affirmed the right of a person to save his life, if no other alternative is open to him, by putting out an eye or lopping off a limb from another person. This view, too, does not find expression in any code of Jewish law, and it appears to have been clearly opposed in an earlier ruling by DAVID IBN ZIMRA.[41]

Among Catholic theologians, the moral stakes involved in the self-mutilation of one person for the benefit of another have been more recently discussed mainly in connection with the problem of organic transplants and grafts.[42] While some earlier moralists regarded such operations "as a violation of the Fifth Commandment and thus as intrinsically unlawful" and as an act just as wrong as to kill oneself for the advantage of one's neighbour,[43] others considered it as "licit and commendable, though not of obligation",[44] and as justified on the grounds of charity and the unity of the human race.[45]

The Jewish sources under review make no reference to mutilations for the therapeutic or cosmetic advantage of others. Jewish law strongly condemns any deliberate infliction of physical injuries (*H.M.*, *cdxx*.1 ff.), even if self-inflicted[46] (*ib.*, 31), including especially suicide[47] (*Y.D.*, *cccxlv*.1-3). The only exceptions sanctioning the violation of the human body's integrity are cases of self-defence (*H.M.*, *cdxxv*.1), the treatment or amputation of diseased parts of the body,[48] an incision in the flesh as a token of mourning for a great saint,[49] the perforation of a Hebrew slave's ear,[50] and the circumcision of Jews and proselytes. Only in one instance was a physical mutilation also sanctioned as an extraordinary penal measure. ISSERLES invested the Jewish court with the right to mete out exemplary punishment to prostitutes, citing with approval ASHERI's mention[51] of an incident, "when a woman who misconducted herself with a non-Jew had her nose cut off [by judicial order] as a mark of disgrace" (*E.H., clxxvii.5*, gloss). The same penalty is also found in other medieval legislations.[52]

While some Jewish authorities, as we have seen, affirm the right, or even duty, of a person to submit to a possible risk of life in an effort to save his neighbour from certain death, no Jewish teacher would go so far as to agree with the "traditional teaching" of the Roman Catholic Church which "admits that one may expose oneself to certain danger of death for the sake of the neighbour, or—as St. THOMAS has it—for the sake of the virtue involved in the act".[53] According to Jewish teaching, a man has no rights over his body[54] or his life which would entitle him to sacrifice it in order to rescue another's life,[55] though it has been suggested that such self-sacrifice may be licit, and even meritorious, if the person to be saved is "a great and saintly man who is required by the community".[56]

The deliberate sacrifice of a human life is unlawful even if it may save many other people from certain death.[57] But this rule may be qualified by some reservations. Thus IS-SERLES, on the basis of the Talmud,[58] decides: "If heathens said to [a group of] Jews: 'Surrender to us one of you and we shall kill him [or else we shall kill all of you]', one shall not hand over any one of them, unless they singled out one and said: 'Give us such and such'; but some hold that, even in that event, one should not surrender him, except if he is under sentence of death, as in the case of SHEVA, the son of BICHRI"[59] (*Y.D., clvii.*1, gloss). MAIMO-NIDES,[60] too, records this law, but he adds that in such cases one refrains from announcing the verdict.[61]

CHAPTER EIGHT

LAW AND PAIN.

RELIGIOUS CONSIDERATION
FOR PHYSICAL SUFFERING

Jewish law, in its concern for the human weal, makes little distinction in principle between proper ill-health and mere physical pain. In the preceding chapters, we have often referred to religious concessions designed to mitigate pain or aches. If we yet add a separate chapter on pain to the illustrations already given, it is only in order to portray the characteristic features of the Jewish attitude to physical suffering, and its comparative background, with the material provided by our sources. The picture thus drawn will supplement, in some important aspects, our earlier investigation into the outlook on the practice of medicine in general.

RELIGIOUS CONCESSIONS FOR PEOPLE IN PAIN

The extent to which pain in general justifies infractions of the law is the subject of some dispute. Although, as a rule, the experience of a localised ache[1] does not warrant the suspension of religious precepts,[2] the codes state expressly in two instances that the rabbis "did not make their decrees [to be valid] in cases of pain"[3] (*O.H.*, *cccxxviii.*33; and *cccxvii.*1, gloss). In the Talmud itself, however, there is no foundation for limiting the validity of rabbinic enactments to persons who are not in pain. Hence, YA'IR BACHARACH[4] concludes that the statement cannot be accepted as an invariable rule and that the specific concessions mentioned apply only in cases of severe pain. On the other hand, AZULAY[5] cites an earlier authority for the view that persons in pain are exempt from the observance of all precepts, but this opinion has been generally rejected as unfounded. Only by reference to specific regulations, there-fore, can the attitude of Jewish law to pain be ascertained.

Pain as a factor in the modification of laws includes mental anguish as well as physical suffering. This is particularly in evidence regarding the obligation to "call the Sabbath a delight" (*Is. lviii.*13). According to the Talmud,[6] this injunction seeks to encourage the enjoyment of physical no less than spiritual pleasures, and the banishment of all sor-row, or the duration of the holy day. Yet, special consider-ation is given to people in distress. Thus, although it is for-bidden to fast on the Sabbath (*O.H., cclxxxviii.*1), a person harrowed when eating food may desist from it, "since it is his pleasure not to eat" (*ib.*, 2 and 3). Similarly, one need not have the Friday evening meal in the glow of the Sab-bath candles, as normally required, if the light is the cause of undue discomfort (*O.H., cclxxiii.*7), and it is allowed to weep on the Sabbath, if this may bring relief from mental stress (*O.H., cclxxxviii.*2, gloss). To visit mourners and the sick may be a distressing experience, and the Talmud[7] saw its way to permitting such visits on the Sabbath only "with difficulty". The codes sanction these calls of comfort and succour, but—to avoid expressions of grief prohibited on the Sabbath[8]—one should not greet the sick with the formula used on weekdays;[9] instead one should say: "It is the Sabbath [to-day] when one refrains from sorrow, and healing is speedy in coming" (*O.H., cclxxxvii.*1; and *Y.D., cccxxxv.*6). For the same reason, all prayers of intercession and lamentation should be eschewed (*O.H., cclxxxiv.*7, gloss), even in the event of national calamities, such as the scourges of blast, locust and drought (*O.H., cclxxxviii.*9; and *dlxxvi.*12). Such a violation of the joyful spirit of the Sabbath is warranted only in the case of a critical economic slump[10] (*ib.*) and for patients in acute danger on that day (*O.H., cclxxxviii.*10 and gloss; and *dlxxvi.*13). While some proscribed the rendering of such prayers in the absence of any immediate threat to life,[11] others even discountenanced petitions in one place for the recovery of a dangerously sick person in another, lest he had meanwhile either returned to health or died, thus leading to an unnecessary agitation of sorrow on the Sabbath.[12]

Marital relations, too, belong to the essential pleasures of the Sabbath.[13] Indeed, scholars are advised to reserve the payment of their conjugal dues for that night (*O.H.*, *cclxxx*.1). It is also permitted to consummate a marriage on the Sabbath, without regard to the wound[14] or the pain caused by the defloration (*ib.*, 2). But if a wife was injured during intercourse, she is entitled to claim damages, including compensation for the pain she endured (*E.H.*, *lxxxiii*.2; and *H.M.*, *cdxxi*.12).

PAIN OF MOTHERS AND INFANTS

The nursing mother enjoys the especial sympathy of Jewish law. To relieve herself of excess milk hurting her she may, the usual Sabbath laws notwithstanding, suckle an inviable child or squeeze the milk by hand[15] (*O.H.*, *cccxxx.* 8); she may also give suck to a heathen infant, even in circumstances in which that is normally not tolerated[16] (*Y.D.*, *cliv*.2, gloss). The same consideration[17] entitles her to overrule her husband's objection to nursing her own child (*E.H.*, *lxxxii*.2). Of special relevance is the following ruling: "If the due alimentation was assigned to [a nursing mother], but she passionately desired to eat more or different food, it is held by one authority[18] that her husband cannot object [to the change in her diet] on account of the danger to the child [which may be caused by the change], because the pain of her body has a prior claim [to consideration over the child's health]; but others[19] maintain that he can restrain her" (*E.H.*, *lxxx*.12). While the former view cannot easily be reconciled with the talmudic passage[20] on which it is based in principle, it evidently justifies a nursing mother in assuaging her own acute discomfort by resorting to food which is definitely harmful to her milk and may thus imperil the life of the suckling.[21] In that case, the husband would presumably be compelled to place his child into the care of a wet-nurse, in the same way as a father of twins must hire a nurse to suckle one child, as the mother cannot be forced to nurse both of them[22] (*ib.*, 13).

Particular concern is also shown for the pain of infants due to circumcision. As we shall see in another chapter,[23] the law counsels special precautions "so as not to harrow [the child]" (*Y.D.*, *cclxiii.*4). There is a view that a postponed circumcision should not take place on a Thursday, so that the most acute pain—which usually occurs on the third day—should not afflict the child on the Sabbath.[24] Sympathy for the infant's pain also accounts for various liturgical usages,[25] as it was felt that the joy of the occasion was somewhat tempered by the knowledge that the child was not free from suffering. The law considers the ordeal of the proselyte, too; between his circumcision and his immersion in a ritual bath required for his conversion there should be an interval to allow for his recovery from the operation (*Y.D.*, *cclxviii.*2), because, in the words of the Talmud,[26] "the water may vitiate the wound before it is healed" and, as JAFFE[27] adds, cause the sore to hurt unduly. Even the "Canaanite slave"[28] had a legal claim to be treated with a gentle regard to his physical sensitivity. Although, when the assessed medical expenses paid by a third party injuring him exceed the amount actually spent on his healing through the use of unusually strong drugs, the excess compensation belongs to his master (*Y.D.*, *cclxvii.*21; and *H.M.*, *dxxiv.*3), "the master has no right to administer strong drugs to the slave in order to take the surplus [payment] for himself; for Scripture consigned him to servitude, not to physical suffering or shame".[29]

PAIN OF ANIMALS

The mitigation of pain in animals, too, occupies an important place in Jewish law.[30] Numerous regulations are designed to guard them against hunger,[31] overwork[32] (*H.M.*, *cclxxii*.1 ff.) and, as we have seen in some detail,[33] disease and distress, and it is a biblical offence to inflict cruelty on them[34] (*ib.*, 9, gloss). Indeed, it is a moot question whether this law against torturing living creatures also includes the infliction of pain on humans. While AZULAY[35] can see no reason for discriminating between man and beast in this respect, YA'IR BACHARACH[36] holds the view that "the *Torah* is concerned only about pain caused to brutes, because they lack knowledge and the intelligence to endure suffering, whereas man can choose to ease his mind and to accept with love whatever befalls him". But this is, of course, only a technical question.[37]

ATTITUDE TO PAIN

The sources we have now considered leave us in no doubt on the attitude of Jewish law to physical suffering. Whether pain is to be looked upon as an instrument of divine punishment or not, it is clearly a curse. Among all the passages we have examined, the suggestion that there is virtue or some desirable *beau ideal* in bodily anguish is entirely absent. There is no trace in rabbinic law of the Christian concept in which "Pathos became Ethos; suffering was a sign of grace, not to be evaded but sought".[38] It is true, the moral codes of the Church also modify many of its principles for the sake of mitigating pain. Thus a leading Catholic theologian permits alcoholic intoxication "to cure typhus and snake bite, and to relieve great pain".[39] But in general, Christianity is distinctly more panegyrical in its commendation of physical suffering than is Judaism.

PANGS OF BIRTH AND DEATH

The issues in which these conflicting views are most realistically illustrated concern the pain suffered at the creation of life and at its termination. The notorious fight of churchmen in the last century against the alleviation of the woman's birth-pangs neither started with the application of chloroform by Sir JAMES YOUNG SIMPSON nor ended with the acceptance of the new drug by Queen VICTORIA at the birth of Prince LEOPOLD in 1853.[40] The *Report of the Joint Commission on Christian Healing*[41] informs us that "before the discovery of anesthesia, a woman in France was detected in an attempt to ease the pain of childbirth with the help of another woman. This was construed as a blasphemous attempt to thwart the curse which God had laid upon EVE,[42] and both women were burnt to death". Towards the end of the last century, a Catholic medical moralist still forbade the use of chloroform at normal births because it might endanger the mother and the child, adding significantly: "Let . . . our women be trained to have courage and resilience, and to the proper appreciation of their high vocation and duties; then I guarantee that they will not cry out for chloroform under the pangs of labour, but cling with redoubled love and sacrifice to the beings whom they bring into existence in pain".[43] It was not, in fact, until 1949 that the Holy Office announced papal sanction for painless births.[44]

In rabbinic writings the question is never raised; as has been remarked, "the prohibition of analgesics would contradict Jewish ideology".[45] Indeed, the sympathy of Jewish law for the sufferings accompanying childbirth is so strong, that some of its leading exponents justify the recourse to contraceptive sterilisation by mothers who fear the pain of further births.[46]

A similar divergence of views concerns the right to induce insensibility before death. A contemporary Catholic moralist states that narcotic drugs must not be given to a patient to relieve his pain, unless he is prepared for death, has made his peace with God and arranged his temporal affairs reasonably well. He adds that some theologians permit such a practice only if "there is danger of the penitent relapsing into sin or committing serious sins of impatience".[47] According to the *Catholic Encyclopedia*,[48] too, the Church is opposed to the administration of narcotic drugs before death—whether natural or by execution—since "they deprive a man of the capacity to act meritoriously at a time when the competency is most necessary". In Jewish law, the consideration for a patient's pain is greater, as we will show elsewhere,[49] than the concern for his spiritual and temporal preparedness to die. Even the criminal walking to his execution was to be saved from unnecessary suffering in compliance with the Golden Rule "thou shalt love thy neighbour as thyself" (*Lev. xix.*18); hence the Talmud,[50] followed by MAIMONIDES,[51] insisted that he had to be drugged into insensibility during the final ordeal so that his feelings might be spared.[52]

CHAPTER NINE

THE SICK AND THEIR TREATMENT — 1.

VISITATIONS AND PRAYERS

In defining the rights of patients and their claims to special favours, Jewish law is not only concerned to remove (within the limits demarcated in the preceding chapters) the obstacles to their healing and comfort which would be raised by the unconditional operation of its religious and moral precepts. The law also provides many detailed regulations on the consideration and acts of kindness due to the sick.

DUTY TO VISIT THE SICK

Foremost among the relevant demands of Judaism is the duty to visit the sick.[1] Such visits are counted among the most meritorious acts of true charity. In a talmudic passage,[2] recited daily by observant Jews,[3] this duty is listed among the ten ethical and devotional exercises " . . . the fruits of which man enjoys in this world, whilst the stock remains for him in the world to come". Indeed, the fulfilment of this obligation belongs to the finest expressions of the *imitatio Dei* ideal,[4] and the law invests it with the character of "a religious precept" (*Y.D., cccxxxv.*1). The Talmud,[5] in fact, likens the refusal to perform this duty to the shedding of blood, since visits to the sick help to restore them to full life. The obligation devolves equally on all, even the great must visit their juniors; coevals, too, must call on each other (*ib.*, 2), although it was believed that they might contract one sixtieth of the disease owing to the accident of their horoscopical identity.[6] Accordingly, the functions of local sick-visitation societies, which were very active in Jewish communities throughout the Middle Ages and after,[7] were mainly performed by the laity. Medieval rabbis did little "parish visiting"; they merely contributed their share like others.[8]

The principal purpose of visiting the sick is not achieved unless the caller is moved to plead for mercy in the patient's behalf[9] (*ib.*, 4 and gloss). Moreover, "by seeing him, one observes his circumstances, [so that] if he requires anything, one will endeavour to obtain it for him, [for instance] to sweep and sprinkle [the sick-room] before him".[10] At the same time, such visits naturally serve to give the patient the pleasure and satisfaction of companionship in his solitude.[11]

The manner of performing this religious precept is carefully defined. There is no limit to the frequency with which the sick should be visited even on a single day; the more often this is done, the more praiseworthy, provided it does not trouble the patient (*ib.*, 2). According to one opinion,[12] even a personal enemy may go to see his sick neighbour; but ISSERLES holds such visits may cause more anguish than comfort to the patient, as he may think his visitor rejoices in his misfortune (*ib.*, gloss). Close relatives and friends may visit the sick at once;[13] distant callers should not come before the lapse of three days,[14] unless the illness struck with great suddenness (*ib.*, 1). Visits during the first and last three hours of the day should always be avoided; for every patient feels abnormally well in the early morning—so that one may not be stirred to seek mercy for him—and abnormally ill at the end of the day—so that one may despair of praying for his recovery[15] (*ib.*, 4). The proper conduct in the sick-room was to sit on the floor, wrapped up in a garment,[16] realising that the Divine Presence rests above the head of the patient[17] (*ib.*, 3). But this applied only when the patients themselves used to lie on the floor; otherwise one may sit on a chair[18] (*ib.*, gloss).

Sick-visits are permitted even on the Sabbath (*O.H.*,

cclxxxvii.1), despite the distress they may cause to the caller.[19] For the promotion of good neighbourly relations, heathen patients, too, ought to be visited (*Y.D.*, *cli*.12; and *ccxxxv*.9). Since visits to the sick constitute a religious act, there is no objection to a patient being visited by a person who took a vow foreswearing the benefit of his services to that patient[20] (*Y.D.*, *ccxxi*.4). But where it is customary to remunerate persons for sitting beside the sick, such a visitor may make the call only if he remains standing (*ib.*), no payment being then due.[21]

In some cases visitors may expose the patient to embarrassment or undue fatigue. One should, therefore, refrain from calling on sufferers from diarrhoea, eye- or haed-diseases, and any other severe conditions which render talking difficult; instead, one should enquire from outside their room about their needs and, listening to their tale of distress, pray for their recovery[22] (*Y.D.*, *cccxxxv*.8). The codes do not list any further categories of patients who need not, or should not, be visited. But the Talmud[23] also warns against calling on any sick person before "the fever has left him".[24] It is not definitely stated whether this precaution is intended to protect the patient from disturbance (as in the cases previously listed) or the visitor from the danger of infection.[25] The propriety of visiting people who suffer from contagious (and particularly pestilential) diseases is, however, discussed in some later rabbinic writings. ISSERLES[26] holds there can be no distinction, in respect of this duty, between ordinary and infectious diseases, with the sole exception of leprosy. But others maintain that no-one can be expected to endanger his life for the fulfilment of this precept.[27] In practice, the latter view prevailed,[28] and approval is expressed for the custom not to assign visitations of plague-stricken patients to anyone except specially appointed persons (who were highly paid for their perilous work).[29] The 17th century records of the Portuguese Congregation in Hamburg indicate that even the communal doctors and nurses were exempt from the obliga-

tion to attend to infectious cases and that the required services were rendered by volunteers entitled to special remuneration.[30] Catholic moralists lay down detailed instructions
on the precautions to be taken by priests when dealing with
cases of contagion,[31] and St. ALPHONSUS LIGUORI in
the 19th century sanctioned certain concessions *"si adsit
periculum infectionis"*.[32]

The sick naturally enjoy priority over other indigent
persons in their claim to private or public assistance. In fact,
KARO records the view[33] that, while contributions to the
erection of a synagogue take precedence over ordinary forms
of charity, even the synagogue's needs must give way to
the requirements of the necessitous sick (*Y.D., ccxlix.*16).
It is, moreover, morally indefensible to refuse to accept
such aid[34] (*Y.D., cclv.*2).

THE SICK IN CIVIL LAW

Out of consideration for the sick, Judaism modifies even
some of its civil laws. Thus, a person detained in a city beyond twelve months by factors outside his control, such as
illness, continues to enjoy the exemption from taxation
granted to temporary residents[35] (*H.M., clxiii.*2, gloss). If
anyone carries on a trade which may cause a nuisance to a
sick neighbor (such as work on blood[36] or carcasses liable
to attract ravens whose screeching may disturb a nearby
patient), he must discontinue his work or remove it to a safe
distance (*H.M., clv.*39). Similarly, people suffering from
headache or other ailments are entitled to object, and to
obtain an injunction, against the continued pursuit in the
neighbourhood of a noisy trade (such as the clattering din
of a workshop) causing them harm (*ib.,* 15, gloss; and *clvi.*2,
gloss), even if the aggrieved party had previously been satisfied to tolerate the noise without protest.[37] Special facilities are also accorded to the sick in court procedure. For
instance, their legal evidence or claims may be deposited

in the absence of the other litigants (*H.M.*, *xxviii*.16), contrary to the usual rule (*ib.*, 15).[38]

PRAYERS FOR THE SICK

The greatest non-medical service to the sick is to invoke the help and compassion of God by prayer. To the general observations already made,[39] we may here add some details on prayers for recovery to health. In the presence of the patient, such pleas for mercy may be expressed in any language; otherwise only Hebrew should be used (*O.H.*, *ci*.4; and *Y.D.*, *cccxxxv*.5) for mystical reasons.[40] When greeting a patient,[41] one should include all "the sick in Israel" in the plea for his well-being (*Y.D.*, *cccxxxv*.6) so as to strengthen the efficacy of the prayer.[42] It is also proper to fast, as well as to pray, for the recovery and safety of individuals whose lives are in danger[43] (*O.H.*, *dlxxviii*.1). The patient himself, too, should deepen his faith in God and in the success of his treatment through prayer[44] (*O.H.*, *ccxxx*.4).

Before and after consuming food or drinks for medical reasons the appropriate blessing should be recited, provided their taste is pleasant[45] (*O.H.*, *cciv*.8), even if they contain forbidden substances[46] (*ib.*, 9; and *cxcvi*.2). But pharmaceutical products not normally taken by healthy people at all require only the blessing usually reserved for mineral or animal substances, even if such products are of plant origin[47] (*O.H.*, *cciv*.11, gloss). We have dealt in a previous chapter with public expressions of thanksgiving for recovery from illness,[48] with physicians' prayers for the success of their cures,[49] and with the proclamation of special days of fasting and intercession in the event of pestilential outbreaks or other public calamities.[50]

CHAPTER TEN

THE SICK AND THEIR TREATMENT — 2.

THE TREATMENT OF WOMEN, ONES PARENTS, AND THE INSANE

Restrictions on the treatment of women by males, particularly in gynecological and obstetrical practice, are among the oldest and most universal features of medical ethics. Throughout antiquity the regular employment of male assistants at births was unthinkable; help in parturition was almost exclusively left in the hands of midwives.[1] Even in ancient Greece, women were usually examined by doctors of their own sex only; male physicians were called in on but the rarest occasions.[2] Only the ancient Hindus permitted doctors to assist in confinements, as shown in the *Susruta* writings.[3] The aversion to the admission of men underwent little change in the Middle Ages. The practice of gynecology and obstetrics remained almost entirely with women from Byzantine times[4] to the 16th century.[5] As late as 1522, a physician in Hamburg, who dressed as a woman to attend and study a case of labour, was still burnt to death for his impiety.[6] It was not until the 17th century that male midwifery by accoucheurs was introduced; previously doctors had been called in only for cases requiring embryotomy.[7]

Even when physicians were allowed to attend women for medical consultations or services, they were subjected to strict precautions against any lewdness in thought or deed. A law of the Visigoths prohibited surgeons from bleeding any free woman except in the presence of the husband or some other properly appointed witness.[8] The Salernitan treatises of ARCHIMATHEUS, following in the traditions of the Hippocratic Oath, ordered the doctor " . . . not to diminish his professional status by ogling the patient's wife, daughter or maid servants",[9] and the 16th century oath, which the physicians compelled every apothecary in France to take, included the promise " . . . never to examine women privately, unless by great necessity, or to apply to them some necessary remedy".[10]

Medieval Islam and Christianity were equally concerned to carry the segregation of the sexes, as far as possible, into medical practice. The Arabian physician AVENZOAR thought that no religious doctor should even view the genitals, let alone operate on them.[11] According to ABULCASIS, no surgeon should examine, or operate on, a woman; any essential treatment should be performed by a midwife or an expert woman on the advice of the surgeon,[12] for Islam required all confinements to be left in the charge of women.[13] Christianity, too, shared these views. Among the motives for the oft-repeated Church council edicts debarring priests from the practice of medicine was the anxiety to prevent them from treating women.[14] The earliest of these decretals (Clermont 1130) referred specifically to the *"impudicus oculus"* in this context.[15] The Catholic opposition to meetings in private between physicians and female patients is maintained to the present day. A Catholic moralist advises women submitting to internal examinations to take witnesses with them to the doctor,[16] and the *Catholic Encyclopedia*[17] states that physicians in charge of convents for nuns should not be under fifty years of age nor be alone with their patients.

In comparison with this background, the Jewish attitude is strikingly liberal. Neither the Talmud nor the codes mention any law which imposes restrictions on the physician in the treatment of his female patients.[18] Indeed, it is claimed that "since the examination of the genitals is also often undertaken by men among the Jews of the Talmud, . . . they differ in this respect from all the peoples of antiquity; for, with the others, this was always done by midwives".[19] This claim, endorsed by one Jewish scholar[20] against the doubts of another,[21] has been qualified, but only because the Hindus, too, permitted men to render obstetrical assistance.[22] It is probably right to assert that there is no conclusive evidence in the Talmud for the existence of professional gynecologists or male accoucheurs among the Jews of antiquity any more than among the Greeks,[21] but the remarkable—and in our context, decisive—fact remains that the Talmud and its legislative successors are singularly free from any condemnation of such a practice.

Voices urging the need for the utmost chastity on medical practitioners are, of course, heard in Jewish sources, too, even if these counsels are not reinforced by special enactments. In general, these warnings were issued, significantly, by the representatives of medicine, not theology. The Talmud[23] holds up ABBA, the bleeder, as an example of piety and charity,[24] and it records that this 4th century sage had separate consulting rooms for men and women. He also gave his patients a special dress for venesection to ensure that no part of the body would be exposed except what is required for the operation. The regard for the bashful modesty of women was so high, that the eminent rabbi and physician SAMUEL paid a sum of money to a female slave as indemnity for the shame imposed on her when he examined her breasts to ascertain the signs of puberty for legal purposes.[25]

The first Hebrew medical writer, ASAF JUDAEUS of the 7th century, abjured his pupils: "Let not the beauty of women arouse in thee the passion of adultery".[26] A thousand years later, the noted rabbinical and medical writer JACOB ZAHALON warned in a similar vein: "When the physician visits women, he should be modest and should not follow the evil thoughts of his heart",[27] and in his prayer for physicians to be recited weekly, he exclaimed: "Cleanse my mind and purify my thoughts that I think no evil about any woman, whether virgin or wife, when I visit her, that I do not go after my own heart and my own eyes".[28] While women were sometimes chosen by the community to undertake sick-visits to women,[29] there is nothing to suggest that Jewish male doctors shunned the treatment of women, or that either they or their female patients were subjected to any religious limitations on their medical freedom in this respect. Our records speak of a fair number of Jewish woman-doctors in the Middle Ages, but their professional activity—in any case very often as oculists[30]—does not appear to have been fostered by the reluctance of physicians to attend women or by the preference of female patients for doctors of their own sex.[31] Of all the Jewish doctoresses mentioned by various historians,[32] only one is referred to as having "performed operations on women",[33] whilst most are expressly stated to have treated men, too.[34]

Legally, then, there are no special restrictions on physicians or their female patients in their professional relationship. Like the Talmud,[35] the codes presume that women consult doctors not only on general medical problems—for instance, on the use of wine as a hair-lotion[36] (*Y.D.*, *cxcix*.2, gloss)—but also on gynecological abnormalities and their cure (*Y.D.*, *clxxxvii*.8). The commentators agree that Jewish physicians have always been accustomed to feel the pulse of women and to give them any other medical treatment, even if such female patients were married and even if a non-Jewish doctor was available.[37] The early 18th century scholar, JONATHAN EYBESCHUETZ,[38] adds that it was the accepted practice of every competent physician to attend to women for gynecological examinations when necessary, because "we raise no objection [to such action] performed as part of his professional work". Some subsequent opinions veered towards a stricter interpretation of the law. In a responsum dated 1863, JACOB ETTLINGER[39] expressed some doubt on whether it was altogether right for men to assist at births, unless the mother was in danger and the Jewish doctor could not be replaced by a non-Jew; but he admitted that the more lenient view permitting such a practice without any qualification was also founded on good authority. On the whole, however, neither the rabbis nor the Jewish physicians showed any tendency towards excessive prudery. Significant, though perhaps not typical, may be the story related of the famed poet and physician, IMMANUEL of Rome (the friend of DANTE), who lived at the turn of the 13th century. Asked by a beautiful prude, whom he was attending, to feel her pulse through her dress, he mocked: "I took a brick, placed it upon her right hand and, holding a fire-pan in my own, I felt her pulse with it and thus made sport of the lady".[40]

The freedom granted to Jewish physicians to treat women, even for conditions peculiar to them, does not imply, however, that this was always, or even generally, the actual practice. Following once again in the talmudic tradition, the codes appear to assume that gynecological examinations, particularly routine tests to ascertain virginity, infertility or the duration of the menstrual cycle, were not usually carried out by men. Thus, when a husband disputes his wife's virginity against her claims of innocence, "one examines her" (*E.H.*, *lxviii*.4) by the "wine-barrel" test[41] (*ib.*, gloss) prescribed in the Talmud.[42] The fact that this test is recommended, though other, more direct methods to establish virginity are equally admissable,[43] may betray a reluctance to have women medically eaxmined for this purpose. There is also no mention of physicians in the investigation recommended for verifying a husband's claim that he found no virginal bleeding in his wife. In such cases, his claim for legal redress[44] is dismissed if she comes from a family whose members are known to lack such bleeding;[45] otherwise "one tests her [to find out] whether a serious illness attaches to her, whereby the moisture of her limbs is dried up, or whether she is starved by hunger", and if, following recuperative treatment, she fails to discharge any blood for the second time, his plea is admitted (*ib.*, 5).

In some instances, such examinations are specifically delegated to women. They are mentioned as ascertaining (for legal purposes) the symptoms of barrenness[46] in women who show no signs of puberty[47] (*E.H.*, *clv*.15); as determining the regular dates of menstruation in women who are deaf-dumb, insane or of disturbed mind through illness[48] (*Y.D.*, *cxcvi*.8); and as certifying that women to be granted a "levirate divorce"[49] have reached their physical majority[50] (*E.H.*, *clxix*.10). It is assumed that for assisting at childbirths, too, female midwives are generally called in (*O.H.*, *cccxxx*.1). Even at the delivery of twins, none but woman-assistants are presumed to be present[51] (*H.M.*, *cclxxvii*.12).

In all these cases, the law merely assumes, but does not require, that women are employed. Only in one instance is there a legal impediment to the attendance on women by (non-professional) men. Following an early talmudic ruling[52] not recorded by MAIMONIDES, some codes rule: "In the case of a sickness affecting the digestive system, a man should not attend on a woman, but a woman may attend on a man" (*Y.D.*, *cccxxxv*.10). A similar regulation restrains men from dressing dead women, while it permits women to carry out such rites on males (*Y.D.*, *ccclii*.3). KARO[53] and JAFFE[54] attribute the discrimination against men attending on female patients to the fear that their superior strength, set against the defencelessness of a sick woman, may lead them to succumb to temptation, whereas women are not likely to misconduct themselves with sick men whom they are nursing.[55] But ISSERLES,[56] JOSHUA FALK[57] and JOEL SIRKES[58] reject this interpretation, since the law is limited to sufferers from one particular ailment only. They assume that the law merely seeks to prevent the obscenity of men, whose sensual lusts are more easily aroused, having to attend to the hygienic requirements of women suffering from indigestion.

SURGICAL TREATMENT OF PARENTS

A unique feature of medico-religious legislation is the virtual ban on the surgical treatment of one's parents in Jewish law. The Talmud[59] defines the injunction "And he that smiteth his father or his mother shall surely be put to death" (*Ex. xxi.*15) to embrace any deliberate act causing a flow of blood. Hence, it is a capital offence to inflict a bleeding wound on one's father or mother; and, lest a loss of blood ensue, it is forbidden to treat one's parents for the removal of a splinter, the opening of an abcess, venesection (*H.M., cdxxiv.*1) or any other surgical operation, even when the operator is a professional barber or surgeon (*Y.D., ccxli.*3), unless no other competent person is available to relieve the pain (*ib.*, gloss). According to NACHMA-NIDES,[60] the fear underlying this law is merely that the wound inflicted on the parent may exceed the minimum necessary for the cure (which would be a deadly sin), not that the incision may prove fatal. For every serious operation, whether on a parent or others, involves some risk of life (which might likewise lead to capital peccability); yet such outcome need not be apprehended, as the law expressly sanctions the practice of medicine.[61]

TREATMENT OF THE INSANE

The stringent regulations on the respect due to parents are compromised neither by their moral depravity (*Y.D., ccxl.*18) nor by their mental deficiency (*ib.*, 10). Accordingly, "he whose father or mother has become mentally unbalanced must demean himself fittingly with them, as far as their capacity will permit, until compassion [and relief] will be vouchsaved to them; but if they have turned so excessively insane that he can no longer stand it, he may go away and leave them, as long as he instructs others to look after them properly" (*ib.*). This ruling first appears in the code of MAIMONIDES,[62] but its logic has been disputed by his glossator ABRAHAM IBN DAUD[63] followed by others.[64] They contend that, if the parents' condition is such that other people can still care for them, surely their own child—who knows their desires best—cannot be absolved from this duty; if, on the other hand, even he is unable to control and protect them, others certainly must find such a task impossible. Similar considerations govern the treatment of an insane wife,[65] and the husband's legal obligations to her. Her insanity does not free him from the duty to provide for her maintenance and medical expenses (*E.H.*, *lxx*.4). Moreover, "if she turned insane and is not capable to look after herself,[66] he cannot divorce her until she recovers;[67] [this enactment was made] so that people should not treat her as an outlaw"[68] (*E.H.*, *cxix*.6).

These laws shed a revealing light on the treatment of lunatics among the Jews. Of particular interest is the abovementioned view of MAIMONIDES—accepted in the codes against the objections of his opponents—concerning one's duty to insane parents. It assumes that even the most obstreperous maniac must not be left without due care and that, when children are no longer capable of giving the necessary attention to their parents, they must find and provide others—presumably trained experts[69]—to do so on their behalf. The brutality, starvation and indignities to which lunatics were exposed up to modern times are notorious.[70] The Talmud knew nothing of such cruelties. Indeed, Jewish legislation not only prohibits the infliction of any injury on a mentally deranged person, but regards such action as a culpable offence for which the victim can legally claim appropriate damages (*H.M.*, *cdxxiv*.8). Yet, the lunatic himself is free from the obligation to compensate others whom he injured (*ib.*). He cannot be held responsible for his conduct, but he can sue others striking him; it is, therefore, as the Talmud[71] puts it, "an ill thing to knock against an imbecile".

CHAPTER ELEVEN

THE DYING AND THEIR TREATMENT.

PREPARATION FOR DEATH AND EUTHANASIA

The predominantly "this-worldly" character of Judaism is reflected in the relative sparsity of its regulations on the inevitable passage of man from life to death. The rabbis, as we have noted,[1] placed a severely practical emphasis on the axiom that the ordinances of God exist so that man "shall live by them" (*Lev. xviii.5*). A theology which sees no contradiction between the statement "Better is one hour of repentance and good deeds in this world than the whole life in the world to come" and the accompanying antithesis "And better is one hour of blissfulness of spirit in the world to come than the whole life in this world",[2] can with equal ease reconcile the fundamentally pragmatic character of Jewish law with the thought "This world is like a vestibule before the world to come; prepare thyself in the vestibule, that thou mayest enter into the hall".[3] Life in this world is indeed but to serve as a preparation for the eternal bliss of the hereafter. But this only reinforces the urgency of focussing man's attention on the ideals to be attained during his mortal existence on earth and on the need to prolong that life to the maximum possible.

Even in the final phase of animation, therefore, the consideration for the physical welfare of the patient remains supreme. Judaism urges every caution to ensure that his last preparations for death shall not aggravate his condition or compromise his will or ability to live. Among these preparations, the ordering of his temporal affairs features as prominently as the reconciliation with his Creator. According to a talmudic directive,[4] he is first to be told to "set his mind on his affairs—if he left a loan or a deposit with others, or if he held a loan or a deposit from others—but let him on no account be afraid of death" (*Y.D.*, *cccxxxv*.7). Following some versions, the patient should actually be told: "For words can neither cause life nor cause death".[5] Later, "when he feels death approaching, one tells him 'Confess!', and one [also] tells him 'Many have confessed but did not die, while many who did not confess died; and as a reward for your confession you will live, for whoever confesses has a portion in the world to come" (*Y.D.*, *cccxxxviii*.1). The order of the confession prayer, too, seeks to reassure the patient: "I acknowledge before Thee, o Lord, my God, and the God of my fathers, that my recovery and my death are in Thine hand. May it be Thy will to heal me with a perfect healing; but if I die,[6] may my death be an atonement for all my sins . . . which I have committed before Thee . . . "[7] (*ib.*, 2). Moroever, the patient should not be instructed in these matters in the presence of uneducated people or of women and children, "lest they will weep and break his heart"[8] (*ib.*, 1). Before the end actually draws near, the mention of death is to be altogether avoided, so as not to make the patient aware of the seriousness of his condition and thus sap his strength.[9]

INFORMING PATIENTS ON DEATHBED

When the Syrian King BEN HADAD asked HAZAEL to enquire from the Prophet ELISHA whether he would survive his sickness, the Prophet sent word: "Go, say unto him 'Thou shalt surely recover'; howbeit the Lord hath shown me that he shall surely die" (2 Kings *viii*.10). Following this precedent, the rabbis insisted on maintaining the patient's hopefulness not merely by withholding information of his imminent death, but by positive means to encourage his confidence in recovery. The Midrash[10] remon-

strates with the Prophet ISAIAH for telling King HEZE-
KIAH, when he was "sick unto death": "Set thy house
in order; for thou shalt die and not live" (2 Kings *xx.*1).
On the contrary, "even when the physician realises that his
patient approaches death, he should still order him to eat
this and not to eat that, to drink this and not to drink that;
but he should not tell him that the end is near".[11] The
same attitude is also found in GALEN[12] and medieval
sources.[13]

According to the teaching of the Church, the doctor is obliged *"ex precepto charitatis"* personally to inform the patient of the hopelessness of his condition if the latter finds
himself in a state of mortal sin or in need of ordering the affairs of his estate. Any failure to do so involves the doctor in
grave sin, since he allows spiritual or material damage to occur which he could have prevented.[14] Even when no such
damage is likely to ensue, frankness is to be preferred so as to
enable the patient better to prepare for death.[15] Patients were
to be so informed even if such knowledge might so depress
them as to endanger their life.[16] This attitude led to the
decree of INNOCENT III, at the 4th Lateran Council
in 1215, forcing the physician, under pain of excommunication, to induce the patient to confess, and to the insistence
of some theologians that the patient's treatment must be
discontinued if he refused to confess.[17]

TREATMENT OF THE DYING

When death is thought to be imminent, the patient is
called *"Goses"*[18] in rabbinic sources, because he then "brings
up a secretion in his throat on account of the narrowing
of his chest"[19] (*E.H., cxxi.*7, gloss; and *H.M., ccxi.*2, gloss).
Even in that state the patient is still to be treated as a living
person in all respects[20] (*Y.D., cccxxxix.*1). One must not
tie his jaws, anoint him[21], wash him,[22] plug his open organs,[23]
remove the pillow from underneath him,[24] or place him on

sand, clay or on the ground[25] (*ib.*). It is also forbidden to lay a vessel or salt on his belly,[26] and to close his eyes before he breathes out his last; "for whoever closes the eyes with the onset of death is [regarded as] shedding blood" (*ib.*).

The reference to the removal of the pillow, and the reason for this law, is further amplified by ISSERLES: "It is forbidden to cause the dying to pass away quickly; for instance, if a person is in a dying condition for a long time and he cannot depart, it is prohibited to remove the pillow or the cushion from underneath him following the popular belief that feathers from some birds have this effect [*i.e.*, to prevent the patient from dying easily]" (*ib.*, gloss.) PORTALEONE still complained in 1612 that he had been unable to abolish this practice despite energetic protests. PREUSS concludes, however, from a contemporary work[28] in which no mention of Jews occurs, that this superstition cannot be considered specifically Jewish. Another forbidden practice is to "place the keys of the synagogue under his head, so that [the soul] can depart" (*ib.*). The belief that such an act helps to remove any impediments to an easy death is first mentioned in a 16th century commentary on ALFASI's code.[29] MORDECAI JAFFE[30] regards it as a "magical remedy".

All these acts are prohibited because they may hasten the patient's death by moving him; for, in the words of the Talmud,[31] "the matter can be compared with a flickering flame; as soon as one touches it, the light is extinguished".[32] Hence, any movement of the dying body must be avoided[33] (*ib.*), even for the purpose of returning a shifted limb to bed[34] or of relieving pain,[35] except in order to save the patient from a fire.[36] This uncompromising opposition to any deliberate acceleration of the final release is well exemplified by the martyred sage HANINA BEN TRADYON who, whilst the Romans burnt him at the stake, refused to follow his disciples' advice to open his mouth to the flames (in order to speed his death) with the defiant exclamation: "It is better that my soul shall be taken by Him Who gave it than that I should do any harm to it on my own".[37] A similar motive prompted an anonymous Jewish author and physician in the 13th century to keep the dosage of one of his medicines secret, so that those who are wanting in faith should not use it for suicidal purposes to shorten their sufferings[38]—a "mercy-killing" device quite often facilitated by present-day doctors.[39] DAVID IBN ZIMRA,[40] in the 16th century, extended the ban on speeding the extinction of life even to the unborn foetus; he records that he warned women against the practice prevalent in Egypt of beating on the abdomen of mothers who died in childbirth in order to kill the fruit, since its end must not be expedited even if its certain death is anticipated.

But there is one qualification to this attitude. ISSERLES permits the removal of "anything causing a hindrance to the departure of the soul, such as a clattering noise near the patient's home (produced, for instance, by chopping wood) or salt on his tongue . . . , since such [action] involves no active [hastening of death], but only the removal of the impediment"[41] (*ib.*). Indeed, the *Sepher Hasidim*[42] (on which this law is based) *prohibits* any action which may lengthen the patient's agony by preventing his quick death, such as to make a noise in his neighbourhood or to place salt on his tongue. The same 13th century work also forbids those attending at the moment of death to cry, lest the noise may restore the soul to the deceased.[43]

EUTHANASIA

It is clear, then, that, even when the patient is already known to be on his deathbed and close to the end, any form of *active euthanasia* is strictly prohibited. In fact, it is condemned as plain murder. In purely legal terms, this is borne out by the ruling that anyone who kills a dying person is liable to the death penalty as a common murderer.[44] At the same time, Jewish law sanctions, and perhaps even demands, the withdrawal of any factor—whether extraneous to the patient himself or not—which may artificially delay his demise in the final phase. It might be argued that this modification implies the legality of expediting the death of an incurable patient in acute agony by withholding from him such medicaments as sustain his continued life by unnatural means—an issue also considered in Catholic moral philosophy.[45] Our sources advert only to cases in which death is expected to be imminent; it is, therefore, not altogether clear whether they would tolerate this moderate form of euthanasia, though that cannot be ruled out.[46]

That Jewish teachers were not out of sympathy with every effort to deliver incurables from their agony is shown by the sanction to seek death as a release from suffering by resorting to prayer[47] or to occult devices.[48] The significance of these concessions can only be appreciated if one considers the often unfailing efficacy commonly attributed to the power of prayer and mystic prescriptions. According to TOSAPHOTH,[49] self-destruction is also permitted as a means to escape from sin under the pressure of violence by heathen oppressors. Some Christian moralists tolerate a similar exception.[50]

Although the term "euthanasia"[51] to denote the "action of inducing gentle and easy death" was first used by LECKY only in 1869,[52] the advocacy of this measure is by no means an innovation of modern times. Already in the 4th century B.C.E., PLATO[53] held that invalids ought not to be kept alive, though he may well have been less concerned with their sufferings than with the social and economic burden on their supporters.[54] There are also good reasons for believing that euthanasia was directly attacked by the clause in the Hippocratic Oath: "Never will I give a deadly drug, not even if I am asked for one, nor will I give any advice tending in that direction", as suggested by one scholar.[55] He considers that euthanasia "was an everyday reality" at the time and that its condemnation in the Oath was influenced by Pythagorean doctrines which, alone in Greek thought, outlawed suicide unconditionally. But another authority[56] denies that euthanasia had any importance for the ancients; he regards the passage in the Oath as referring to murder by poisoning. It is certainly significant that the Alexandrian pioneer in anatomy, ERASISTRATOS of the 3rd century B.C.E., is recorded to have taken poison—to end his sufferings from an incurable cancer—with the words: "It is well that I should remember my country"—a sentiment which may indicate that the practice was not uncommon.[57] In the Middle Ages, too, voices vindicating euthanasia were occasionally heard, and Sir THOMAS MORE approved of it, at least theoretically, in his *Utopia*.[58]

The practice has always been sternly opposed by the Church as a violation of the Sixth Commandment—from the Church Father St. AUGUSTINE[59] in the 4th century to the philosopher St. THOMAS AQUINAS[60] in the 13th century and even to the pronouncement in 1940 of the Roman Holy Office which condemned all direct euthanasia as a breach of the "natural and divine positive law".[61] The Archbishop of Canterbury, however, expressing the views of the Anglican Church during a debate in the British House of Lords in 1936,[62] qualified his opposition to the practice by stating: "If there be extreme cases where it is legitimate to shorten a life of pain, they should be left to be dealt with by the medical profession". Meanwhile, British law, in common with most modern criminal codes, continues to brand "mercy-killing" as an act of "murder or other homicide", according to the circumstances of its administration.[63]

CHAPTER TWELVE

THE DEAD AND THEIR TREATMENT.

THE ESTABLISHMENT OF DEATH, THE DISPOSAL OF INFECTIOUS AND PREGNANT BODIES AND THE DISSECTION OF HUMAN CORPSES

When the patient dies, his body generally passes from the attention of the physician into the care of the undertaker and the religious officials who attend to its interment. With that passage it is also removed from the sphere of medio-religious considerations, and it ceases to be of concern to us in our present work. We shall not, therefore, here discuss the numerous Jewish regulations on what is to be done with the human body after death. But there are some circumstances in which the physician's interest in the body is required, or desired, even beyond its demise, and this chapter will consider these cases insofar as they may concern religious issues.

ASCERTAINING THE MOMENT OF DEATH

Religious literature has devoted much attention to the problem of ascertaining the exact moment of death. In Judaism, however, unlike Christianity, this problem has little or no purely religious significance, since there are no sacramental rites to be accorded to the dying prior to the soul's final departure from the body. From the ritual point of view, the only practical distinction in Jewish law between a live and a dead body concerns the rules of defilement whereby Jews of priestly descent must not, by biblical decree (*Lev. xxi.*1 *ff.*), be within four cubits of a corpse (*Y.D.*, *ccclxxi.*5) or under a common roof with it (*ib.*, 1 *ff.*). But

Cohn

even in regard to these regulations, there was no need to define the division between life and death in precise terms, because priests are in any case forbidden to enter a house containing even a dying person[1] (*Y.D.*, *ccclxx*.1). Moreover, the susceptibility of a body to ritual defilement is determined partly by legal factors unrelated to the purely physical symptoms of death. Thus, "he whose neck is broken together with the greater part of its flesh, or he whose neck is split [lengthwise] like a fish—even if he be still alive—is [legally] regarded as dead and liable to cause defilement"[2] (*ib.*).

These considerations explain why Jewish law does not define the onset of death in connection with the regulations on the treatment of the dead at all. Altogether, the issue is raised only on two occasions—both among the Sabbath laws and both dealing with quite unusual circumstances. In the first reference, the codes, in strict accord with the Talmud,[3] rule that the Sabbath may be violated to free a person buried under a pile of rubble, even if found crushed in such a way that he could only live for a short while (*O.H.*, *cccxxix*.4). These operations should be continued until one reaches the victim's nose, whether the head or the feet were first to be discovered; and only when no signs of life can be felt at the nose[4] is certain death to be presumed (*ib.*). In the second reference, ISSERLES altogether denies our competence "nowadays" to ascertain the exact moment of death; hence he is against following the talmudic directive[5] —still endorsed by KARO (*O.H.*, *cccxxx*.5)—of performing the caesarian section on a woman who died during childbirth in the hope of delivering the child alive (*ib.*, gloss). But even ISSERLES modifies the demarcation line between life and death as fixed in the Talmud only to a very slight extent. He merely doubts our expertness in tracing that line with sufficient accuracy to enable us to know the exact moment of the mother's death while her fruit is possibly still alive (*ib.*). He agrees, however, that the talmudic definition of the onset of death can be accepted for all other practical purposes.

The problem is of particular relevance to the minimum and maximum time which should elapse between the cessation of life and burial. The Talmud[6] extends to all corpses the biblical law, originally applicable to some executed criminals only, according to which it is mandatory to inter the dead and an offence to leave the body unburied overnight (*Deut. xxi.*23). The codes, too, insist on the immediate burial of the dead; a delay **overnight is sanctioned** only if it serves to enhance "the honour" of the deceased—for instance, to await the provision of shrouds or a coffin, or the arrival of relatives[7] (*Y.D., ccclvii.*1). As already noted,[8] the treatment of the body in preparation for its burial may be commenced almost as soon as life appears to be extinct; only the momentary instant of the "departure of the soul" must be allowed to pass undisturbed (*Y.D., cccxxxix.*1), lest the body was then merely in a swoon.

The Jewish insistence on immediate burial has been vigorously defended in the face of considerable opposition by some Jewish reformers as well as the civil authorities.[9] Already in 1612, "an early and valuable protest against the outrageous practice . . . of hasty and premature burials" was made by the eminent physician ABRAHAM PORTALEONE when he ordered his body to be buried only three days after his death.[10] But the controversy did not become acute until 160 years later, when the Duke of Mecklenburg-Schwerin issued a civil decree forbidding the burial of the dead before the lapse of three days. This innovation was warmly endorsed by MOSES MENDELSOHN,[11] who sought to adduce talmudic support[12] for the then current medical belief that the onset of death could not be definitely established until signs of the body's putrefaction had appeared. These claims, together with the alleged evidence from the Talmud, were sharply refuted by his contemporary JACOB EMDEN[13] and later, in a responsum dated 1837, by MOSES SCHREIBER[14] who maintained that "all the spirits of the world . . . will not dislodge us from the position of our holy Law" regarding the establishment of death by the cessation of breathing.

While the earliest rabbinic sources usually speak of death as the "going out of the soul",[15] they also concede the view that the association between body and soul is not altogether severed until three days after death.[16] According to the Midrash,[17] the soul hovers over the grave for three days, hoping to be restored to the body and departing only when the face begins to change with the onset of decomposition; hence it was believed that the mourners' grief reached its climax on the third day. But this belief has no bearing on the insistence on immediate burial. The only related considerations in Jewish law are to disallow evidence on the identity of a person taken more than three days after his death[18] (*E.H., xvii.*26) and to permit, notwithstanding the ban on heathen practices, the watching of graves for three days in case the interred body is still alive (*Y.D., cccxciv.*3), but this applied "only in ancient days when they used to place the dead in sepulchral chambers which could be uncovered to reveal the corpse".[19]

In the moral theology of the Church the problem has received frequent and detailed attention,[20] mainly to determine the maximum limits within which the last sacraments may be administered, at least conditionally. It is also raised to define the moment at which the embalming of a corpse may begin. Most Catholic moralists hold that the only absolutely reliable sign of death is the onset of the body's corruption. They generally agree that there is a time between apparent death and the departure of the soul—a period called "latent life". It may vary from between half an hour or an hour, in the case of death from a long and wasting illness, to three or even seven hours, if death had occurred suddenly.

Neither the Talmud nor the codes make any reference to the treatment of infectiously diseased corpses and their disposal. ISSERLES, as already mentioned,[21] waives the ordinary laws of mourning for plague-victims (*Y.D.*, *ccclxxiv*.11, gloss), and on this basis a rabbi recently concluded that the laws on burial, too, might be modified in cases of contagion as required.[22] According to an earlier view, it is permitted in times of pestilence to corrode the bodies by strewing them with quicklime as an alternative to having them buried "in the forests at a place where no human settlements exist".[23] In similar circumstances, the *Sepher Hasidim*[24] sanctioned searching the dead for tokens which, in the popular mind, might cause the visitations to spread and endanger the survivors, since "anything required to save life may be done with the dead". Catholic theologians, too, are prepared to license certain concessions in such cases; they specifically permit, for example, the private interment of people who died from infectious diseases without bringing them into the church.[25]

DISPOSAL OF GRAVID CORPSES

The law on the treatment and disposal of women who died whilst pregnant has a long and controversial history. Insofar as it affects mothers who died in childbirth, we have surveyed the various views expressed in the Talmud, the codes and other Jewish writings in our Introduction.[26] It now remains to consider the different opinions on what should be done with a gravid corpse, a problem to which a great many responsa have been devoted since the 16th century.[27] While it was, by common consent, regarded undesirable, or even ominous and dangerous, to inter a woman and her child together,[28] there were widely divergent views on what measures might, or should, be taken to avoid this. Some authorities insisted that even in such cases the law against keeping a body unburied overnight should not be violated.[29] Others sanctioned a delay of twenty-four hours,[30] or even of a period not exceeding three days,[31] in the hope that a posthumous delivery of the child might occur during that time. Some rabbis recommended the recitation of certain magical formulae and various manipulations by doctors and midwives, including the bathing of the corpse in hot water, in order to induce it to surrender the child.[32] Others, again, objected to such practices.[33] But all are opposed to any surgical interference, since that would constitute an unwarranted desecration of the dead.[34] The *Shulhan 'Arukh* merely mentions the custom to bury women who died in childbirth without shrouds[35] (*Y.D., ccclxiv.*4, gloss).

Among Christian teachers, opinions are even more widely divided. Already in 1175, Bishop ODON of Paris decreed that the child must be removed from the mother by operative treatment,[36] and this provision was endorsed by several Church Councils.[37] Pope BENEDICT XIV issued detailed rules on the purpose of the operation and the precautions to be taken.[38] Other measures, too, were recommended to rescue the child alive. Thus, the Council of Cologne ordained in 1280 that on the sudden death of a mother in labour her mouth should be kept open with a gag, so that her child would not suffocate during its removal.[39] But occasionally the Church was opposed to these practices, as shown by the rule of the Icelandic Bishop JON SIGURDSON in 1345, ordering child-bearing women to be buried like other people without removing the child.[40] The Roman ritual of 1584, too, merely spoke of *"De Benedictione foetus in utero matris"*.[41] This view, however, did not prevail. CANGLIAMILA, in his authoritative *Embryologia sacra* first published in 1763,[24] went so far as to make it compulsory for priests to perform a post-mortem caesarian section when necessary,[43] a decision approved by several later moralists[44] but rejected by others.[45] As late as 1860, one authority[46] still branded as "weaklings" those priests who regarded such an operation as "unfitting" for them. According to another moralist,[47] the duty to extract the foetus by surgical means is binding only if the mother died after the end of the 28th week of gestation (when the fruit begins to be viable).[48]

Among the medico-religious problems affecting the dead, we have to consider above all the very extensive field of anatomical dissection. The religious opposition to this practice is hardly less old than the first scientific incursions into the human body are themselves. In fact, that opposition may well have anticipated, and delayed, the birth of anatomical studies. The first rudimentary attempts at gaining some knowledge of man's body by dissecting it after death go back to very ancient times indeed. But almost every enquiry into this field was accompanied by religious restraints of one form or another. In Egypt the obscure beginnings of anatomical investigations may go back to 4000 B.C.E. when, as MANETHO related, ATHOSIS (the son and successor of MENES, founder of the first dynasty) wrote on anatomy and human dissection.[49] It is claimed that the oldest anatomical treatise extant is an Egyptian *papyrus* which may date from 1600 B.C.E.[50] PLINY, too, asserted that Egyptian physicians conducted post-mortem examinations to ascertain the cause of death at a very early date.[51] But as soon as we leave the vague evidence of primeval times and reach more reliable data, we invariably encounter religious objections. Even the Egyptian practice to embalm and disembowel the dead did not lead to an expansion of anatomical knowledge owing to religious scruples. Although, as the Bible expressly states, JACOB's body was embalmed by "the physicians" in Egypt (*Gen. l.*2), the belief that it was an act of gross impiety eventually militated against the employment of doctors for carrying out the operation. Consequently, the incision of the corpse was entrusted to special functionaries, the *"Paraschite"*, who became an object of universal execration and who had to flee after their work amid a hail of stones.[52] Dissesctions in the cause of pure science ceased altogether in deference to religious feelings.

In Greece—and we here include the important contributions to anatomy of the Ptolomaic school at Alexandria under the influence of Hellenism—the history of dissection was not fundamentally different. The inception of the science of anatomy has been variously attributed to ARISTOTLE,[53] to several writers of the Hippocratic school, and in particular to ALCMAEON of Croton (PYTHAGORAS's younger contemporary) at about 500 B.C.E.[54] and to DIOCLES of Athens 150 years later.[55] But any sustained advances were rendered impossible not only by the failure to appreciate the importance of dissection for medical purposes, but by social and religious prejudices,[56] especially the insistence on immediate burial.[57] OSLER[58] maintains that, until the rise of anatomy at Alexandria early in the 3rd century B.C.E., the study of the structure of the human body was "barred everywhere by religious prejudice". At that Egyptian outpost of Hellenistic culture the new anatomical science, probably founded by HEROPHILUS and ERASISTRATOS,[59] flourished for a time virtually unhampered by religious restrictions. But even that single break in the deep-seated tradition of religious opposition to dissection was only of short duration. SINGER[60] claims that the practice ceased half a century before GALEN began his medical education in 146 C.E. and that he consequently saw none. Although various scholars have adduced some evidence to modify this view,[61] it is certain that from GALEN's time until over twelve centuries later there is not even the faintest trace of any practical research into the human body.

As we move East in the ancient world, we find essentially the same conditions. The occasional references to human dissection in the Syriac *Book of Medicines*[62] are no doubt due to the impact of the Alexandrian school where its author had studied in the 2nd century B.C.E.[63] In ancient India, where medicine and surgery had developed to a high standard, the dissection of the human body was opposed on religious grounds,[64] at least when it involved the use of the knife.[65] The first dissections in China are ascribed to the great and legendary physician PIEN

CH'IAO many centuries before the Alexandrian exploits in this branch.[66] But there, too, the practice came to be regarded as incompatible with religious piety and was, with rare exceptions, discontinued until modern times.[67]

With this background of practically universal religious antagonism to dissection, it is rather remarkable that the Jews of antiquity, far from expressing any hostility to the practice, appear in fact to have engaged, or at least acquiesced, in it. PHILO of Alexandria, in a significant passage generally overlooked by medical historians, speaks of " . . . physicians of the highest repute who have made researches into the construction of man and examined in detail what is visible and also, by careful use of anatomy, what is hidden from sight in order that, if medical treatment is required, nothing which could cause serious danger should be neglected through ignorance".[68] This statement may, of course, reflect local influences rather than Jewish teachings, but its enthusiastic support of dissection for medical ends is nonetheless notable.

Although the allegation first made early in the 19th century,[69] and later endorsed,[70] that the Babylonian talmudist RAV of the 3rd century "bought cadavers and dissected them" has rightly been dismissed as a "phantasy" lacking every foundation,[71] there is some evidence to support the claims by several historians[72] that dissections and autopsies on humans were carried out by the authors of the Talmud,[73] albeit only very occasionally. Yet, it would be an exaggeration to assert that "dissection in the interests of science was permitted by the Talmud".[74]

The main talmudic references to the subject can be listed quite briefly. In one passage,[75] the Palestinian teacher, R. YISHMAEL of the 1st century, relates that the Alexandrian Queen CLEOPATRA once delivered her female slaves, who had been sentenced to death, to the king for anatomical investigations; upon opening their bodies he discovered that the form of the male embryo was completed on the 41st day following conception and that of the female on the 81st day. This talmudic account shows "serious discussion on scientific method and the planning of an experiment".[76] A similar report of dissections by Egyptian kings is mentioned quite independently by the Roman historian PLINY.[77] In a more important statement,[78] the Babylonian sage and physician SAMUEL records that the disciples of the same R. YISHMAEL once boiled[79] the body of a prostitute, who had been condemned to death by the king, to ascertain the exact number of bones in human beings (to solve a religious question requiring these data). KATZENELSOHN[80] argues convincingly that SAMUEL could not have recorded such an operation unless it had actually occurred, because human dissection was then no longer undertaken in Alexandria or elsewhere. He concludes that these Palestinian Jewish disciples must have been first to reintroduce anatomical investigations on human corpses since the days of HEROPHILUS and ERASISTRATOS. KATZENELSOHN also assumes that practical researches must be presupposed for the detailed list of human bones given in the Mishnah,[81] particularly since the figure given by the Greek physicians is at variance with the more accurate number listed by the rabbis.[82] Elsewhere, the Talmud speaks of "hands soiled through [handling] blood, fetal growths and placentas" for ritual enquiries,[83] and of a sage who was once a grave-digger who admitted that he "used to bury the dead and to observe the bones of the dead", whereby he studied the osteological effects of alcoholism.[84]

None of these statements deal specifically with anatomical experiments for purely medical purposes,[85] nor can any of them be taken to imply an unconditional sanction of human dissection. But it is noteworthy that no voice of protest was raised against these practices or their description in the Talmud, a fact all the more remarkable if it is remembered that Jewish law in general rigorously upholds the inviolability of the human body in death as well as in life[86] and that it condemns any undue interference with the corpse as an execrable offence against the dead.[87] It could be inferred from a discussion in the Talmud[88] that post-mortem autopsies would not be tolerated even if they would facilitate the verification of evidence in criminal proceedings. But the circumstances in the case under discussion were such as would in any event render the findings of an autopsy, had it been permitted, irrelevant to the incrimination of the suspected offender and insufficient for his acquittal from capital guilt. It does not necessarily follow, therefore, that talmudic law would rule out post-mortem examinations for forensic purposes if the results might yield crucial information to the courts. In fact, the trend of the argument certainly suggests that the ban on disfiguring the dead would be lifted if an autopsy could save the life of a person on trial for murder.[89] In civil litigations, however, even the exhumation and inspection of a corpse as evidence in support of a party's claims is prohibited as an unwarranted sacrilege.[90] But it must be emphasised that a sharp distinction was generally made between such autopsies and scientific dissections. The experiments at Alexandria, and later at Bologna and elsewhere, were quite independent of medico-legal dissections which developed as a separate discipline and not as a branch of scientific anatomy.[91]

Judaism, then, became heir to a distinctly tolerant attitude to dissection. Yet, as we shall see, it eventually evolved an outlook which, in its modern rabbinic formulation, was increasingly unfavourable to the utilisation of the dead in the service of science.

The development within Christianity followed just the reverse pattern. Although it had for long inherited a tradition of latent, and often overt, opposition to dissection, the Church ultimately reconciled herself completely with the demand of science for human bodies. The history of this development has been befogged by much, and sometimes bitter, controversy; for it is closely bound up with the contentious issue of the relations between the Church and science in general. But the main outlines of the course pursued by the Church are fairly clear. Leading medical historians, whose testimony we have already adduced,[92] agree that the emergence of Christianity, with its disparagement of the body and its needs, was one of the major factors in bringing the ancient spirit and achievements of scientific enquiry to an abrupt end and in replacing empiric experimentation by dogmatic submission to authority for almost a millenium and a half. In the field of medical research, no branch was more completely atrophied than anatomical dissection. For well over a thousand years, there is no trace of any human dissection at all—that science receded into absolute oblivion.

While the decline of anatomy at the beginning of the Common Era could hardly be ascribed to the as yet quite insignificant influence of the new faith,[93] the Christian tradition of its disapprobation was set quite early. Already in about 400, St. AUGUSTINE had declared: "With a cruel zeal for science, some medical men who are called anatomists have dissected the bodies of the dead, and have inhumanly pried into the secrets of the human body in order to learn the nature of the disease and its exact seat and how it might be cured".[94] TERTULLIAN, two centuries later, is said to have "hated dissection".[95] Although the early Church never issued a formal ban on anatomy, the idea of dissection "must have outraged Christian sentiment".[96] It was regarded as a violation of man's dignity and as incompatible with the belief in bodily resurrection. Even the dissection of animals was not always possible, as the student was in danger of being taken for a magician.[97]

As we enter the second millenium, we find little change in this outlook. At the School of Salerno in the 11th century, often described as the first university, the ape used by GALEN for anatomical experiments was replaced by the pig,[98] because it was thought internally to resemble man most.[99] But human corpses were still excluded, probably due to the opposition of the Church.[100] Only in the 13th century do we encounter the first incipient revival of the scientific interest in the human cadaver. In 1238 FREDERICK II ordered that a corpse should be dissected every five years in the presence of physicians and surgeons for study purposes.[101] This decree is the first mention of dissection as an established practice,[102] even though the instruction probably was merely nominal.[103] At Bologna the practice of dissection began in the third quarter of the same century.[104] The first frank reference to a post-mortem examination dates from 1286, when a physician at Cremona opened a corpse to find the cause of the pestilence raging in Italy that year. In 1302 a court ordered a post-mortem investigation on a victim of suspected poisoning, and in 1316 MONDINO DE' LUZZI published the first "modern" work on anatomy, following public dissections at Bologna University.[105] Thenceforth, the renewed interest in dissection spread very slowly. It was officially sanctioned—with certain safeguards which usually restricted the subjects to criminals—at Venice in 1368, at Montpellier in 1375, and at Lerida in 1391.[106] But these experiments had as yet little scientific value.[107] Their purpose was to illustrate ancient medical texts rather than to serve independent research. The public displays of "anatomies" were often turned into "academic feasts" as shown in many contemporary pictures,[108] and—to quote from the statutes of Florence—"food and wine and spices were to be provided to keep up the spirits of professors and students during these unwonted ordeals".[109] Anatomical demonstrations did not commence in Paris, Vienna and Prague until the 15th century,[110] while at the University of Padua the medical curriculum made no provision for the study of anatomy in the middle of that century.[111] Even in the 16th century dissections were not common.[112] PARACELSUS still "despised anatomy and failed to see how any knowledge could be gained from the dead body"; only a little later the entire outlook was changed by VESALIUS.[113] In Italy, Holland and France dissection as a means of teaching anatomy became popular only in the 17th century; in Germany and England it was introduced later still.[114] At most European universities regular anatomical instruction on cadavers was not commenced until early in the 18th century,[115] and only then did the students begin to participate actively in the dissections, instead of relying on the demonstrations of special officials as had been the practice previously.[116]

This picture of the slow evolution of modern anatomical studies shows many lacunae indicating the frequent reverses encountered by the new science in its tedious progress. As we now proceed to fill in these gaps in the picture, we shall discover that the religious prejudice against dissection, if not direct theological opposition to it, faded only very gradually. By far the most important, and also the most contentious, Church document quoted on this issue is the Bull *"De Sepulturis"* of Pope BONIFACE VIII dated 1300.[117] It decreed that " . . . persons cutting up the bodies of the dead, barbarously cooking them in order that the bones, being separated from the flesh, may be carried for burial into their own countries are by that very fact excommunicated". This papal ban on boiling human corpses (presumably of crusaders who had died far from their homes) to facilitate their transport to consecrated ground is of particular interest to us. For at about the same time, the Jewish savant ADRETH[118] gave a ruling permitting the corrosion of dead bodies through quick-lime in order to ease the removal of the remains for interment beside the graves of the deceased's family. Both pronouncements, so strikingly similar in their timing and subject matter, are the first medieval utterances to be later used in determining the official religious attitude to dissection of Christianity and Judaism respectively, though ultimately that attitude was reversed by both religions.

The leading medical and social historians are about equally divided in their views on the relevance of BONIFACE's Bull to human dissection for anatomical purposes. The scholars VIRCHOW,[119] PARK,[120] BAAS,[121] PUSCHMANN,[122] WHITE,[123] ALLBUTT,[124] STERN,[125] and SINGER[126] broadly agree that, while the edict was not specifically directed against anatomists, it certainly fortified the public abhorrence of dissection and was, in fact, largely responsible for delaying the progress of anatomical research. On the other hand, HAESER,[127] PAGEL,[128] NEUBURGER,[129] WALSH,[130] GARRISON,[131] RASHDALL[132] and CASTIGLIONE[133] do not see any essential relationship between the Bull and the history of anatomy. Whereas WINDLE[134] calls the allegation "a hoary fable", ALSTON[135]—who recently subjected the whole subject of the Christian attitude to dissection before 1500 to a searching analysis—admits that the Bull did, in effect, discourage anatomy, at least when it involved the boiling of corpses. Some Catholic authors have suggested that the misunderstanding as to the Bull's intentions is due to a biased interpretation of it in the 16th volume of the *Histoire litteraire de la France* which was mainly written by the French historian PIERRE CLAUDE FRANCOIS DAUNON soon after the French Revolution.[136]

Support for the claim that BONIFACE's Bull actually hindered anatomical studies is usually found in the following passage by MONDINO: "The bones which are below the *'os basilare'* cannot well be seen unless they are removed and boiled, but owing to the sin involved in this I pass them by".[137] But ALSTON[138] has shown that the only express statement indicating that the Church in fact forbade dissection was made in the *Anatomy* by GUIDO DE VIGEVANO[139] in Paris around 1340. During the following centuries the indications of Church opposition or interference are erratic; so is the evidence that the practice enjoyed theological sanction. RASHDALL[140] regards "religious prejudice" as responsible for the objections to dissection until it was introduced at the various European universities. PUSCHMANN,[141] too, believes that in the 16th century the general bias against the practice was religiously motivated rather than of a social nature. MACMURRICH[142] reports that in 1519 Pope LEO X denied LEONARDO DA VINCI admission to the hospital at Rome, where he wished to pursue anatomical studies, because he had engaged in dissection. A little later VESALIUS complained that "the ecclesiastical caucus would not countenance the vivisection of the brain"[143] and that in Madrid he could not lay his hands on so much as a dried skull.[144] SIGERIST[145] also finds that the real birth of anatomy occurred only with the Renaissance, after the religious bands had loosened.

On the other hand, the Church authorities occasionally granted express licences for the dissection of human cadavers, and the bodies of popes and other Church dignitaries were often opened and embalmed, sometimes perhaps even dissected, in the Middle Ages.[146] In 1482 a brief of Pope SIXTUS IV authorised dissections on condition that ecclesiastical sanction was first obtained, and the practice was again confirmed by Pope CLEMENT VII in 1524.[147] When in 1556 CHARLES V referred complaints that dissection was sinful to the theological faculty at Salamanca, he received the reply: "The dissection of human cadavers serves a useful purpose and is therefore permissible to Christians of the Catholic Church".[148] But even in later centuries, permission to dissect had to be obtained from the popes as an indulgence.[149] On the other hand, Protestant cities in Germany were more ready than others to admit anatomical experiments.[150] Occasional protests against dissection continued to be voiced up to modern times,[151] and the undercurrent of theological misgivings did not finally disappear until PROSPERO LAMBERTINI, later Pope BENEDICT XIV, expressed the official attitude of the Catholic Church as favouring the practice for the advancement of the arts[152] and sciences in unequivocal terms in 1737.[153] That year, by another striking coincidence, was also the year in which, as we shall see, the first authentic Jewish pronouncement on anatomical dissection was made. The present-day Code of Canon Law, although it regards the "dishonouring of the bodies of the dead by theft or other crimes committed on the bodies or graves of the deceased" as a penal offence,[154] does not ban dissection, as the

Code deals only with the violation of the body for evil purposes.[155]

The stagnation of medieval anatomy and surgery is also sometimes attributed to the negative attitude to human dissection in Mohammedan and Jewish thought. Thus, one scholar argues that it was "the superstitious horror of mutilating a corpse" among the Arabs and Jews which stifled scientific progress in the earlier Middle Ages,[156] while another has claimed that "the Jewish tenets, adopted by the Mohammedans, compelled students to be satisfied with making their observations on the carcasses of brutes".[157] Among the Arabs, religious opposition to dissection was certainly explicit and sustained, as attested by many modern scholars.[158] The *Koran* itself expressly forbids the opening of a corpse, even if the person should have swallowed the most valuable pearl not belonging to him.[159] This clearly negates the assertion by ALSTON[160] that there is nothing in Islamic scriptures which could be interpreted as opposing dissection and that the backwardness of Western anatomy could not, therefore, be attributed to its influence. In fact, the koranic prohibition was always applied in support of the ban on anatomical dissection at Turkish,[161] Persian and other Mohammedan universities.[162] Though the law was amended in 1838 to permit the dissection of Christian and Jewish bodies,[163] in practice the religious prohibition of anatomical research was usually upheld even in very recent times.[164]

It is evident that the Jews, too, did not make any significant contribution to the advancement of anatomical studies in the Middle Ages. But whether, as has been alleged even by so knowledgeable a master of Jewish medical history as FRIEDENWALD,[165] their failure to examine human cadavers for scientific ends was in any way due to religious inhibitions is difficult to establish. Certain it is that there is no substance whatever in the charge, first made by JEAN ASTRUC[166] early in the 18th century and later often repeated by others,[167] that the biblical laws of ritual defilement (*Nu. xix.*11) militated against the dissection of human bodies.[168]   Neither these laws nor their talmudic ramifications prohibit the touching of a dead body (except to Jews of priestly descent[169]); they merely lay down the conditions of impurity resulting from such contact, and the procedure to be adopted to regain ritual cleanliness.   Nor can the allegation of Jewish religious opposition to dissection be sustained by any direct reference to the subject on the part of a single Jewish physician or rabbi before the 18th century.   On the contrary, there is some evidence to suggest that a few Jewish physicians did, in fact, carry out post-mortem examinations very occasionally.   While the claim that MAIMONIDES may have made practical tests in anatomy[170] can be dismissed as altogether conjectural, there is clear proof of the participation in dissections by other Jewish and Marrano doctors.

Thus, the celebrated Marrano physician of the 16th century, AMATUS LUSITANUS—in whom his parents had "implanted . . . an attachment to Jewish religion, tradition and customs"[171]—himself performed twelve dissections at Ferrara to confirm the discovery of the valves in the azygos veins made by him in conjunction with his friend, the papal physician CANANO, in 1547.[172]   Again, ABRAHAM ZACUTUS LUSITANUS, the Marrano who joined the Jewish Congregation at Amsterdam in 1625,[173] is said to deserve "special praise for the frequency with which he made autopsies at a time when they were rare".[174]   The famous religious and medical writer of the 17th century, JACOB ZAHALON, too, appears to have at least condoned dissections; for he refers with evident approval to a post-mortem examination carried out by a non-Jewish doctor on a Jewish victim of the plague in 1656 to discover if death was due to a bubo or to an intestinal hernia.[175]   Of interest, too, is the anatomical illustration which serves as the frontispiece to TOBIAS COHEN's *Ma'asei Tuvi'ah*, a popular medico-religious work first published in Venice in 1707. It depicts the body of (what appears to be) a Jew opened to expose the inner organs and compares their function to the divisions of a house.[156] There was even a *"Prosektor"* at the *"Koenigsberger Anatomie"* who was a Jew named Dr. LEWIN JOSEPH HIRSCH (1758-1823).[177] Another Jewish anatomist who attained some eminence in the 19th century was M. L. HIRSCHFELD in France.[178]

These few instances are obviously too isolated to admit of any general conclusions on the Jewish religious attitude to dissection in those times. But one may regard as more significant, if not conclusive, the complete lack of any rabbinic sources on the subject prior to the 18th century. As we have observed, practical studies in anatomy began to be well established at many European universities in the 17th century and, on a more limited scale, even before then. It can hardly be assumed that the many Jewish physicians and students did not occasionally face the problem created by the necessity to participate, at least passively, in the "anatomies" regularly performed at the medical schools. The absence of any rabbinic protests against the growing practice is all the more remarkable as Jewish corpses were often especially favoured by the anatomists. An anonymous "Address to the Public" published in London in 1829 informs us that, "as the Jews bury early, their cemetery formerly produced the best and freshest subjects [for dissection], equal in freshness to the body sent to the venal undertaker . . . ".[179] The Jewish community at Padua were vexed by this problem already in the 17th century, when students at the famous university demanded the use of all Jewish bodies for anatomical work.[180] Jews certainly objected to this wretched "body-snatching" no less bitterly than their neighbours did on many similar occasions;[181] yet, despite their specially close concern with this problem, there is no record of any condemnation of dissection itself in the prolific rabbinic writings during those centuries.

If there existed, then, no explicit rabbinic stricture on anatomical studies, they were never unequivocally sanctioned, either. It was only in comparatively modern times that ADRETH's permission to use lime for hastening the cadaver's decomposition[182] was adduced as corroborative evidence to justify the legalization of dissection.[183] Unlike BONIFACE's Bull which gave an unfavourable verdict in very similar circumstances at the same time, ADRETH's ruling was merely applied to the kind of case actually envisaged in the responsum, or to almost identical contingencies. ISSERLES, for instance, simply codified it thus: "It is permitted to place lime on [the dead] in order to consume the flesh quickly, so as to [be able to] bring [the body] to the place as willed [by the deceased]" (*Y.D.*, *ccclxiii*.2, gloss). A little earlier, DAVID IBN ZIMRA,[184] on the basis of the same ruling, stated that he could see no objection to the use of quick-lime for speeding the admission of the soul to Heaven (which, according to the Midrash,[185] must await the body's decomposition), but he added that he would nevertheless advise against such interference with the ordinary course of nature. By a curious reversal of effects, ADRETH's sanction was utilised by a leading scholar in the 19th century to frustrate the anatomists' avid rapacity in securing Jewish bodies for dissection; he counselled a questioner from America to bury the bodies with lime in order to render them unfit for anatomical examination.[186]

It was not until 1737—the very year in which the Roman Church finalised its attitude in favour of dissection[187]—that the problem of anatomical research was submitted to rabbinic judgment for the first time. In that year, a Jewish medical student at the University of Goettingen[188] asked R. JACOB EMDEN, a leading authority of his age, whether he could participate on the Sabbath in the dissection of dogs used in the absence of human material. The rabbi replied that such operations on the Sabbath involved many prohibitions, whether carried out on humans or on animals; in the case of human corpses, even if they were not Jewish, it was in any case forbidden to derive any benefit from them.[189] For this latter statement he referred to a decision by ADRETH[190] also recorded by KARO (*Y.D.*, *ccclix*.1). In the same century the question was treated again by

EZEKIEL LANDAU,[191] the widely recognised scholar who died at Prague in 1793. He had an enquiry from London where permission was sought for an autopsy on a Jewish patient, who had died after an unsuccessful operation for calculus in the bladder, to ascertain the proper surgical treatment for similar cases in the future. In his reply, which did not refer to the ban on benefiting from a human corpse (EMDEN's principal concern), LANDAU stated that any disfigurement of the dead was an act of gross indignity strictly prohibited in Jewish law.[192] The respect due to the dead could be set aside only if there was a reasonable and immediate prospect of thereby saving human life. But as the patients to be cured through the experience gained from the post-mortem examination were not yet at hand, its object was too remote to warrant disgracing the dead. Moreover, "even non-Jewish doctors do not make experiments in anatomy on any corpses except those of judicially executed criminals or of people who had given their consent in life; and if we were—Heaven forfend!—to be lenient in this matter, they would dissect all [our] dead in order to study the arrangement of the internal organs and their function so as to determine the medical treatment of the living".[193]

From the 19th century, the problem of dissection is discussed by almost all leading rabbis in innumerable responsa. Previously the question arose only in individual cases. But as the practice became increasingly general and the religious problem it created more pressing, a number of new elements were introduced into the discussion. The great Hungarian respondent, MOSES SCHREIBER,[194] in a written judgment dated 1836, accepted the position taken up by EMDEN and LANDAU before him; only he opined that the ban on benefiting from the dead might not apply to the bodies of non-Jews in accordance with their own views and their religious teachings.[195] But he emphatically agreed that the remote possibility of saving life could not override the certainty of desecrating the dead; by the same token all work involved in medical studies would suspend the Sabbath laws

on the assumption that a human life might thereby be preserved at some future date. Hence he regarded it as reprehensible for a Jew to bequeath his body for anatomical
research. In 1852 the German scholar JACOB ETTLIN-
GER[196] further argued that the duty to save life could obli-
gate only the living to disregard their personal rights and
religious duties in the interest of their fellow-men. But as
the dead themselves were free from any religious obligation,[197] and as the saving of life at the expense of another's
possessions and dignity was in any case questionable,[198] one
would not under any circumstances be justified in disturbing
the dead. Yet he sanctioned the operation if the deceased
had sold or allotted his body for that purpose in his lifetime.
Both opinions were later opposed by MOSES SCHICK,[199]
SCHREIBER's leading disciple. He concluded from the
Talmud[200] that no-one could renounce the respect due to
his body. On the other hand, he held that the Talmudic
rule whereby all laws (except idolatry, bloodshed and incest)
must give way for the saving of life[201] also applied to the
prohibition of disgracing the dead; hence autopsies were
warranted if the lives of other existing patients might thereby be preserved. Two eminent German rabbis at the time
also expressed this view.[202]

In the present century opinions have varied widely.
With the growing and increasingly direct benefits accruing
to medical science from studies on human corpses, some rabbis strongly favoured permitting the practice. The British
Chief Rabbi HERMANN ADLER,[203] in a memorial address in 1905, lauded the late FREDERIC DAVID
MOCATTA for having directed that, should he die from
an obscure disease, an autopsy be performed at the expense
of his estate "for the advancement of medical science".
While ABRAHAM ISAAC KOOK[204] advised the purchase
of non-Jewish bodies for anatomical studies, BENZION
UZIEL,[205] another Chief Rabbi of the Holy Land, saw
no objection to the dissection of Jewish bodies, provided it
was carried out with due care and respect; but he dis-

approved of persons selling their bodies before death. Another rabbi even suggested a popular campaign to persuade people to grant their written consent for their posthumous service to medicine.[206]

In favour of the sanction it was argued that to study anatomy by observation did not constitute a forbidden "benefit" from the dead;[207] that any intrinsically forbidden act performed for study purposes was altogether exempt from the original prohibition;[208] that there was no disgrace to the dead when the welfare of the living was at stake;[209] that a ban on anatomical studies would "close the door to medical science";[210] and that, with hospitals everywhere full of patients actually awaiting the findings of anatomical research and with the speed of modern communications, the objections raised by LANDAU no longer held good.[211]

Nevertheless, many rabbinic authorities remained implacably opposed to any general sanction of dissection, particularly on the bodies of Jews who were summoned to consecrate their lives to the service of God in a special way and therefore merited special respect.[212] An American scholar[213] has listed an impressive array of rabbis who were adamant in their refusal to countenance autopsies, let alone anatomical experiments, on human bodies. He himself caustically suggested that those desiring their sons to study anatomy or advocating the use of Jewish bodies should bequeath their own bodies for dissection. He would not allow even Jewish suicides and criminals to be delivered to the anatomists, since the Bible stressed the respect due to the dead specifically in regard to executed persons.[214] Exceptions might be made only in the case of people afflicted by some hereditary disease if an autopsy could help in the proper diagnosis and thus benefit the next-of-kin. A London rabbi,[215] too, advised relatives not to give permission for post-mortem inquests, though they need not resist the demand for autopsies required by law. Even a scholar as modern in outlook and secular training as DAVID HOFFMANN,[216] late Rector of the *Rabbiner Seminar* in Berlin, was not prepared to go beyond the restrictive position taken up by LANDAU nearly two centuries earlier.

The opposition became especially bitter when rabbinical authorities were faced with the problem on a communal scale. For instance, when the "Prosectorium" in Warsaw demanded the supply of Jewish bodies for anatomical studies in 1924, the local rabbinate fiercely resisted the demand.[217] Many rabbis insisted on the ban even if that meant the exclusion of Jews from medical schools or their estrangement from the Jewish faith, unless such an attitude might provoke measures against the Jewish community in general.[218] The actual delivery by the Warsaw Burial Society of a Jewish woman's corpse for dissection led to a great upheaval at the time.[219] When the question was raised by a tuberculosis hospital in Denver, Colorado, the leading American rabbis likewise took an uncompromising stand against the supply of Jewish bodies for dissection.[220]

Among the arguments advanced to justify these objections—widely upheld right up to the present—were that dissections involved a proper "benefit" from the dead since they included acts and not merely observation,[221] and since they directly promoted the doctors' material interests,[222] that the motive for disturbing the dead was not the honour of the living but their physical advantage;[223] that all talmudic concessions on those grounds were in any case limited to keeping the dead unburied for a maximum of twenty-four hours;[224] that the burial of all parts of the body, required in Jewish law, could not be assured after its dissection;[225] that the indiscriminate renunciation of Jewish bodies would publicly shame the Jewish name;[226] and that any general sanction would lead to many abuses which could not be controlled.[227]

The problem became really pressing with the foundation of the Hebrew University in Jerusalem and the planned establishment of a medical school there. Already in 1924 the difficulties were widely discussed in rabbinical circles.[228] For two decades religious objections to dissection remained an insuperable obstacle to the realisation of the project. The University simply had to carry on without a medical school, just as had been the case at several Moslem universities and as is still the case in the State of New Jersey, where anatomical experiments continue to be banned to this day.[229]

But with the rise of Israel as an independent state the pressure became so great that some adequate compromise between the religious and medical claims had to be found. Negotiations ensued between Chief Rabbi ISAAC HERZOG, acting on behalf of the Chief Rabbinate of the Holy Land, and the "Hadassa" University Hospital of Jerusalem, and these led to an agreement whereby post-mortem examinations were sanctioned when (i) they are legally required, (ii) the cause of death cannot otherwise be ascertained, provided this is formally attested in writing by three physicians (as designated in the agreement), (iii) they may help to save the lives of other existing patients, as similarly attested, (iv) they are required in cases of hereditary diseases to safeguard the health of the surviving relations; provided always, among other stipulations, that the hospital authorities will carry out the autopsies with due reverence for the dead and that they will deliver the corpses and all parts removed therefrom to the burial society for interment after use.[230] Regarding the use of bodies for medical teaching purposes, the Chief Rabbi further issued the following statement: "The Plenary Council of the Chief Rabbinate of Israel . . . do not object to the use of bodies of persons who gave their consent in writing of their own free will during their lifetime for anatomical dissections as required for medical studies, provided the dissected parts are carefully preserved so as to be eventually buried with due respect according to Jewish law".[231] A few years later, in 1953, similar provisions were embodied in the Anatomy and Pathology Act passed by the Israeli Parliament.[232]

In the discussions which led to these decisions, it was emphasised that there could be no distinction in Jewish law whereby "the body of an honoured or rich person must not be dissected, whereas that of a poor or forsaken person could be so used; the sole foundation of a sanction could only be the saving of human life, and in that consideration no difference could be made between one or another".[233] This attitude, as has been pointed out,[234] is in direct contrast with, for example, the English Warburton Anatomy Act of 1832 which released for anatomical study all bodies that were unclaimed and therefore regarded as *res nullius* in civil law.[235] In Jewish law it is, on the contrary, the body of a person left without relatives whose burial imposes a special obligation on the whole community; even the High Priest—otherwise forbidden to defile himself even for his closest next-of-kin—must ignore his sanctity by personally attending to the immediate burial of such a person.[236]

With the concordat reached between the highest religious and medical authorities in Israel the argument over those no longer able to speak for themselves was by no means resolved. Several religious doctors, too, have joined in the debate. To the growing list of medical articles on "Post-mortem Examinations among the Jews"[237] have lately been added polemical contributions by two Jerusalem physicians, SUSSMAN MUNTNER and JACOB LEVY, defending the more extreme views of the devotees of anatomy and the traditionalists respectively. Both doctors claim the main debate to be now only of academic interest: the former because he believes the rabbinical opposition to be at an end; the latter because he considers the medical need for bodies at an end. To MUNTNER it appears that, in regard to autopsies, "all arguments have already ceased and everyone has now been reconciled to the sanction even from the religious point of view".[238] Virtually all the talmudic and rabbinic sources he has collected lead him to the conclusion that there never existed any objection to anatomical dissection; if some Jewish scholars did express a contrary opinion, it was only "because they wished to introduce the heathen concept of the honour of the dead and the ban on dissection into our literature".[239] For LEVY, on the other hand, "the star of anatomy is now sinking". With the important facts about human anatomy already known, the present tendency is for anatomical research to be replaced by various physical methods in the diagnosis and treatment of disease. Thus he refers to the three most recent and revolutionary advances in medicine—the discovery of penicillin and other antibiotics, heart operations and polio vaccinations—as owing their development to biological, chemical and X-ray research, not to dissection.[240] LEVY denounces the Israeli Anatomy and Pathology Act—which permits any autopsy on medical certification without regard to the wishes of the deceased or his family—as an affront to the freedom of conscience, unparalleled in other civilised countries. In Israel, he protests, 90% of all who die in hospitals are subjected to autopsies, as against only 30% at Columbia University. Even with this wholesale violation of the dead, he argues, no commensurate advantages either in prestige or in scientific discoveries have accrued to medicine in Israel which would vindicate the disregard for the sanctities of Jewish law.[241]

In respect of medical training, LEVY admits that some facilities may have to be sacrificed for the maintenance of the highest moral and religious standards in the Holy Land. But he suggests that practical anatomy can now be studied on drawings and plastic models, on tissues removed in live operations or imported from abroad, and—if necessary—by a short course at a foreign university.[242] For, in practice, the conditions under which even the more lenient authorities approved of dissection simply cannot be carried out: there can be no respect for the dead in the anatomy room (often there is levity instead), and it is impossible to ensure that all parts of the corpse are ultimately buried.[243]

And so the debate continues unabated.

CHAPTER THIRTEEN

CONTROLLING THE GENERATION OF LIFE—1

EUGENICS, STERILISATION AND CONTRACEPTION.

In no department of medical ethics have the claims of religion been pressed with greater consistency than in the wide fields of genetics and procreation. In the ordinary course of his practice, the physician often has to make decisions involving some risk of life. In such cases he is usually justified in being guided by purely medical considerations, provided his ultimate object is to preserve his patient's life or health. But when a human life is deliberately set at stake, or its generation restricted, to protect another life, or for lesser reasons, grave religious and moral problems are raised. Any decision in such issues demands a reliable evaluation of life, in absolute as well as relative terms—a task altogether outside the purview of medical science.

EUGENICS

The principles defining the right, and its limitations, to interfere with the generation and maintenance of life find their broadest application in the realm of eugenics. The scientific study of measures to preserve and improve the quality of the human stock is of comparatively recent origin. The very term "eugenics", in its modern connotation, was coined only in 1883 by Sir FRANCIS GALTON,[1] the pioneer of this science. But already in ancient times attempts at preventing the birth or growth of defectives were not wanting. In Greece, for instance, these endeavours ranged from PLATO's advocacy of drastic measures "to safeguard the highest quality of the human herd"[2] to the barbaric practice of exposing crippled children to die in the woods.[3] Eugenic factors may also account, at least in part, for the ban on consanguineous marriages which most nations of antiquity embraced to some extent.[4] In general, however, the safeguards against the degeneration of the human race were haphazard and isolated, seldom reinforced by legal enactments and never religiously motivated. On the contrary, the outlook fostered by religion was usually quite antipathetic to any conscious control of human generation, particularly in the Middle Ages when the eugenic concept became virtually extinct.

Jewish law certainly went very much further than any other in ancient and medieval times in cultivating the eugenic ideal by prudent legislation and counsel. MAX GRUNWALD, in his study of biblical and talmudic sources on eugenics, summarises the attitude of Judaism thus: "It quite consciously strives for the promotion of the quality as well as quantity of the progeny by the compulsion of matrimony, the insistence on early marriage, the sexual purity of the marital partners and the harmony of their ages and characters, the dissolubility of unhappy unions, the regulation of conjugal intercourse, the high esteem of maternity, the stress on parental responsibility, the protection of the embryo, etc. To be sure, there can be no question here of a compulsory public control over the health conditions of the marriage candidates. But that would positively be in line with the principles of Jewish eugenics: the pursuit after the most numerous and physically, mentally and morally sound natural increase of the people, without thinking of an exclusive race protection."[5] These objectives inform many explicit regulations in Jewish law, as we shall now briefly set out.

In the codes an entire chapter (*E.H.*, i) is devoted to the obligation to marry and to propagate the race. To refuse to do so is tantamount to bloodshed and to expelling the

Divine Presence from Israel (*ib.*, 1). The fulfilment of this duty is enforceable by the courts (*ib.*, 3); but it is no longer the practice to exercise compulsion in matrimonial matters,[6] provided there is no legal impediment to the proposed marriage (*ib.*, gloss). A man has performed the biblical precept to "be fruitful and multiply" (*Gen. i.*28) if he has at least a son and a daughter[7] (*ib.*, 5); yet he should seek further to augment his natural increase beyond his minimum duty[8] (*ib.*, 8). Of particular interest are some of the regulations in the chapter on the obligation "to endeavour to take a fitting wife" (*E.H.*, ii). Special emphasis is placed on the choice of a partner equipped with the highest intellectual and moral virtues; a detailed list sets forth the order of preference in the selection of a wife, relative to the father's record of service to the community (*ib.*, 6), and the verse "Cursed be he that lieth with any manner of beast" (*Deut. xxviii.*21) is applied to him who marries the daughter of an ignoramus (*ib.*, gloss).

These and many similar provisions in Jewish law are clearly motivated by eugenic considerations for the moral excellence of the progeny. The Talmud[9] recognises the hereditary element in the determination of character and virtue when it counsels a man seeking worthy children to examine the brothers of his prospective wife, "since most children take after their maternal uncles". Stress is also laid on physical compatibility in marriage. There should be no undue discrepancy in the ages of the parties (*ib.*, 9). In size, too, the Talmud[10] insists that they should be so adjusted to each other as to prevent the formation of a phenomenally tall or tiny offspring.

Most important, from the eugenic point of view, is the ruling that one should not marry into a leprous or epileptic family—that is, a family thought to be predisposed to these conditions following their manifestation among three family members[11] (*ib.*, 7). According to RASHI,[12] any (hereditary) disease is evidently included in this category. This ruling may well represent the first eugenic enactment, and the only legislative bar to the procreation of a diseased progeny, in ancient and even medieval times. Compulsory medical examinations before marriage are, of course, only a very modern innovation adopted in a few countries.[13] But since the earliest talmudic times, Jewish law granted men the right to reassure themselves that their partners were free from any serious physical defects.[14] For this purpose women to be married were expected to visit the public baths in the presence of the grooms' female relations (*E.H.,* *cxvii.*5) or friends (*ib.,* 6, gloss), and the mere existence of such baths in a town was taken as sufficient proof that the husband was aware of any physical blemishes in his wife before their marriage (*ib.,* 5; *cf.* 4, gloss). Under certain conditions, the discovery of physical defects or ailments in either the wife (*E.H.,* *xxxix.*3, 4; and *cxvii.*4) or the husband (*E.H.,* *cliv.*1) even entitles the other party to dissolve the marriage.

Insane persons cannot contract a valid marriage at all[15] (*E.H.,* *xliv.*2). While the marriages of the deaf-and-dumb[16] are effective, albeit only rabbinically (*ib.,* 1), the rabbis refused to make any provision for the legalisation of marriages with or between lunatics. The declared reason for this refusal is the conviction that such marriages could never be happy or peaceful[17] and not, as has been suggested, "because they would produce backward children",[18] but this law is obviously still of great eugenic interest.

STERILE MARRIAGES

Important, too, in this context is the compulsory dissolution of marriages which have proved sterile. Although marriages between impotent or sterile parties are valid (*E.H., i.*8, gloss; *xxiii.*5, gloss; and *xliv.*4), it is a husband's duty to divorce his wife if she had born him no children after ten years (*E.H., cliv.*10), excluding the periods during which marital relations were impossible due to illness or separation[19] (*ib.*, 11). Originally, the court was to compel the husband to dissolve such a marriage even against the will of both parties (*ib.*, 10 and 21), but ISSERLES remarks that this was no longer done in his day[20] (*ib.* 10, gloss; and *i.*3, gloss). The divorce serves to enable the husband to fulfil his duty of procreation by marrying another woman (*E.H.*, *cliv.*10), but his former wife, too, is entitled to be remarried (*ib.*, 16) on the assumption that the barrenness of the first marriage may not have been due to her.[21] The practical importance attached to this provision in the Middle Ages can be gauged from the many instances of royal, civil and rabbinic dispensations authorising Jewish husbands "to marry another wife or other wives" if the first wife remained without progeny after ten years of married life.[22]

A eugenic motive may also underlie the regulation regarding the "lethal woman". This describes a woman who was bereaved successively of two husbands and who must not be married for a third time, as it is then presumed that her husbands are bound to die (*E.H.*, *ix.*1). The talmudic authors of this precautionary enactment are divided in their explanation of the reason for her misfortune. One view attributes the death of her husbands to the influence of "her bad luck"; the other ascribes it to "the well [of her womb]",[23] that is, to a deadly venereal disease afflicting her. According to the second opinion, therefore, the restriction does not apply to a woman whose husbands died by violence or through a plague (*ib.*, gloss). AZULAY[24] presumes that, following this view, the men's death is due to hereditary traits in the wife; consequently, the precaution may be necessary even if the two husbands who died had been married, not successively to a single woman, but simultaneously to two sisters whose bereavements thus revealed their lethal propensity.[25] On this assumption, it clearly follows that Jewish law would ban the marriage of women who are medically certified to suffer from a grave venereal infection. MAIMONIDES,[26] on the other hand, explains this law mainly in psychological terms: The mere knowledge that a wife has been widowed twice may so haunt the third husband—if he is physically or mentally weak—as to prove fatal to him. Hence, he rules[27]—as does KARO (*ib.*, 1) after him—that, if she was yet married for a third time, the union need not be dissolved. But none of these considerations are held to apply to a man who has successively lost two wives; he is invariably free to remarry (*ib.*, 2). This discrimination in favour of men may be due to the same rational factors as restrict the hereditary predisposition to haemophilia (recognized in the laws on circumcision) to female carriers.[28]

These regulations illustrate the lengths to which Jewish law is prepared to go in safeguarding marital partners and their children from the prospect of contracting crippling or deadly afflictions and in protecting society from an avoidable increase in physical and mental disabilities. But Judaism enacts, recommends or sanctions eugenic precautions only by limiting the right to contract or maintain marriages which may prove dangerous. It does not recognise the right to interfere with the natural relations of lawfully wedded partners to prevent the birth of defective children. This is completely in line with the law's insistence on celibacy or divorce, but never on sexual abstinence, in cases of any permanent medical or religious impediment to a normal relationship within marriage.[29] Even with this vital qualification, the Jewish approach to eugenics reveals an awareness of the individual's responsibility to society and the generations yet unborn which was altogether unknown in any preceding or contemporary system of religious thought or social medicine.

The Roman Catholic Church does not concede to the state the right to ban the marriage of defectives to the present day. Only in 1930, Pope PIUS XI confirmed in his encyclical *Casti Connubii* that, while such persons may be dissuaded from entering into matrimony, they commit no crime by marrying even if they give birth only to incapacitated children.[30]

By contrast, the attitudes of the two religions to sterilisation, and particularly castration, are almost completely reversed. While operations to deprive men of their generative powers have been tolerated by the Church for very long, in Judaism they have been strongly and absolutely condemned since the earliest times. In fact, the Hebrews were the only nation of antiquity to impose a religious prohibition on the emasculation of men and animals[31] alike[32]—a prohibition which was not endorsed by BUDDHA, CONFUCIUS, CHRIST or MOHAMMED.[33]

The practice itself is very ancient. In China, where various methods were employed,[34] castration was performed both as a penal measure[35] and as a means to produce eunuchs for the imperial court before 1000 B.C.E.[36] The Romans claimed that SERIRAMIS, a mystical queen of Babylon, was the first to use castration—as a precautionary measure on all male infants in the royal nurseries after her husband's death to prevent any claims on her throne. According to CICERO, the practice is of even higher antiquity, having figured in Greek mythology, when OURANOS was castrated by his son KRONOS. There is a similar story in the Egyptian *Book of the Dead*. In more historic times, special operating centres to supply eunuchs were found in the island of Delos and, according to HERODOTUS, on Chios. In Roman society, as JUVENAL testified, eunuchs were often employed by aristocratic ladies. The practice persisted until the time of the Emperors CONSTANTINE and JUSTINIAN, when laws banning castration made it equivalent to homicide.[37]

Whether the Hippocratic Oath specifically proscribed the operation has been much debated. The ordinary rendering of the relevant clause is: "I will not use the knife even on sufferers from stone"; but this has been amended to: "I will not castrate even persons who are not grown up"[38]—an interpretation which is accepted, with some minor qualifications, by LITTRE[39] and PUSCHMANN[40] (who regards the whole Oath as belonging to the ante-Hippocratic period). The Oath continues to demand of physicians that they "leave this to those people who make a business of it . . . ". Consequently, W.H.S. JONES[41] doubts whether, in view of the Greek abomination of castration, its performance would be simply delegated to others, as that would amount to "compounding a felony". He therefore suggests that the entire clause is probably a later insertion, particularly since it is not mentioned in the Christian version. EDELSTEIN,[42] on the other hand, rejects the reference to castration altogether. He believes that the phrase is directed against lithotomy and that it is intended to exclude all surgical operations from the physician's work. This would again reflect the influence of the Pythagoreans who valued surgery less highly than dietetic and pharmacological remedies.[43] In any case, it is likely that no formal enactment against castration existed in Greek times, and that, if physicians did not supply eunuchs, they were produced in considerable numbers by practitioners who did not belong to the Society of the Asclepiadae.[44]

With the advent of Christianity eunuchs were no longer required for service in the harems of kings and princes or in the households of wealthy ladies. But they began to satisfy the altogether new demand for saintliness and sexual abnegation in the nascent Church. Already the Gospel of St. MATTHEW speaks of "eunuchs which have made themselves eunuchs for the kingdom of heaven's sake", adding "He that is able to receive it, let him receive it" (*Matth. xix*.12). Although the patristic commentators usually interpreted this passage in a spiritual sense, it was often used to vindicate the early votaries of voluntary castration for the avoidance of sensual passions.[45] Such self-emasculation was practised by the Church Father ORIGEN and by many Patriarchs of Constantinople.[46] The tradition set by the Byzantine Patriarchs also found expression in the statement of the early Christian physician, PAUL of Aegina: "Although the aim of medicine is to correct and not to corrupt nature, the physician nevertheless at times finds himself compelled by those in authority to perform castration".[47] The significant fact that the Christian version of the Hippocratic Oath omitted reference to castration has already been mentioned. In Western Christianity, the practice often became very prevalent until checked by some ecclesiastical edict, sometimes only to reappear with a different motive a little later. The Valesians of the 3rd century castrated themselves in large numbers "thinking thereby to serve God" (in the words of St. AUGUSTINE[48]); then, in 325 the Council of Nicea banned voluntary castrates from priestly offices.[49] In medieval Italy, many ecclesiastics emasculated themselves "because of cupidity" until the practice gradually disappeared following a prohibition by Pope CLEMENT XIV.[50] Later many parents in Italy had their children castrated to preserve their soprano voices as choristers, particularly in churches—a practice only abolished by Pope LEO IX.[51] As late as in the middle of the 18th century, self-emasculation was again renewed by a Christian sect in Russia, and then in Roumania, known as Skoptzy.[52] Present-day Canon Law regards castration as an "irregularity", though it is not clear whether vasectomy is included.[53]

The Roman Catholic Church has defined her attitude to sterilisation for eugenic, therapeutic and punitive ends only in recent times. The earlier traditions notwithstanding, a Holy Office reply of 1940 condemned any direct sterilisation as a contravention of the natural law.[54] Catholic moralists are unanimous in rejecting the validity of the eugenic motive and in sanctioning the operation for medical reasons "when no other provisions can be made for the good of the whole body".[55] But opinions are still conflicting on the right to use sterilisation as a penal measure.[56] During the present century, a number of European countries and American states have introduced legislation providing for the compulsory sterilisation of defectives,[57] and the movement in favour of extending these provisions is steadily growing except among the Latin nations where the opposition of the Church is considerable and effective.[58]

Judaism has consistently objected to every form of castration and surgical sterilisation in the most uncompromising terms (except for urgent medical reasons). The biblical proscription of castration was originally mentioned only in regard to the exclusion of maimed animals from serving as sacrifices on the altar (*Lev. xxii.*24), but the Talmud[59] widely extended the scope of this prohibition, so that it was formulated in the codes thus: "It is forbidden to impair the reproductive organs, whether in man or in domestic animals, beasts or birds, whether these are clean or unclean . . . , and whoever performs a castration transgresses a biblical offence for which he is liable to corporal punishment" (*E.H., v.*11). The same offence is committed by a person who castrates one who is already impotent,[60] so that "if one comes and cuts off the penis, and then another comes and cuts off the testicles or lacerates them, and then yet another comes and severs the seminal cords; or if one comes and crushes the penis, and another comes and lacerates it, and then another comes and cuts it off, they are all liable to corporal punishment" (*ib.*). The prohibition also includes any indirect sterilisation of males, for instance, by freezing the generative organs until they become impotent; but such acts are not actionable under biblical law[61] (*ib.*, 13). The same limitation applies to the surgical sterilisation of females, whether human or animal[62] (*ib.*, 11).

The mutilation of the reproductive organs by physical means is only one of the methods to induce permanent sterility considered in Jewish law. A purely medical treatment is to drink the "cup of sterility", also known as the "potion of roots".[63] Such drinks, commonly consisting of a concoction of various herbal ingredients mixed in wine,[64] occur freely in the Talmud and midrashic literature, as indeed in many other ancient sources[65] and medieval collections of popular medical recipes.[66] All rabbinic codes, even up to modern times,[67] legislate on this sterilising agent which is thought to be effective on both males and females. But in 1894 a German rabbi satisfied himself by medical evidence from qualified physicians that such a contraceptive potion was "no longer known in our time" and that it had "surely been forgotten in the course of time".[68] That no drink taken by mouth is at present known to be effectively contraceptive is also confirmed by N.E. HIMES,[69] the modern medical historian of contraception. The persistence with which the rabbis in all ages nevertheless dealt with the "cup of sterility" may support the conjecture that it was perhaps meant to refer euphemistically to a kind of vaginal spermicide, though its application to males—equally taken for granted, albeit far less frequently, in these sources—would still require explanation.

Regarding such a sterilising potion, MAIMONIDES[70] and KARO simply rule that, whereas it is an offence — though not punishable[71]—to give it to a man or any other male creature so as to produce sterility, it is permitted for a woman to consume it "for the purpose of making herself sterile so that she cannot bear children" (ib., 12). From the wording of this ruling it may be inferred that any sterilisation of males not involving an operation on the genitals themselves is prohibited only if calculated to produce sterility;[72] but it is a matter of dispute whether such non-surgical sterilisation constitutes a biblical or merely rabbinic offence.[73] Most authorities, however, including ACHAI Gaon,[74] TOSAPHOTH,[75] ASHERI[76] and his son JACOB in the *Tur* code,[77] assume that the prohibition holds good even if the potion is taken as a cure for some ailment, with the undesired but inevitable result that the patient is thereby sterilised.[78]

In any event, it is generally agreed that such sterilisation, as indeed even any direct castration, is lawful if performed to obviate any danger to life.[79] Only one late authority dissents from this view, holding that the rule whereby the saving of life overrides every law does not operate "when the destruction of the world is [at stake]"[80]—an opinion which has been vigorously refuted "since the world will not perish if that individual will not beget children".[81]

The only reference to sterilisation for religious or moral reasons is found in a ruling by the early 14th century talmudist YOMTOV ISHBILI,[82] repeated by AZULAY and others.[83] The ruling forbids a man to drink a sterilising potion to facilitate his single-minded pursuit of religious studies, but it sanctions the act if it is intended "to rid him of his lusts and lewd thoughts", provided he has already fulfilled his duty of procreation. But there is, of course, no question of tolerating castration or any other physical interference with the genital system for such a purpose.[84] Indeed, already in the 13th century the *Sepher Hasidim*[85] warned: "A man should not sin in order to prevent further sins, as the one who, having misconducted himself with women, made himself sterile so that he should sin no more." How obviously Judaism recoiled from the notion of castrating priests or ecclesiastics for the promotion of their spirituality is manifestly demonstrated by the fact that the very basis for the opposition to *human* castration lies in the biblical exclusion from priestly services of a man who "hath his stones crushed"[86] (*Lev. xxi.*20). The Talmud extends this disqualification to all priests who are castrated or impotent,[87] and it also debars men with such disabilities from being appointed as judges in capital cases[88] and—according to one opinion[89] (*O.H., liii.*9)—as public readers in the synagogue.

In the case of women, on the other hand, the administration of a sterilising potion is, as already mentioned, not forbidden at all. The distinction between men and women is due to the recognition that castration proper—the principal offence—is not applicable to females at all[90] and that, moreover, the precept of human propagation is not technically incumbent on women[91] (*E.H., i.*13). In KARO's view, the sanction is evidently unconditional[92]— a view endorsed by his commentators DAVID HALEVY[93] and SAMUEL URI.[94] But SOLOMON LURIA,[95] followed by JOEL SIRKES[96] and others,[97] holds that such an action can be countenanced only if the potion is taken for independent medical reasons or, in particular, to avoid acute pain in confinement following previous experiences of difficult labour.[98] MOSES SCHREIBER[99] in an exhaustive responsum dated 1821, ruled that—in view of the accepted ban on polygamy and on a divorce against the wife's will—such sterilising treatment might be applied only with the consent of the husband (as he would thus be precluded from having any further children). But if his wife fears excessive pain or danger in childbirth, she may disregard his objections, because "she is not bound to torment herself on account of her submission to her husband" and because "one need not destroy oneself in order to populate the world".

To these motives as a valid indication for the sterilisation of women by non-surgical means LURIA[100] also adds one eugenic consideration. He permits a woman to take the potion "if her children do not go in the right way, and she fears she may bear more such children". This corresponds to the reasoning of BEN SIRAH who considered it better to be childless than to have godless children (*Ecclus. xvi.*3). The Midrash,[101] expressing a similar sentiment, tells that ABRAHAM and DAVID prayed to God that they might die without children rather than to leave a godless progeny behind them. But, in general, the Jewish outlook is not at all in sympathy with this argument. The Talmud, for instance, relates that the Prophet ISAIAH reproved King HEZEKIAH because he had excused his refusal to marry and to have children by his fear that his progeny would (as he foresaw) be wicked. Said the Prophet: "What do you care for the secrets of God? You should perform your duty, the pleasure of God".[102] Similarly, the Midrash[103] chides the sons of AARON, and justifies their punishment with death, because they had remained unmarried, claiming they were unable to find maidens worthy of their priesthood.

According to biblical law, "he that is crushed or maimed in his privy parts shall not enter into the assembly of the Lord" (*Deut. xxiii.*2)—that is, into matrimonial relations with a Jewish party, though he is permitted to marry a proselyte (*E.H., v.*1). Men are so disqualified by certain injuries to the penis, the testicles or the seminal cords, as defined in the Talmud[104] and listed in the codes (*ib.*, 2-9). The defect in the testicles includes the absence of, or injury to, one of them (*ib.*, 7). ISSERLES confirms this ruling against those who declare a man as fit if his left testicle only was removed; but he adds that he knows of decisions in accordance with that more lenient opinion, though the majority view disagrees with it (*ib.*, gloss). The belief that a man with a single testicle could be fecund is already represented in the Talmud[105] by the rabbi-physicians YISH-MAEL and SAMUEL. In the 13th century, this view was endorsed by R. TAM[106] and MORDECAI[107] who observed: "It happens every day that men who have had one testicle removed by the physicians (in operations on the abdomen or for stones which obstruct urination) beget children . . . ; but it is proper to warn the doctors to excise the left testicle,[108] if possible". Nevertheless, the view that both testicles were indispensable prevailed in the *Shulhan 'Arukh*—as it did in the edict of Pope SIXTUS V at about the same time (1585) providing for the dissolution of all marriages of men who did not possess two testicles.[109]

But in Jewish law, these regulations—which apply to genital defects in the male only[110]—are greatly limited by one important qualification: the impairment must be caused by an act of man, "for instance, by deliberate mutilation or by injury through a thorn", not by an act of Heaven (*ib.*, 10). According to MAIMONIDES,[111] the latter includes any condition brought about by illness as well as by any congenital abnormality, whereas RASHI[112] and ASHERI[113] restrict it to conditions found at birth or "caused by thunder and storms". KARO records both views (*ib.*). While MAIMONIDES's interpretation is the generally accepted ruling,[114] it is a moot question—often discussed in the more recent responsa—whether a man whose genitals were surgically removed or impaired for medical reasons is exempt from the ban. Present-day rabbinic opinion seems inclined to sanction the marriage of such a person, at least if the disease necessitating the operation had already rendered him completely impotent.[115] It is clear, then, that we are here dealing with a biblical precept which defies a fully satisfactory rationalisation;[116] there is no consistent relationship between the conditions defined in these regulations and the medical diagnosis of complete sterility. A man's infecundity is not in itself a bar to marriage[117] any more than the permanent sterility in women presents an impediment to legitimate conjugal relations (*E.H.*, *xxiii.5*, gloss). The ban merely proscribes the matrimonial union of *certain types* of castrates with *certain types* of women (*i.e.* only with those of Jewish birth).

THERAPEUTIC CONTRACEPTION

Far more widespread than the recourse to permanent sterilisation is, of course, the practice to induce temporary sterility by measures taken during or after intercourse to prevent conception. The history of man's endeavour to frustrate the generative act is very ancient indeed, and so are the records of religious and moral opposition to this practice. But as the problem of contraception has always been raised in a social rather than medical context, we will not here discuss its long history in general. The following short survey will be confined only to the relatively few sources on the medical aspects of the subject and the religious approach to them.[118]

The Roman Catholic Church, fortified by a tradition of unremitting warfare on all forms of contraception going back at least to St. AUGUSTINE,[119] refuses to consider therapeutic indications[120] as firmly as any other motive. Her theologians regard continence as the sole licit means to prevent births which may prove dangerous to the mother's life or otherwise undesirable.[121] Lately they have, however, given very much thought to the so-called "safe-period" calculation, based on the OGINO-KNAUS theory of the infertile cycle,[122] and to the legality of disseminating information on using this to prevent births by periodic recourse to abstinence.[123] The Anglican Church, on the other hand, would not to-day object to contraceptive safeguards used for medical reasons. Although birth-control had been denounced as "dangerous, demoralising and sinful" at various Lambeth Conferences, a resolution passed in 1930 permitted the use of methods other than continence "where moral obligation to limit parenthood is felt".[124]

In medieval Arab writings, there are but few references to medical indications for contraception. The 12th century physician ISMA IL AL-JURJANI mentions a woman of "tender years" as one that should be so protected against the danger of conception.[125] In general, the Islamic religion did not condemn abortion outright, much less anti-conceptional measures; consequently, Mohammedan doctors had no compunction in recommending contraceptive safeguards to women who might be endangered on becoming pregnant.[126] A thousand years earlier, the famous Roman physician SORANUS, too, advocated the use of abortifacients, or preferably contraceptives, when a "birth threatens to become dangerous, or when the uterus is too small . . . , or when any other hindrance to birth exists".[127]

In virtually all Jewish sources on the subject of contraception, the consideration of its legality is limited to cases when it is medically indicated. All rabbinic rulings on the practice are largely based on a talmudic statement[128] permitting[129]—and, according to some interpretations, requiring[130]—wives who are minors, pregnant or lactating to take contraceptive precautions by the insertion of a tampon during intercourse, because a conception in such circumstances may prove fatal to the mother,[131] the existing embryo,[132] or the suckling[133] respectively. But another view recorded in the same passage counsels—or, according to others, tolerates[134]—reliance on divine protection on the strength of the verse "The Lord preserveth the simple"[135] (*Ps. cxvi.*6). Several authorities[136] assume that this dispute applies only to these particular cases, where the danger of a conception is in any event rather remote; hence, they infer that, in cases of a more definite threat to the mother's life arising from a pregnancy, there would be no objection at all to the use of contraceptives. Others[137] hold that the three women are mentioned to illustrate the attitude to cases of resultant danger to life in general; while yet others[138] regard the entire sanction as limited to these three women only.

Although the codes, rather surprisingly,[139] omit any direct reference to contraception altogether,[140] the problem received considerable attention in almost every rabbinic responsa work of the last century or two. The opinions for and against the use of some artificial methods to prevent conception where danger to life may otherwise ensue are about equally balanced. The most lenient view is first put forward by SOLOMON LURIA[141] in the 16th century. He permits a wife to apply a tampon before intercourse, and so do many authorities who agree to this action if a conception may prove dangerous.[142] AKIVAH EGER,[143] again, almost two centuries later, followed by his son-in-law MOSES SCHREIBER,[144] leads those who will not tolerate any impediment to operate during intercourse. Some later authorities add that, when a pregnancy constitutes a permanent danger to life, X-ray or surgical contraceptive treatment is to be preferred to devices requiring constant use.[145] But under no circumstances is the husband permitted to do anything to render his act ineffective.[146] Nor are mere considerations of health, as distinct from life, usually sufficient to warrant active precautions on the part of the wife. Already in the 18th century, it is true, a rabbi recognised that it might be advisable to space the arrival of children; but the recommended means to achieve this did not include recourse to contraception.[147]

CHAPTER FOURTEEN

CONTROLLING THE GENERATION
OF LIFE — 2

ABORTION AND EMBRYOTOMY

The practice of criminal abortion, it has been claimed,[1] is older than any civilisation. It is found on a surprisingly widespread scale among the most primitive peoples as well as in the most advanced societies.[2] Although the artificial interruption of a pregnancy is a far more complex and dangerous operation than the prevention of conception during intercourse, abortion was for very long practised more frequently than contraception. The reason is obvious. The latter presupposes a knowledge of techniques and, indeed, of the elementary facts about human generation unfamiliar to many primitive and uneducated people. Moreover, the frustration of the conjugal act at its inception requires, apart from skill, anticipatory precautions against a contingency so often only realized after the act has been performed. Yet, neither the hazards nor the moral and legal wrong in criminal abortions have succeeded in raising an effective barrier to the operation. According to an estimate made in 1939, 100,000 to 150,000 cases occurred annually in England and Wales alone, 40% of them criminal.[3]

The moral revulsion against interfering with the natural process of gestation has varied considerably in different ages and civilisations. Only seldom did the human conscience offer no resistance at all to foeticide, even though there were often no legislative restraints on the practice. In antiquity the people of the more remote East were, on the whole, firmer in opposing abortion than those of the West. Buddhism proscribed the practice for purely religious reasons and punished offenders with special severity, as the souls of unborn children were considered vicious and dangerous.[4] In India the law books of the *Aryas*[5] and the *Manava Dharma-Sastra*[6] condemned abortion as homicide for the Hindus and Brahmas respectively at a very early age. Among the Parsees, too, the induction of abortion was strictly forbidden by the Avesta religion.[7] According to the Assyrian code, women responsible for procuring abortions were to be impaled, and it was not permitted to bury their bodies.[8]

But as we turn West, we find no trace of any enactments against abortion before 200 C.E.—with the possible exception of Egypt, where the law appears to have punished the practice severely,[9] though abortifacient prescriptions occur quite freely in the *Ebers Papyrus*.[10] Neither the code of HAMMURABI[11] nor the Bible legislated on abortion except in relation to the payment of compensation in the event of an assault on a pregnant wife resulting in the loss of her fruit (*Ex. xxi*.22). But we may assume that "abortion was strictly against the spirit of the Bible", though there is no evidence for the claim that it "was undoubtedly severely punished".[12] It is more likely that in biblical times, as in later ages, such operations with criminal intent were generally unknown among the Jews.[13]

In Greek and Roman society abortion was very widely practised. LECKY has summed up the position in these words: "No law in Greece, or in the Roman Republic, or during the greater part of the Empire, condemned it . . . A long chain of writers, both pagan and Christian, represent the practice as . . . almost universal. They describe it as resulting, not simply from licentiousness or from poverty, but even from so slight a motive as vanity which made mothers shrink from the disfigurement of childbirth . . . At the same time, while OVID,[14] SENECA,[15] FAVORINUS[16] (the Stoic of Arles), PLUTARCH[17] and JUVENAL[18] all speak of abortion as general and notorious, they all speak of it as unquestionably criminal".[19] ARISTOTLE[20] recommended abortion in certain circumstances, but he considered it "incompatible with holiness" after the foetus had attained animal life.[21] The Platonic and Stoics—like others who held that animation began only at birth—raised no objection to abortion at any stage of the pregnancy.[22] But according to the Pythagoreans, the human foetus was animate, and therefore inviolable, from the moment of conception.[23] This attitude, argues EDELSTEIN,[24] eventually prevailed in the 4th century B.C.E., when it found its way into the Hippocratic Oath which declared: "I will not at any time give to a woman any drug or instrument for the purpose of causing abortion". But SINGER[25] and JONES[26] consider this passage to be of late, perhaps early Christian, origin. GARRISON[27] has pointed out that the pagan version of the Oath (*Urbinas MS*) limited the interdict to the use of pessaries, whereas it was only in the Christian reading (*Ambrosian MS*) that abortion was forbidden by any process.[28]

The ethics of Greece had advanced more rapidly than the laws of Rome. In Roman law and society the father for long enjoyed absolute rights over the members of his family, so that it could not be wrong to kill a foetus which in any case was regarded as "a part of the mother".[29] The law — superficially following the earlier Semitic pattern — exacted punishment from offenders only on account of the injury done to the father or the mother in cases of attacks leading to a miscarriage.[30] This was the legal attitude. But moral protests were quite often made. OVID condemned "women who thrust and pierce with the instrument, and give dire poisons to their children yet unborn" which, he added, even the wild beasts did not do. But the punishment was still left for nature to exact: "She dies herself and is borne to the pyre with hair unloosed, and all who behold her cry 'It's her desert!' "[31] Judicial penalties were not introduced before 200 C.E.,[32] though CORNELIA had imposed deportation or the confiscation of goods on anyone selling aphrodisiac or abortifacient beverages.[33] Similar provisions were embodied in Justinian law.[34]

THERAPEUTIC ABORTION

Meanwhile, abortion, and particularly embryotomy, also began to serve medical ends. In India the *Susruta* prescribed the dismemberment of an embryo if attempts at its version to facilitate a normal birth had proved unsuccessful.[35] The Greeks practised embryotomy only on a dead fruit.[36] Among the Romans the operation became quite frequent, and it was discussed in detail by all ancient surgeons.[37] SORANUS,[38] the leading obstetrician of antiquity, though he preferred contraceptives to the interruption of pregnancies (since it was man's duty to "maintain what nature has created"[39]), resorted to abortion, too, when it was medically indicated. But he strongly deprecated its practice when it was motivated by a desire to preserve the woman's beauty or to hide the consequences of adultery.[40] He also refused to employ mechanical means, recommending "safe medical methods" instead.[41]

Christianity embraced a completely different outlook. A mere glance at the voluminous literature of the Church on abortion — by far its most extensively treated medical subject—will indicate that in no field of medical ethics are the Christian teachings more unique and at greater variance from any other widely accepted system of ethics, past or present. Tracing the origins of this attitude, PLOSS and BARTELS[42] declare, perhaps somewhat polemically: " . . . the distinctive Christian doctrine about abortion is founded neither on Roman law nor Hebrew. It has been formed and formulated under the influence of the Hellenistic Schools of Greek thought, the Peripatetics, Neo-Platonics, and Neo-Pythagoreans. Their confused mysticism appealed strongly to the uneducated masses who were primarily attracted to Christianity; and Christianity absorbed this influence all the more readily in that it lacked the intellectual background for a constructive system of ethics". The Christian attitude, continue the authors, was further consolidated by a crucial mistranslation in the *Septuagint*[43] which TERTULLIAN, ignorant of Hebrew, blindly accepted. His teaching was perpetuated by St. JEROME, though he rendered the biblical passage correctly. The *Septuagint* clearly sought to impose the death penalty for foeticide, provided the embryo had assumed human form. The fruit was then legally protected by the rule "a life for a life". The attitude of the Church was, moreover, vitally determined by two further considerations: the entry of the soul into man, and the need for baptism as a prerequisite for salvation. Christianity[53] through the teachings of TERTULLIAN who argued: "Whatever is dead [*viz.*, any still-birth] must

ENTRY OF SOUL INTO BODY

There is a very large literature on the problem "*de animatione foetus*".[44] Speculation on the moment when the soul enters the human body has "continued without cessation from the time of AKHNATON (*c.* 1400 *B.C.E.*), reaching a climax perhaps in Christian times with CANGIAMILLA's *Embryologia Sacra,* and living on embedded in Roman Catholic theology up to our own day".[45] ARISTOTLE[46] distinguished between three stages: the foetus was endowed with vegetative life at conception, with an animal soul a few days later, and with a rational soul on the 40th or 80th day of gestation in the cases of males and females respectively.[47] The Romans believed that animation occurred on the 40th day in all cases,[48] but they regarded an embryo merely as "*spes animatis*" and not as being entitled to human rights.[49] The Stoics, again, denied the existence of a soul before birth,[50] while another widely held Hellenistic theory refused to attribute human status even to infants if they had not yet partaken of human food.[51] The Pythagoreans, finally, taught that the soul infused the body from its conception.[52] It was this last doctrine which originally prevailed in Christianity[53] through the teachings of TERTULLIAN who argued: "Whatever is dead [*viz.*, any still-birth] must

— 174 —

have lived _once_".[54] He even regarded the prevention of a birth as murder, reasoning: "He is also a man who is about to be one".[55] This teaching was confirmed by St. GREGORY of Nyssa in the 4th century.[56] St. AUGUSTINE[57] then introduced the distinction between formed and unformed foetuses first made in the *Septuagint*—treating only the killing of the former as homicide. This distinction was embodied in Canon Law as well as in Justinian law, which accepted the Aristotelian definition on the animation after 40 or 80 days.[58] The entry of the soul into man during his foetal development remained the subject of much discussion in the literature of the Church; it was even given artistic expression. The actual process was described, for instance, in a striking vision by St. HILDEGARD in her mystical work, the *Scivias*, in the middle of the 12th century, and illustrated in a miniature of the *Wiesbaden Codex*.[59]

Added to these considerations as a crucial factor determining the attitude to abortion was the teaching, firmly enunciated by St. AUGUSTINE[60] and St. FULGENTIUS,[61] that the embryo was included among those whose souls were condemned to eternal perdition if they died unbaptised. Although THOMAS AQUINAS later suggested the possibility of salvation for an infant that died before birth,[62] the original doctrine long retained great practical importance. It led to regarding the death or murder of an unborn child as a worse calamity than that of a baptised person,[63] to the insistence on the extraction of a foetus from a dead mother's womb by a priest if necessary,[64] and to the invention of a "baptismal syringe" for the intra-uterine administration of baptism.[65] Present-day Canon Law still requires all living foetuses to be baptised.[66] The distinction between killing a baptised and an unbaptised child gradually lost all but its theological significance (the Council of Metz in 852 still imposed a heavier penance on the latter crime[67]). But the outlook engendered by this teaching certainly fortified the Catholic opposition to any form of abortion down to our time.

Accordingly, the Church always condemned abortion as a grave sin. The heavy canonical penalties imposed by the Council of Elvira in 305 were somewhat mitigated by the Council of Angora (Ancyra) nine years later. The original view, branding the killing of even inanimate foetuses as murder, was upheld by the Councils of Byzantine in 692 and of Worms in 868. During the following centuries, however, a clear distinction between formed and unformed foetuses was generally made, the killing of the latter being punished by a fine only. This position, embodied in the *Gratian Decretals*, was maintained by INNOCENT III and GREGORY IX in the 13th century. But in 1588 SIXTUS V renewed all previous censures on abortions at any stage of gestation, adding the penalty of excommunication even on advisers. This rigid decree was a little relaxed by GREGORY XIV in 1591. Yet the difference between animate and inanimate foetuses was never introduced again. It is omitted in the penal codification *Apostolicae Sedis* by PIUS IX in 1869 as well as in the current code of Canon Law which came into force in 1918.[68]

The destruction of the human fruit for therapeutic reasons, though at first apparently tolerated by the early Church[69] and still recommended by the Christian physician AETIUS,[70] was already condemned by TERTULLIAN[71] as an act of "barbarity". Throughout medieval and modern times, the Roman Church consistently forbade any "surgical operation which is directly destructive of the life of the foetus or the mother", to quote from the Holy Office decrees of 1884 and 1888.[72] Therapeutic abortion was explicitly condemned in a further decree of 1895.[73] But especially since the somewhat equivocal decree of 1898 on abortion in cases of ectopic gestation,[74] Catholic moral theologians have debated and written much to define the limits of "direct abortion"—alone held to be unlawful. It is argued, for instance, that in an ectopic pregnancy the foetus may be regarded as "a materially unjust aggressor", because "it is not in a position in which it had a right to be", and that its death may therefore be hastened at least indirectly.[75] But the present tendency is to reject the validity of this argument.[76] Again, some moralists permit, as "indirect abortion", to pierce the amnion to empty the pregnant uterus and expel the foetus in order to save the mother from immediate danger.[77] But others aver that "every interference which must necessarily cause the expulsion of the inviable fruit is permissible under no circumstances, no matter how ethical the object may be".[78] Accordingly, "when [certain] grave complications . . . occur in the early months of pregnancy . . . , the Catholic physician . . . must withdraw from the case. If there is no other physician to attend to the woman, he must let her die".[79] This applies even "when both mother and child will perish if the pregnancy is allowed to continue".[80] These rulings, which govern Catholic medical practice to the present day,[81] are justified by the assertion that potential life, even in the earliest stages of germination, enjoys the same value as existing adult life; hence "Better two deaths than one murder".[82]

Outside the literature of the Church, references to abortion, therapeutic or otherwise, are relatively few in the Middle Ages. The decadence of surgery, and the standards of professional ethics fostered by the Hippocratic Oath, combined with the influence of the Church, all but eliminated such operations. Apothecaries, like physicians, were abjured not to abet in abortions. In the 13th century, they had to swear " . . . never to administer an abortive potion . . . ".[83] In 16th century France, the physicians compelled them to take an oath which included the promise " . . . never to administer poisons . . . nor to give drinks to procure abortion, without the advice of a physician".[84]

ABORTION IN CIVIL LAW

The civil law codes mentioned abortion but rarely. TACITUS[85] while he deprecated the limitation of the offspring as morally wrong, had admitted that there was no punishment for abortion among the early Teutons. Under the impact of Christian teachings the attitude gradually hardened, but this evolution continued to be very slow. The Visigothic Code denounced the ancient practice as "heathenish".[86] In the Frisian Code (*c.* 800) no fine was imposed for abortion or infanticide, though it insisted that children must be kept alive after baptism. In the 11th century the Longobardi edict (*Edictum Rotharis*) laid down a fine only if an abortion was performed without the consent of the mother or guardian. The German legal codes of the 13th century (*Schwabenspiegel* and *Sachsenspiegel*) did not mention abortion at all.[87] The first German code to brand abortion as a criminal offence, treating it as murder if the foetus was animate, was the ordinance of the Bishopric of Bamberg in 1507. This was incorporated in the code of CHARLES V (*Constitutio Criminalis Carolina*) enacted at Regensburg in 1532. By the 18th century most German states had adopted similar laws, dating animation halfway through gestation.[88] The same position prevailed in Austria until 1787, when the Josephinian Code reduced the penalty for abortion to five years' imprisonment. Similar modifications were made in the Prussian code of 1794.[89] In England, the induction of abortion was threatened with death already in the 13th century *Fleta*[90] (a commentary on the common law), and the supreme penalty was abolished only in 1837. But it was not until 1803 that the practice first became a statutory offence by an Act of Parliament.[91] In the intervening centuries, when abortionists were almost everywhere simply hanged,[92] the crime was dealt with by the ecclesiastical courts and therefore omitted from the civil codes.[93]

Following the French Revolution, and particularly the protests of eminent physicians and jurists against granting full human rights to the unborn products of conception,[94] the harshest features of the medieval laws were eventually removed from all civilised codes.[95] But the penalties imposed for criminal abortion at present still differ widely in European countries.[96] The distinction between animate and inanimate foetal life, too, gradually disappeared.[97] More recently, therapeutic abortions became officially sanctioned by law.[98]

ABORTION IN JEWISH SOURCES

The only Jewish authors, apart from the Samaritans and Karaites,[99] to suggest even vaguely that abortion may be a capital offence are PHILO and JOSEPHUS. But their statements on the subject are somewhat confused, if not plainly inconsistent. PHILO, clearly under the influence of the *Septuagint* and its Hellenistic background, interprets the biblical law on assault leading to a miscarriage thus: If the fruit is "unshaped and undeveloped", the attacker must be fined "both for the outrage and for obstructing the artist Nature in her creative work . . . ". But if it is already "shaped and all the limbs have their proper qualities . . . , he must die, for that which answers to this description is a human being . . . , like a statue lying in a studio requiring nothing more than to be conveyed outside . . . ."[100] Yet, elsewhere in the same work PHILO calls only a person who has killed a child already born "indubitably a murderer", and he speaks of the embryo as part of the mother as long as it is united with the womb.[101] In another work, again, he evidently regards abortion as a capital crime without distinguishing between the formed and unformed state of the fruit.[102] It may be assumed that PHILO probably "knew of induced abortion as a solution of the problem of birth-control . . . Knowing PHILO as we do, it is impossible to think that he would not have been bitterly opposed to it on moral grounds, but that the practice was legally actionable in his courts seems highly questionable".[103] Another suggestion is that PHILO, whilst polemising against the Stoic view which regarded the foetus as part of the mother, deliberately overstates the Jewish position to impress the moral circles among the heathens.[104]

In JOSEPHUS's writings we meet with a similar discrepancy. In his *Antiquities*[105] he fully subscribes to the rabbinic view, adding only that, apart from the compensation due to the husband for the loss of his offspring, a fine is also imposed for diminishing the population. But in *Contra Apionem*[106] he regards a woman causing an abortion as guilty of infanticide, "because she destroys a soul and prevents the increase of the race". While WEYL,[107] LOEW,[108] and PLOSS and BARTELS[109] consider this a reference to the death penalty as exacted by the courts, ZIPSER[110] and HEINEMANN[111] believe it is an apologetic defence against non-Jewish attacks on Judaism. But APTOWITZER,[112] opposing these views, assumes that the opinion expressed in *Contra Apionem* reflects merely JOSEPHUS's assessment of abortion as morally tantamount to murder.

According to the rabbinic interpretation of the assault in the Bible,[113] compensation is payable to the husband for the loss of his offspring only if the mother survived. Otherwise the attacker suffers the death penalty for killing the mother, but he is not liable to any fine for aborting her fruit, because in Jewish law the death penalty always absolves the offender from the payment of any compensation or fine.[114] The only other talmudic reference to abortion occurs when the Palestinian sage R. YISHMAEL includes the killing of an embryo among the offences for which the Noachides (*i.e.* Gentiles) are liable to the death penalty.[115] This teaching is based on rendering *Gen. ix.*6: "Whoso sheddeth the blood of *man within man*,[116] his blood shall be shed". This 2nd-century teacher, as already noted,[117] revived the traditions of the Alexandrian schools. His ruling may represent an effort to check excesses in the experiments on foetal anatomy which he sanctioned, or it may reflect the outlook of the *Septuagint* and PHILO. The assumption that it indicates the influence of the Roman penal legislation on abortion[118] is rejected convincingly on the ground that the Roman laws against abortion only date from 200 C.E.[119] Another view is that this extension of the Noachidic laws was intended, on the contrary, as a protest against the widespread Roman practice of abortion and infanticide.[120] The ruling is still codified by MAIMONIDES;[121] according to TOSAPHOTH,[122] against the view of some later rabbis,[123] it is also binding on Jews on the talmudic principle that "there is nothing permitted to Jews which is forbidden to Noachides".

Outside these peripheral sources, criminal abortion is not treated in Jewish religious literature before the 12th century, when it received a casual mention. There is no reference to the subject in the codes, and even the responsa do not discuss it until the 17th century. The omission seems all the more glaring in view of the extraordinary attention given to abortion by Christian authors and other legislators at all times.

This silence can hardly be due to the ignorance of criminal abortion among the Jews in the talmudic era, as has been suggested.[124] To at least some of the talmudists who lived for so long within the orbit of the Roman Empire the malpractices rampant there—a scholar has rightly retorted —could scarcely have been unknown.[125] In later ages, too, knowledge of the evil was sufficiently widespread to prompt some of the leading Jewish and Marrano medical writers— such as ASAF JUDAEUS[126] in the 7th century, AMATUS LUSITANUS[127] in the 16th, and JACOB ZAHALON[128] in the 17th—to denounce in their works any complicity in the practice. The explanation seems to be, rather, that foeticide was virtually non-existent in Jewish society at any time.[129] Even to the present day, as the Catholic medical historian WALSH[130] has testified, there are hardly any abortions among poorer Jews, and none among the orthodox. But that some isolated aberrations did occur occasionally is shown by an enactment of the Communal Conference at Candia in 1238. It forbade a fiance to enter the house of his father-in-law except under special safeguards, in order "to prevent premature pregnancies which sometimes led to abortions and infanticide".[131] The few references to similar incidents in rabbinical works of the time

Religion + Health P. 316 1920

S. W. Baron
Jewish Community v[?]II[?] p315
1942

will be given later, as we survey the Jewish religious attitude to criminal abortion.

Therapeutic abortions, too, though generally sanctioned in Jewish law (as we shall see), are but rarely mentioned in Jewish historical sources. Yet, there can be little doubt that Jewish physicians resorted to them, and particularly to embryotomy, no less freely than did their Arabian colleagues, among whom the operation was performed quite frequently, even on living children.[132] Their tradition goes back to RHAZES (850-932) who counselled embryotomy whenever other methods to save the mother failed. But with the decline of the Arab-Jewish era in medicine, the practice probably became altogether defunct. The operation is completely ignored in the two leading medico-rabbinic works, JACOB ZAHALON's 'Otzar Hahayim (Venice, 1683) and TOBIAS COHEN's Ma'asei Tuviah (Venice, 1707).[133] There is also hardly any mention of Jewish midwives procuring abortions.

ABORTION IN JEWISH LAW

In Jewish law, the right to destroy a human fruit before birth is entirely unrelated to theological considerations. Neither the question of the entry of the soul before birth nor the claim to salvation after death have any practical bearing on the subject. The Talmud[134] and the Midrash,[135] it is true, mention an argument between the Emperor ANTONIUS and R. JUDAH (the compiler of the Mishnah) in which the time of the soul's entry is variously fixed at the moment of conception, of the body's formation, and of birth (the first view ultimately prevailed). The Talmud[136] also records many conflicting opinions on the moment from which an infant is "fit to enter the world to come" or, according to NISSIM,[137] to share in the resurrection of the dead—ranging from conception or birth to circumcision or the ability to speak and respond "Amen". But both discussions are mainly of academic interest[138] and quite irrelevant

— 182 —

to the legal rights and status of unborn children. Similarly inconclusive are the talmudic statements attributing personal functions and discernment to embryos—such as their participation in the Song of MOSES[139] and in the acceptance of the divine law,[140] their malediction of sinners,[141] the dispute of REBEKKAH's twin sons within her womb,[142] and DAVID's composition of Psalms before his birth.[143] All these passages occur in purely aggadic contexts and are not related to legal issues.

More indicative of the attitude of Jewish law to the unborn child's claim to life are the various legislative measures to safeguard the foetus in the mother's womb. To this end, as we have detailed in previous chapters, some pregnant women are permitted (or advised) to use a contraceptive tampon during intercourse,[144] divorced and widowed women are debarred from remarriage while pregnant,[145] and even the desecration of the Sabbath is sanctioned.[146] Yet none of these regulations necessarily prove that the foetus enjoys human inviolability. Since, as has been suggested,[147] every danger to the fruit involves a threat to the mother as well, these laws may conceivably have her protection as their primary objective. Furthermore, the right to violate the Sabbath for the saving of prenatal life need not be incompatible even with a direct permission to kill it deliberately;[148] for a similar *non sequitur* applies to the murder of one who is dying "by the hand of man".[149] In any case, the rights assigned to the foetus must be set against the generally accepted legal doctrine that the unborn child is deemed an organic part of the mother, though this doctrine is by no means uncontested in the Talmud.[150] Indeed, we may be correct to assume[151] that even those Palestinian teachers who shared the Alexandrian view that the embryo is a separate being for itself did not reach the conclusion that the deliberate termination of its life constituted murder and was punishable by death. Nor did either these talmudic savants or their opponents make any legal distinction between formed and unformed foetuses.[152]

— 183 —

The only direct reference to therapeutic abortion in the Talmud is the following mishnaic ruling: "If a woman is in hard travail, one cuts up the child within her womb and extracts it member by member, because her life has priority over its life; but if the greater part of it was already born, it may not be touched, since one does not set aside one life for [the sake of] another".[153] The point at which human life commences to be inviolable and of equal value to that of any adult person is thus distinctly fixed at the moment when the greater part of the body—or, according to some versions,[154] the head—has emerged from the birth canal. A further crucial consideration is introduced in the talmudic discussion on this Mishnah.[155] The question is raised, why should it not be permissible, even during the final phase of birth, to set aside the child's claim to life in favour of the mother, as it should be regarded as an aggressor in pursuit of the mother?[156] The answer given is that this case is not altogether analogous to a pursuer who may be struck down in self-defence, since the mother is here considered as "pursued by Heaven". But this consideration does not arise before the main process of birth is complete, because we are not then dealing with two equal lives; or, in the words of RASHI,[157] "whatever has not come forth into the light of the world is not a human life [lit. 'soul']". On the other hand, MAIMONIDES[158] and the subsequent codes (*H.M.*, *cdxxv*.2) resort to the "pursuer"-argument to justify embryotomy even before the major part of the child is born: "This, too, is a negative precept: not to have compassion over the life of a pursuer. Hence, the rabbis ruled that, if a gravid woman is in hard travail, it is permitted to dismember the embryo in her womb, whether by drug or by hand, for it is like a pursuer [intent on] killing her; but if its head was already delivered, it may not be touched, for one does not set aside one life for [the sake of] another, and that is the natural course of the world".

This important ruling appears to be contradictory in its reasoning. On the one hand, it relies on the "pursuer"-

argument to vindicate the operation; on the other, it dismisses its validity because nature, not the child, pursues the mother. Moreover, there seems to be a discrepancy between this ruling and the Mishnah which permits the deliberate sacrifice of the unborn child simply because its life is subordinated to that of the mother and not because she is being "pursued". Several attempts have been made to resolve this difficulty. YA'IR BACHARACH[159] suggests that the absence of human status would not in itself warrant the embryo's destruction. While "He that smiteth a *man,* so that he dieth, shall surely be put to death" (*Ex. xxi.*12) implies, according to the exegesis of the rabbis,[160] that the killer of an unborn child should not be so punished, the embryo is still sufficiently human to render its destruction a moral offence, even if it is not a penal crime. Hence the need for the additional element of "pursuit". On similar lines EZEKIEL LANDAU[161] explains that one could no more kill the embryo to preserve the mother—except by combining the fact that it is of lesser value with its incrimination as a "pursuer" — than one would sacrifice a person suffering from a fatal injury for the sake of saving a normal life, even if the killing of such a person does not technically constitute murder.[162]

There may be a further reason which prompted MAIMONIDES to introduce the factor of "pursuit" into the first case treated in the Mishnah. When an expectant mother is sentenced to death, the Mishnah[163] rules that her execution must be deferred until after the child's birth only if "she already sat on the birth stool" at the time the verdict was announced.[164] The Talmud[165] explains this by arguing that the foetus is regarded as a separate body, whose life must not be sacrificed, as soon as it has "torn itself loose" from its normal uterine position. But before the process of birth has set in, the child, as an organic part of the mother, is liable to share her fate so as to spare the mother the agony of suspense.[166] Once the mother sits on the "birth-stool", then, the unborn child enjoys an intermediate status: it is not yet "a *man*" making its destruction a capital offence; at the same time, it is no longer "a part of the mother" when its dismemberment can be treated like the excision of any other organ which may endanger her life. It is during that stage, when the mother is already "in hard travail", that the threat to the mother's life is not by itself a sufficiently good cause for the child's destruction; only the additional "pursuit" element can justify the operation. But after the major part of the child is born, it assumes human status and even the "pursuit"-element is not enough to warrant its deliberate sacrifice, since the "pursuit" is, after all, not wilfully intended by the child but caused by nature.[167]

These decisions, then, deal only with embryotomy in two specific cases. In both the mother and her child find themselves locked in mortal conflict with each other during the process of parturition. But these laws do not refer to an interruption of a pregnancy in its earlier stages nor to a situation in which the refusal to intervene, in an attempt to rescue the mother or the child, would lead to the death of both.[168] These problems were raised in Jewish sources only from the 17th century onwards.

The uncertainty regarding the first of these two problems arises from the conditional circumstances in which the Mishnah, as interpreted in the codes, permits the recourse to embryotomy. Since they assume that the "pursuit" of the child must be an essential element in the threat to the mother's life to warrant its dismemberment, that ruling does not necessarily determine the law on therapeutic abortion in cases when some extraneous illness, and not the child, would directly lead to the mother's death if her pregnancy were allowed to continue. Hence, while the early 17th century scholar, JOSEPH TRANI[169] of Constantinople, regarded any abortion as lawful when performed in the interest of the mother's health, ISAAC LAMPRONTI,[170] the Italian rabbi-physician of the first half of the following century, could see no justification for the induction of abortion if the mother's life was being attacked not by the child by a disease afflicting her.[171] The later responsa, however, generally endorse the view that a therapeutic abortion—whether the fruit is viable or not[172]—is legitimate, indeed imperative, when the mother's life cannot otherwise be saved.[173] This is entirely consonant with the Mishnah and the codes, since (as we have suggested) they resort to the argument that the child may be sacrificed as a "pursuer" only during the actual process of birth, when the superior value of the mother's life by itself may no longer entitle one to override the child's claim to life. But during the pregnancy, the "pursuit" by the child is not required to justify its destruction for the sake of the mother's survival.

According to the Talmud and MAIMONIDES, as we have mentioned,[174] the Noachidic dispensation regards the killing of an embryo as murder. Consequently, there is some doubt whether the sanction of therapeutic abortions can be extended to non-Jews, too. While TOSAPHOTH[175] tended to recognise no difference between Jews and Gentiles in this matter, TRANI[176] held that a Jew must not be an accomplice to the abortion of non-Jews, unless he charges a professional fee.[177] HAYIM BENEVISTI,[178] an eminent Turkish rabbi of the 17th century, also warned against assisting Gentiles to procure abortions, as that would render one liable to the charge of "putting a stumbling block before the blind" by leading others to sin.[179] Whether a non-Jewish practitioner might perform an embryotomy according to Jewish law was left unresolved by a later authority.[180]

Only in more recent times have Jewish teachers dealt with embryotomy in cases when the refusal to sacrifice the child for the sake of the mother, even after its major part has been delivered, would lead to the loss of both lives. In the rulings of the Mishnah it is always presumed that the abandonment of one life will definitely save the other.[181] Hence, ISRAEL LIPSCHUETZ[182] argues that it would probably be lawful to destroy the fruit even during the final stage of birth, if a failure to intervene would cause it to perish together with the mother. But in the responsa on this problem there are some differences of opinion. One authority[183] suggested that in such an event one would not be justified in interfering with the course of nature, since a deliberately inflicted death could not be weighed against a natural demise; furthermore, "who made [the doctor] a ruler and a judge over this issue?" Another rabbi,[184] though he discountenanced embryotomy even in the case of a breech-birth[185] once the greater part of the child was born, was not certain if the operation could be permitted to prevent the death of both mother and child. MOSES SCHICK[186] conceded to the physician the right, at least in principle, to rescue the mother at the expense of the child (even if otherwise the mother's natural death might help to keep the child alive), provided he was confident of the success of the operation. DAVID HOFFMANN[187] confirmed this ruling during the present century.

In reaching this conclusion, these rabbis gave due weight to a factor which we did not so far mention. When, in the mortal conflict between the mother and the child, the alternative to the loss of one life is the survival of the other, both lives are considered equal as soon as the child assumes human status—that is, following the delivery of its major part; it must not then be destroyed to save the mother. But the balance in the value of the two lives is still not sufficiently even to allow the child's inviolability to outweigh the loss of both lives. If they were completely equal in value, it would, of course, be wrong to prevent the death of both by deliberately destroying one of them; for we then have to apply the principles — already established in a previous chapter[188]—on the surrender of one innocent life for the preservation of even a whole group of persons. In our case, however, the two lives in danger are not altogether equal. That inequality derives, not from any intrinsic inferiority of the child, but from the fact that its viability is not held to be fully established until after the first thirty days of its life.[189] Should the child die within that period, it is regarded legally as a still-birth,[190] because it is then thought to have lacked the vitality to survive from the beginning. Consequently, of the two lives at stake, the one is certain and established, whilst the other is still in some doubt. Yet, this difference in value is too insignificant to justify the child's destruction, unless the alternative is the eventual death of both mother and child.[191]

Jewish references to criminal abortion, as already mentioned, are extremely scarce. The first of them in religious writings dates from the 12th century, unless there is an earlier date for a passage in the *Zohar*[192] which condemns foeticide as "destroying God's structure and His work" in terms reminiscent of the phrase used by PHILO.[193] The *Sepher Hasidim*[194] tells of a prostitute who sought advice on how to abort her fruit. When a man wished to give the required instructions, arguing it was better she destroyed the child before birth than afterwards, he was warned not to be involved in such sinful conduct: "It is better that she should sin against it than [that the offence be committed] through your hand; moreover, it is possible that her child will be rescued from her, or that she will die and the child will live". In the 13th century *Sepher Hayashar*[195] there appears a sympathetic prescription for abortion with the comment that such forbidden cures are described only so that the physician knows how to guard himself against any evil which may occur. The anonymous writer adds there are sometimes licentious women desiring to abort their illegitimate fruit; "moreover, we have seen writings of some leading scholars in our time permitting the practice, but we wish to have no truck with such a thing . . . in the absence of danger to the mother". The contemporaneous work *Toldoth*[196] also records that there were girls who tried to rid themselves of their fruit, and it likewise holds that abortifacients should be taken only when indicated by any risk of life to the mother.

The religio-legal issues involved in such operations were discussed by two German rabbis, YA'IR BACHARACH[197] and JACOB EMDEN,[198] of the 17th and 18th centuries respectively. They were asked whether a Jewess, who had become pregnant following an adulterous relationship, could resort to a dose of ecbolics for the abortion of her bastard fruit. Both agreed there was no formal prohibition to interrupt a pregnancy before the first phase of parturition had set in, but they differed in their final verdict. BACHARACH could find no legal distinction between a bastard[199] and a legitimate embryo in this respect; yet he maintained that such operations could not be tolerated in practice, because their sanction would open the floodgates to immorality and debauchery. EMDEN, on the other hand, considered the case of an adulteress to be different insofar as she had been guilty of a capital offence (*Lev. xx*.20); since in Jewish law her execution would involve the death of her fruit, too,[200] he could see no objection to its destruction in these circumstances. But in a later responsa work the abortion of an illegitimate embryo is distinctly forbidden.[201]

The Jewish attitude to the destruction of foetal and nascent human life, then, is complex and but sparsely defined in our chief sources. We may therefore here summarise the principal conclusions of our survey. There are four distinct legal phases in the development of man: (i) Up to the moment when the first signs of parturient labour set in, the foetus is an organic part of the mother. While, according to the consensus of rabbinic opinion, its life is not protected by any definite legal provisions, the artificial termination of a pregnancy is strongly condemned on moral grounds, unless it can be justified for medical or, possibly, other grave reasons. (ii) During the process of birth and until the child's head or the greater part of its body has emerged, its life is still of inferior value, but nevertheless vested with a certain measure of human inviolability. Its claim to life may (and must) be set aside in the mother's interest only if it is the child (and not some illness) that threatens her life. During these two phases, it would be a criminal violation of the sanctity of human life to let the mother die (in the aforementioned circumstances) by refusing to destroy her fruit. (iii) From the moment the major part of the child is born, it assumes human status in most respects, and the value of its life is practically equal to that of any adult person. But, unless conclusive evidence exists to show that it was carried for a full term of nine months, the child's viability is not fully established or presumed until the thirty-first day of its existence. That uncertainty frees the murderer of such an infant from capital guilt. It also confers the right to save the mother at the expense of the child, when the failure to sacrifice the child would lead to the loss of both lives, but not when it would otherwise be expected to survive the mother's death. (iv) A child born definitely after a full-term pregnancy, or else following the first thirty days of its life, enjoys human rights in every respect. It must not be sacrificed for the preservation of one or even more lives under any circumstances (except those applicable to the surrender of normal adult lives).

This classification deals, of course, only with the child's claim to life, not with any other legal rights or theological considerations (such as the entry of the soul or its title to immortality)—factors unrelated to our subject.

CHAPTER FIFTEEN

CIRCUMCISION
PROCEDURE AND MEDICAL IMPEDIMENTS

As a rule, Jewish law does not presume to offer any guidance on purely medical procedures. But the performance of circumcisions represents an important exception, for the operation was usually entrusted to lay practitioners acting as religious officials. Up to the 19th century, we find physicians acting in this capacity on but the rarest occasions.[1] It is true, mention of a doctor performing a circumcision already occurs in JOSEPHUS's *Antiquities*.[2] But there the subject operated on was an adult proselyte (King IZATES of Adiabene), and the conclusion reached on these premises that physicians were generally employed as circumcisers[3] has rightly been repudiated as being based "on a lack of the requisite knowledge in the fields of theology and philology".[4]

Only in more recent times has the suggestion been urged in some quarters[5] that the operation be entrusted entirely to physicians—a suggestion often frowned upon in rabbinical circles[6] as it may deprive the act of its distinctly religious character. But following a demand first made by a medical college in Prussia in 1799,[7] ritual circumcisers were frequently required to obtain medical certificates before being admitted to the practice; such authorisations are now demanded in most Jewish communities.

Jewish law merely disqualifies non-Jews[8] (*Y.D.*, *cclxiv*. 1), women[9] and non-conforming Jews from acting in this capacity, urging one to engage the services of "the best and most pious possible coreligionist"[10] (*ib.*, gloss). The act may, of course, be performed by any surgeon on an infant requiring it before the eighth day for urgent medical reasons, but such an operation does not possess any religious validity[11] (*ib.*). Conversely, it is forbidden for Jews to circumcise Gentiles, except for the purpose of their conversion (*Y.D.*, *cclxiii*.5, gloss), because one thereby helps to obliterate the distinctive mark of Israel's covenant.[12] But when the operation is necessary for healing purposes, it may be carried out in circumstances in which other medical services, too, can lawfully be rendered to non-Jews[13] (*Y.D.*, *cclxviii*.9, gloss).

Ritual circumcisions, then, were usually in the charge of non-medical practitioners. They drew their remarkable competence[14] from an unbroken tradition in this art extending over nearly four millenia, during which the manner of the operation remained virtually unchanged,[15] combined with their mastery of the rabbinical teachings on the subject. It was therefore left to the legal codes and commentaries to provide these lay surgeons with precise instructions which would render any recourse to independent medical advice unnecessary. These directives detail the procedure in normal cases as well as the conditions of ill-health under which the operation must be varied, deferred or altogether abandoned.

PROCEDURE

The method to be adopted is laid down thus: "One excises the foreskin, [that is,] the entire skin covering the glans, so that the corona is laid bare. Afterwards, one tears with the finger-nail the soft membrane underneath the skin, turning it to the sides until the flesh of the glans appears. Thereafter, one sucks the membrum until the blood is extracted from the [more] remote places, so that no danger [to the infant] may ensue; and any circumciser who does not carry out the sucking procedure is to be removed [from his office]. After sucking [the wound], one places on it a compress or a plaster or some medicinal powder to stop the bleeding" (*Y.D.*, *cclxiv*.3). ISSERLES adds that one should take care to tilt any seam of the plaster outwards, lest it stick to the wound and thus endanger the child (*ib.*, gloss). The operation itself, then, consists of three distinct acts: the excision of the prepuce; the laceration of the mucous membrane covering the glans, and its retraction to the outer skin layer; and the sucking of the blood from the interior of the wound . All three acts are already mentioned —without, however, being clearly defined—in the Talmud.[16] The two last acts are specifically Jewish; they are not known among the Moslems (and the Karaites) who simply retain the membrane over the glans[17] or wait until it breaks on its own, thus lengthening the healing process.[18] But even among the followers of rabbinic Judaism, these two rites have been the subject of various interpretations and, more lately, of considerable controversies.

The tearing of the mucosa is, according to the Mishnah,[19] an indispensable part of the operation, and "whoever performs a circumcision without [the act of] tearing is as if he had not carried out the circumcision" (*ib.*, 4). The talmudic term for this act (*Peri'ah*) can be rendered either "tearing" or "uncovering".[20] The first interpretation is accepted by MAIMONIDES[21] and others[22] who, moreover, insist that the act must be performed with the finger-nail.[23] The term may, however, refer merely to the "exposure" of the corona,[24] and this is evidently supported by so early an authority as HAI Gaon. This 10th century scholar speaks of the excision and the (*Peri'ah*) done by a single act as "a long-established statute" in Babylonia.[25] He also mentions the use of a knife if the inner skin is too hard to be broken by hand.[26] Accordingly, Z.H. CHAJES[27] suggested that the reference to the finger-nails merely reflected the custom at the time, but that the use of an instrument, if necessary, was equally lawful. He added, nevertheless, that the parted membrane must be folded over by hand only, "since the employment of a knife or a forceps [for this act] causes great pain to the infant, whereas by using his hand the operator can sense how much pressure to apply so as not to increase the pain unduly". Since early in the 19th century, the opinions for and against the replacement of the nails by instruments have found vigorous protagonists. While the traditional method was opposed for hygienic reasons in some quarters,[28] JACOB ETTLINGER[29] and other rabbis[30] went so far as to disqualify circumcisers using instruments in normal cases, unless no other operator could be found. The recent invention of various hemostat-clamps (to crush the inner and outer linings of the skin together prior to the excision of the foreskin)[31] is further extending the field of this controversy. But the present tendency is to continue to act in strict accord with the traditional practice.

Far more widespread and often bitter has been the conflict of views on the subsequent sucking of the wound by mouth. The Talmud,[32] which insists on the act without stipulating that it must be done by mouth, simply remarks that "there is danger" if it is omitted. The explanation that the suction serves to bring out the blood from the interior of the organ is first mentioned by MAIMONIDES,[33] but neither this nor any other fact justifies the statement that "MAIMONIDES improved the method of circumcision ... and introduced several precautionary measures".[34] JACOB HAGOZER,[35] the first to write a special work on the subject (and like MAIMONIDES of the 12th century), demanded the sucking act "so that the blood shall not congeal in the mouth of the penis, which is dangerous". On the other hand, two important compendia of Jewish law of the 13th and 14th centuries, *Sepher Hahinnukh* and *Kol Bo*, do not mention the act at all. The omission, while not necessarily implying any dissent in practice, does appear to suggest that the oral suction was not regarded as an essential part of the religious ritual. But it was only since the beginning of the last century that the traditional procedure was challenged in practice as well as in principle. The argument that the physical contact between the operator and the child exposed both to the danger of infection often leading, it was alleged,[36] to fatal results eventually induced some civil authorities to ban the act,[37] and a growing number of circumcisers resorted to various appliances specially invented for the purpose.[38] At present many circumcisers simply press a cotton swab against the fresh wound.[39]

Although the contention that the suction by mouth did not belong to the essential constituents of the ritual[40] and that any effective means to prevent the danger envisaged by the Talmud was legally admissible was founded on good authority,[41] many rabbis—led by ETTLINGER[42] and other eminent scholars[43]—expressed and organised strong opposition to these innovations. ISRAEL LIPSCHUETZ[44] held that, in this respect, the established tradition should be upheld even against the claims of medical experts.[45] Some physicians, too, rallied to the defence of the time-honoured practice.[46] The traditionalists firmly denied that the method they advocated had been responsible for any deaths.[47] The divergencies of opinion and practice are common to the present day. But the original method of sucking by mouth tends to be increasingly confined to the most orthodox circles only.

Whenever it is physically impossible to perform a ritual circumcision—owing either to the congenital absence of the foreskin[48] (*Y.D.*, *cclxiii*.4) or to its previous removal in circumstances which rendered the act religiously invalid (*Y.D.*, *cclxiv*.1, gloss)—a drop of blood must be drawn from the organ as a symbolic token of initiation into the "covenant of ABRAHAM".[49] But exceptional care is urged in the gentle performance of this operation, and especially in examining the penis; this should be done by hand and not with any metal instrument, "so as not to harrow [the infant]"[50] (*Y.D.*, *cclxiii*.4). On the Sabbath, however, this act must not be carried out (*Y.D.*, *cclxvi*.10). Similarly, it is necessary to postpone from the Sabbath to the following day the circumcision of a child born with certain abnormalities or delivered by a caesarian section[51] (*ib.*; and *O.H.*, *cccxxxi*.1 *ff.*).

Otherwise the normal date for the circumcision of a Jewish child is the eighth day of its life. This must not be altered except for reasons of health. Jewish law defines the pathological impediments to the operation with much precision, always interpreting illness in its broadest meaning, and it counsels the utmost caution in deciding on these issues—affecting, as they do, human lives that can never be restored once lost[52] (*Y.D., cclxiii.*1).

Accordingly, it is forbidden to circumcise a sick child before its recovery[53] (*Y.D., cclxii.*2). If the illness affects the whole body, a complete week must elapse following the recovery before the operation may be carried out[54] (*ib.*). Such illness is, for example, "the fever"[55] (*ib.*). But if the complaint is limited to a single organ, such as a slight eye-ache, the circumcision can take place immediately upon recovery (*ib.*). Various authorities assert that a child is unfit for the operation even if it is merely in pain, whether due to illness or to any other cause.[56] ISSERLES adds that an acute eye-ache[57] is to be regarded as a disease of the whole body (*ib.*, gloss) necessitating a further delay of seven days. According to several responsa,[58] an infant's general weakness is also a legitimate ground for deferring the circumcision, but they make no reference to the attainment of a minimum weight before the operation can be carried out.[59]

Apart from these general provisions, the law details some specific symptoms in this connection. "If a child is yellow (or green?[60]), it is a sign that its blood has not yet descended into it,[61] and one does not circumcise it until this occurs and its colour is restored to that of other infants; similarly, if the child is found to be red, it is an indication that its blood has not yet been absorbed in its limbs but [remains] between the skin and the flesh,[62] and one does not circumcise it until the blood is [properly] absorbed in it"[63] (*Y.D., cclxiii.*1). These regulations, entirely of talmudic origin, have been variously interpreted. Both the excessively and insufficiently red colouring evidently betokens, it is considered, a blood disease or some failure in the function ing of the neo-natal circulatory system. KATZENEL-SOHN[64] discusses the theory that the first condition may be identified as *icterus neonatorum* and the latter as *erythema neonatorum,* but he comes to the conclusion that the first description can only indicate a deficiency of blood. PREUSS[65] and KRAUSS[66] also think of the first symptom as a green-ish paleness — hence anaemia, like theχλωρὸς of the Greeks. EBSTEIN,[67] however, cannot decide whether the reference is to jaundice or anaemia (chlorosis), according as the oper-ative term means "yellow" or "green". In any case, the rabbinical responsa are agreed on demanding a postpone-ment of the operation if the child suffers from any form of jaundice,[68] though it is not certain whether another seven days must then be allowed to elapse as after other diseases.[69]

HAEMOPHILIA

Historically of particular interest is the following fur-ther law: If a mother lost two sons through weakness (from bleeding) following their circumcision, it is assumed that her children are predisposed to die from the operation; hence her third son must not be circumcised until he grows up and becomes strong (*ib.,* 2). In the application of this law it makes no difference whether the brothers have a common father or not (*ib.*). While KARO grants the exemption also to brothers who share only a common paternity but have different mothers (*ib.*), ISSERLES records a dis-senting view; but he adds that in such capital cases any doubt is to be resolved in favour of the more lenient inter-pretation (*ib.,* gloss). All authorities agree, however, on extending this law to maternal cousins, too; so that if the death (due to circumcision) of one woman's son was fol-lowed by the death of her sister's son, the remaining sisters must defer the operation on their sons until they are adults (*ib.*, 3). This law, in its talmudic sources,[70] probably marks the first recognition in medical history of haemophilia,[71] on which the first clinical observations were published only in 1784.[72] Moreover, ISSERLES's view that a common maternity conditions the operation of this law—because, as the commentators explain, "the blood derives from the mother"[73] —accords with the experience that the disease is usually transmitted through matrilinear consanguinity. The contrary view held by KARO is not, in fact, found in the Talmud.[74] Nor is the ruling that the circumcision of the third son should be performed later in his life mentioned there. This is first recorded by MAIMONIDES,[75] against the opinions of ALFASI and ASHERI who omit it, and to the misgivings of Z.H. CHAJES[76] and EZEKIEL LANDAU[77] who question its authority and insist on special caution in such cases. KATZENELSOHN,[78] however, justifies the decision of MAIMONIDES as being in harmony with the claims of modern medicine that the disease definitely becomes quiescent after the twenty-second year of life.

CIRCUMCISION OF DEAD INFANT

A child that died under the age of eight days should be circumcised with a flint or a reed over its grave and given a name as a memorial (*Y.D.*, *cccliii*.6), "so that it will be shown compassion by Heaven and live when the dead are resurrected" (*Y.D.*, *cclxiii.*5). This practice, though not mentioned by MAIMONIDES, is of geonic origin.[79] KARO's explanation, first recorded by ASHERI[80] in the name of NACHSHON Gaon, is based on a teaching in the Midrash[81] that ABRAHAM will sit at the entrance of *Gehenna* and prevent the admission of any circumcised Jew.[82] The same passage also states that excessive sinners, to make their entry into *Gehenna* possible, will be given the foreskins of infants who died without being circumcised.[83] Hence, some early authorities suggest that the posthumous circumcision of such children serves as "a measure for the benefit of sinners", the foreskins being wasted to save the sinners from being condemned to perdition.[84] According to yet a third view, a still-born or dead infant should be circumcised simply "to avoid his burial with his foreskin, for that would be a shame unto him".[85] In the responsa opinions are divided on whether such circumcisions may be carried out on festivals[86] and whether a child already buried without the operation may, or ought to be, exhumed to have its foreskin removed.[87] Naturally, whenever it is possible to circumcise a child before its expected death, this should be done.[88]

CHAPTER SIXTEEN

THE PHYSICIAN — 1

HIS STUDIES, STATUS,
PROFESSIONAL ETHICS AND PRIVILEGES

As a rule, it can be assumed that the physician's standing in society reflects the place occupied by his art in the popular repute, and any inconsistency in this relationship can be regarded as exceptional. It is therefore "a strange anomaly that as in the later Empire [from the 3rd and 4th centuries] medicine deteriorated, physicians . . . were many and held in higher and higher esteem".[1] Consequently, our estimate of the medical profession, with its rights and duties, in this and the succeeding chapters will partly serve to supplement the material on the general attitude to medicine treated in our first chapter.

As an outline of the literary and social background to the medico-religious regulations to be surveyed in these chapters, we shall preface them by some observations on the appreciation of the physician. He has long been a favourite subject for the most exaggerated expressions of panegyric and disparagement alike. How often have satirists re-echoed the sentiments inspiring these lines of an unknown Spanish-Jewish poet of the 15th century:—

"The countenance of the doctor is like that of angels, exalted
In the eyes of the patient; while the pains are increasing,
His words are sweeter than dripping honey . . . ,
And when health returns
And the doctor asks for his gold pieces
He becomes like unto Satan in the form of man . . . !"[2]

More frequently praise and contempt for physicians comes from separate authors. Like others, Jewish writers, too, have supplied their quota of complimentary and derogatory sayings. Two centuries before the Common Era BEN SIRAH, in one of the earliest and finest tributes to the medical fraternity, devoted an entire chapter (*Ecclus. xxxviii*) to their eulogy, starting with the famous verse: "Honour the physician according to thy need of him with the honours due unto him; for verily the Lord hath created him".[3] But then again, a few hundred years later, the Mishnah declared: "To hell with the best of the physicians!"[4]

The impulse to laud the healing art and its practitioners is natural enough. The reason for their at least equally frequent exposure to obloquy and ridicule may be less obvious. Yet, one could adduce innumerable parallels to the mishnaic statement from other literatures.[5] During the period of the Mishnah none other than GALEN himself had said of his colleagues: "Between robbers and physicians lies this difference only, that the misdeeds of the former are performed in the mountains, but those of the latter in Rome itself".[6] Completely identical with the taunt in the Mishnah was the proverb *"Optimus inter medicos ad Gehennam"* which "enjoyed unquestioned currency in the learned world" together with the by-word *"Ubi tres medici, tres athei"*.[7] In a similar vein, when the Emperor SIGISMUND decreed in 1496 that every Imperial State in Germany should appoint a public medical officer to be paid from Church revenues and to attend the poor gratis, he explained: " . . . for the high masters and physicians never do this and therefore they go to Hell".[8] As our final sample, this is what the famous essayist ADDISON wrote in his *Spectator* of March 24, 1711: "We may lay it down as a maxim, that when a nation abounds in physicians, it grows thin of people".[9]

But more instructive, in our context, are the numerous interpretations[10] which have been offered to explain the statement in the Mishnah. The Talmud did not comment on the pasage at all, which is as significant as it is unusual.

RASHI[11] held that the stricture simply applied to a doctor "who does not subdue his heart to trust in Heaven, who sometimes causes the death of his patients, and who is in a position to treat the poor [free] but does not do so". Most commentators accepted RASHI's views that the curse was directed against physicians who were overconfident in their craft or guilty of unduly commercialising their profession.[12] According to the ethical treatise *'Even Bohan* (1322) by the Provencal writer and philosopher KALONYMUS BEN KALONYMUS, the reference was not to genuine physicians but to quacks, because their art was lying and deception.[13] The 15th century Spanish author and rabbi-physician SOLOMON IBN VERGA[14] thought the mishnaic saying was intended to warn physicians to be cautious in their treatment; they were always to see hell opened before them should their negligence lead to fatal consequences. SIMON DURAN,[15] about a century later, believed the phrase sought to castigate only those doctors who maintained their own views in the presence of greater experts and who relied on their own experiments. A similar explanation was given by the talmudist SAMUEL EDELS[16] in the 17th century. But JONATHAN EYBESCHU-ETZ,[17] in the following century, related the dictum to his theory that the divine sanction of healing applied only to external injuries, whereas attempts to cure internal diseases were deprecated.[18] His contemporary, ISAAC LAM-PRONTI,[19] on the other hand, suggested that the condemnation was aimed at the surgeons, "because they vary the instructions of the wise [physicians], and in particular they exceed, or fall short of, the proper measure when letting blood, according to their limited intelligence, thus killing their patients; and many times have I seen . . . such evil . . . "

"To hell with the best of the physicians!", then, was never understood as a denunciation of the conscientious practitioner in general.[20] Any such interpretation would already be ruled out by the inclusion, in an early talmudic passage,[21] of "the best of the physicians", together with the local judge, scribe, clerk and sexton, in the group of communal servants who "have no share in the world to come", i.e. among those who have heavy public responsibilities and who are warned against the danger of negligence or error.[22] It is also quite plausible that the association of physicians with hell was—as has been suggested[23]—"in its original form . . . nothing but a pun, based on the assonance of 'Roph'im', physicians, and 'R'pha'im', the dwellers of the nether world".[24] The occasional sallies at the medical profession in later Jewish works, too, were hardly meant to denigrate the honest physician. FRIEDENWALD, who has written a whole chapter on "Wit and Satire about the Physician in Hebrew Literature",[25] concludes from the numerous selections given by him "that the physician was often made the target of wit and satire . . . — but only the ignorant, the unscrupulous, the pretentious and the quack".[26] In fact, most of these statements only endorse, in one form or another, the old maxim quoted by ISAAC ABARVANEL: "The knavish doctor is the colleague of the angel of death".[27]

HIGH REGARD FOR PHYSICIANS

If medieval Jewish writings can be searched in vain for the type of sayings assembled in WITKOWSKI's *Le Mal qu'on a dit des Medecins*, or in CHARLES L. DANA's *The Evil Spoken of Physicians*,[28] they are replete with expressions of admiration and praise for the "faithful physician"—a term reverently applied to God Himself.[29] We shall here confine ourselves to giving a few illustrations of the high, and often enviable, station occupied by medical men and studies in Jewish medieval life. Thus, the medical writer LEON JOSEPH of Carcassonne made an illuminating comment on conditions in France at the end of the 14th century when he stated that "he studied medicine because he saw that only Jewish physicians had any standing in the community, while the rest of the members of his race were constantly humiliated".[30] There was evidently no change in the high place accorded to medicine in 1490 when JACOB BEN DAVID PROVENCAL, a talmudist and maritime trader at Marseilles, addressed a letter to DAVID BEN JUDAH MESSER LEON of Mantua in which he strongly urged the advantages of joining the medical profession than which there was no more honourable livelihood, since rabbis were ill rewarded, little honoured and unable to maintain their families in reasonable comfort.[31] If up to the 18th century the status of the physician was generally better than it is to-day—in some countries he wore a sword, and people commonly took off their hats to him[32]—it was particularly so in Jewish society. In medieval England he, as well as the rabbi, enjoyed the title *"Magister"*,[33] just as the term "doctor" was used for members of both professions in Polish-Jewish documents of that time.[34] In many communities, physicians usually held leading communal positions, and they were honoured with the rabbinical title *"Morenu"* ("our teacher") when called up to the reading of the Law in the synagogue.[35] Most medieval rabbis, disdaining to be paid for their ecclesiastical services, had to engage in other pursuits for their subsistence. Among the careers they chose medicine was by far the most popular— partly, no doubt, by reason of the dignity attaching to it.[36] In the Middle Ages no less than one half of the best known rabbis—as well as poets and philosophers—were physicians by profession.[37] The two vocations were so closely associated that respected Christians often repaired to rabbis as patients asking for advice and medicines.[38]

MEDICINE AS EDUCATION

There were certainly also other factors, apart from the quest for honour and lucre, which attracted the Jewish intellectual to medicine on such an extraordinary scale, and which caused the Jews to be so prominent in medieval medicine. One suggestion is that the principal lay physicians in the Middle Ages were Jews owing to the persecution of rational medicine by the Church.[39] The Italian rabbi-physician, DAVID DE POMIS of the 16th century, explained "the fame of the [Jewish] physician" as due to the fact "that we Jews are considered to enjoy God's providence —as indeed we do; more than that, we are judged to be expert in the prognosis of disease".[40] These considerations may account for the popularity of Jews in medicine, but not for the popularity of medicine with Jews. An important element in this relationship was undoubtedly the pre-eminent place medicine occupied in medieval education and learning outside religious scholarship. Already in classic Rome medical knowledge had formed part of general culture, as shown in the writings of PLUTARCH, PLINY and many other authors.[41] As books and scholasticism progressively ousted empiric observation from the curriculum of medical instruction,[42] the tendency to treat medicine as an academic arts subject rather than as a practical science became even more pronounced. It was not until more recent times that the position was virtually reversed; in fact—as a historian[43] has complained—it is now the "serious defect" of modern civilisation that the cultured layman knows a good deal about medicines and almost nothing about medicine.

To the medieval Jew, therefore, the study of medicine provided the key to a world otherwise barred to him. Physicians were the chief representatives of secular scholarship in the ghettos; moreover, the acquisition of medical knowledge was often the means enabling Jews to enter the universities and to study other arts and sciences.[44] When Jewish students in considerable numbers trekked across half the face of Europe—from Poland to Padua, for instance—in search of a university which would admit them,[45] they could hardly have been baited only by the prospect of finding some professional employment and recognition on their return after so many years of struggle and privation.[46] It was the essence of culture, as understood in those days, they were after when they applied themselves with such zeal to reading and translating the classic texts of medicine or to joining medical schools in distant lands. In an age when knowledge, outside medicine, was almost entirely of a religious character and mostly under ecclesiastical control,[47] the pursuit of medicine (often through private instruction[48]) offered to the Jew the only escape from the social and intellectual confines into which he was driven by popular prejudice and hostility.[49]

These factors will help us to appreciate why the study of medicine was so specially encouraged by the leaders of Jewish religious thought and why it became a privileged subject enjoying a religious sanction not granted to other secular branches of education. The tradition of combining medical with religious studies may indeed go back to the talmudic academies in Babylonia, and perhaps in Palestine.[50] Throughout the Middle Ages, particularly in Spain, medicine was always the most prominent subject in the secular syllabus, usually well ahead, in the order of precedence, of philosophy, astronomy, mathematics and the natural sciences.[51] Medicine was acccorded pride of place, next to religious studies, in the educational programmes drawn up by JOSEPH BEN JUDAH IBN AKNIN[52] (a disciple of MAIMONIDES) in the 12th century, by JUDAH BEN SAMUEL IBN ABBAS[53] in the 13th century, and by ELEAZAR ASHKENAZI[54] in the 14th century. Its pursuit was strongly encouraged in a moral poem attributed to HAI GAON,[55] in the ethical will of JUDAH IBN TIB-BON,[56] in the *Sepher Hasidim*,[57] and in a favourite moralist work by MEIR ALDABI[58] of the 14th century. Whether the chief object of the urge to study medicine was to broaden the student's cultural horizon (as implied by HAI and IBN TIBBON), or to enable him to mitigate human suffering (as suggested in the two last-mentioned works), or "to perceive the greatness of the Holy One and His wonderful deeds" (as advocated by GEDALIAH IBN YACH-

YAH[59] in the 16th century), or to help preachers to make their sermons more popular (as recommended by the Jerusalemite rabbi-physician RAPHAEL MORDECAI MALKI[60] at about 1700)—none of these religious guides, however dispersed in time and place, sought to promote such study for mainly professional ends. It is also significant that medicine featured as a chief subject of instruction at all the Jewish universities — we know of at least four such projects in Europe between 1000 and 1600[61]—which had been planned or established to provide religious and secular training.

The bias in favour of medical studies found a secure place in Jewish religious law, too. When ADRETH[62] issued his famous ban on the study of philosophy, metaphysics and allied subjects by people under the age of twenty-five years (cf. Y.D., ccxlvi.4, gloss), he expressly excluded medicine, as its pursuit was clearly sanctioned in the Bible. He also exempted medical books from the edict against reading secular literature on the Sabbath[63] (cf. O.H., cccvii.17). Altogether, even during the 17th and 18th centuries, when the rabbis generally disapproved of university education, they invariably favoured the indulgence in medical studies.[64] JACOB EMDEN,[65] for instance, in a discussion on the value of secular studies, particularly emphasised the importance of medical knowledge, since the life of all creatures depended on it. Caution was urged only if these studies were carried to excess at the expense of religious pursuits.[66] Medical books, too, were regarded as specially valuable.[67] They should not be seized as a pledge on a loan, for the doctor's inability to consult them might lead to a patient's death.[68] In the codes, however, there is no specific reference to either medical books or studies.

THE OATH OF HIPPOCRATES

In medieval times and up to our own day, medical students were generally required to take the Hippocratic Oath on the completion of their training. Although the Oath is, surprisingly, never mentioned by GALEN, allusions to its popularity already occur in the writings of several Roman authors of the 1st century *C.E.*,[69] and it has moulded the outlook of the medical profession ever since.[70] The original pagan version was subsequently revised, mainly in its introductory phrases, to suit the religious terminology of the Arabs and Christians using it. The Arab form of the Oath goes back at least to the 13th century.[71] In the Christian version the opening sentence "I swear by . . . " is altogether omitted. This may be due to the Christian reluctance to take any oath, following the injunction "Swear not at all" (*Matth. v.*34).[72] Yet, academic oaths were frequently taken at the medieval universities, and they were (subject to the papal power of dispensation) absolute and eternal; their violation doomed the deponent to perpetual perdition should he die unabsolved.[73]

In view of the religious sanction given to the Oath and of the important role played by the Hebrew language[74] and Jewish physicians in medieval medicine, it seems strange that there is no trace of any Hebrew or Jewish version.[75] Nor is there any mention of a physicians' oath in rabbinic literature. This omission may well be due to the same reason as has been given for the peculiar form of the Christian version. The Jewish aversion to oaths is, if anything, even more emphatic than the Christian. According to the Talmud[76] and the codes, "whoever makes a vow, even though he fulfils it, is called a wicked person and . . . a sinner" (*Y.D., cciii.*1); he is "as if he builds an [illegitimate, private] altar"[77] (*ib.*, 3). One should refrain from taking formal oaths, "so as not to take the Name of Heaven in vain", even in business or at court (*O.H., clvi.*1), submitting to financial loss rather than to the necessity for swearing.[78] Nevertheless, it can hardly be doubted that Jewish students, on graduating from the medical schools, were not exempted from taking the Hippocratic Oath.[79] Indeed, sometimes the Christian manner of taking oaths prevented Jews from obtaining their degrees.[80] At Leghorn, for instance, medical degrees were granted to Jews only after 1728, when they were allowed to substitute the Pentateuch for the crucifix at the swearing ceremony for admission.[81]

Although the Hippocratic Oath "made a profound impression" on Jews as well as on Moslems and Christians,[82] there may also be a more significant reason for its absence from Jewish sources and the failure of the rabbis to provide the physician with a formula setting forth the standards of professional propriety. Strictly speaking, a Jewish code of medical ethics (in the technical sense of professional rules of etiquette and moral conduct) cannot be said to exist at all. Jewish law lays down *special* moral qualifications only for religious officials.[83] For physicians, however, there are no specific ethical directives on the lines set out in the Hippocratic Oath. Its principal provisions—on the respect due to teachers, the protection of human life, abortion, sterilisation and chastity—are in any case covered by laws which are incumbent on any Jew and which could not, therefore, be designated as professional rules of conduct. Even statements deposed by litigants, defendants and witnesses in Jewish civil or criminal proceedings need not usually be confirmed by oath.[84] There could be no more justification for abjuring physicians to observe laws binding on them and others alike.

The only clause in the Hippocratic Oath altogether ignored in Jewish law concerns the undertaking to guard professional secrets,[85] unless this can be regarded as covered by the many warnings against all manner of gossip[86] based on the injunction "Thou shalt not go . . . as a talebearer among thy people" (*Lev. xix*.16) and the Preacher's advice "Reveal not the secret of another" (*Prov. xxv*.9). It is, no doubt, due only to the influence of the Hippocratic Oath that doctors are warned against betraying secrets with more demonstrative jealousy than their brothers in the theological and legal professions, though their work might be expected to be of an equally confidential nature.[87] Jewish ethics could envisage circumstances—when the public interest or some other overriding factor is at stake—in which it would be proper to break the confidence of people in one's professional charge.[88] But there could then be no distinction between ministers of religion, lawyers and physicians.

On the other hand, the medico-religious legislation of Judaism includes some items of professional ethics not mentioned in the Hippocratic Oath. As far as these relate to medical charges, licenses and legal responsibilities, they will be treated in the succeeding chapters. We shall here deal only with the physician's obligation to heal and its limitations. As already stated,[89] it is a religious precept for a competent doctor to practise his art; indeed his refusal to do so is tantamount to shedding blood (*Y.D., cccxxxvi.*1). A withdrawal from medical practice is condemned, even if other physicians are available, "since a man is not [always] destined to be healed by any [random] person" (*ib.*). AZULAY,[90] however, is inclined to sanction such withdrawal if the practitioner is afraid he may err. KARO, too, declares: "Nevertheless, one should not engage in medicine unless one is competent, nor if there is a greater [expert] than oneself [available]; otherwise one is [accounted as] shedding blood" (*ib.*). In the *Tur* code,[91] these reservations are further elaborated by analogy with the right of rabbis to pronounce judgments only in the absence of more competent authorities (so *Y.D., ccxlii.*4, 13 and 31, gloss); "for how may one rule in matters affecting life and death when a greater [expert] than oneself is [available]?"[92] The comparison between the rabbinical and medical professions—repeated elsewhere,[93] too—is highly significant. It shows that both shared common norms of professional conduct in several respects and that they enjoyed a similar status in the community.

RELIGIOUS CONCESSIONS FOR PHYSICIANS

In conclusion, we may detail certain religious concessions granted to physicians in their practice. MAIMO-

NIDES,[94] in a responsum, permits doctors to say their prayers before the statutory time if they have to attend on noblemen early in the morning. ADRETH,[95] followed by KARO, sanctions their handling of receptacles for urine whilst wearing phylacteries, but conscientious practitioners are advised not to do so (*O.H.*, *xliii.*9). Similar points discussed more recently include the physician's right to board a conveyance for visiting the sick on the Sabbath,[96] to use detergents for washing hands on the Sabbath,[97] and to leave the house during the week of mourning (for a close relative) in order to attend a patient.[98] Of historical interest is the ruling, given by JOSEPH COLON[99] in the 15th century and codified by ISSERLES, permitting Jewish physicians to don the distinctive garb usually worn by their Christian colleagues, notwithstanding the general ban on adopting non-Jewish customs and wearing apparel (*Y.D.*, *clxxviii.*1, gloss). Early in the 18th century, the Palestinian scholar MOSES HAGIZ[100] allowed Jewish doctors to carry swords, as was the general practice,[101] except on the Sabbath when this was expressly forbidden (*O.H.*, *ccci.*7). But physicians could not, as a rule, claim the special privileges extended to religious scholars, who were exempt from the payment of taxes[102] (*Y.D.*, *ccxliii.*2) and from conscription to the communal labour corps (*ib.*, 1), and who enjoyed other social benefits (*ib.*, 4). In a law already found in the Talmud,[103] doctors and barbers are expressly precluded from establishing their surgery in a closed alley, if objections are raised by any neighbours on account of the nuisance caused by the comings and goings of the patients (*H.M.*, *clvi.*1). Under such conditions it is also forbidden for a tenant in a corporate housing estate to let his premises for this purpose (*ib.*). Doctors share this disability with secular teachers (*ib.*), whereas religious tutors cannot be thus restrained even if their neighbours claim that the children's noise disturbs their sleep[104] (*ib.*, 3).

According to a talmudic law,[105] codified by MAIMONIDES[106] but omitted in the *Shulhan 'Arukh*, a conscientious

Jew must not reside in a place which has no adequate religious, educational and social functionaries, including a physician and a barber. Following this rule, doctors were, in fact, usually found even in quite small Jewish communities.[107]

CHAPTER SEVENTEEN

THE PHYSICIAN—2

HIS LICENSE TO PRACTICE AND LEGAL RESPONSIBILITIES

Modern medical licensure is a creation of the Middle Ages.[1] But the need for protecting society from the spurious activities of the irresponsible medicaster—by authenticating competent physicians—was already recognised in antiquity, albeit only in comparatively rare instances. The ancient Indian doctors, for example, had to petition the king for permission to practice independently.[2] In the West, too, we find occasional efforts to eliminate unauthorised practitioners. In Rome the *Lex Cornelia* of 88 *B.C.E.* made the unqualified physician liable to arrest if any death was caused through his fault.[3] Yet PLINY[4] still complained that there was no law punishing doctors for ignorance and negligence, the privileges vested in the recognised physician.[6] But this and no licensing system existed before the 2nd century *C.E.*[5] It was only under SEVERUS SEPTIMUS (146-211) that a license of the municipal council was required as a title to safeguard, too, was soon allowed to lapse, and with the disappearance of the great medical schools during most of the 1st millenium there also came to an end any legislative measures aimed at maintaining proper professional standards.

In medieval times we meet with qualifying examinations for physicians occasionally among the Arabs. In 931, for instance, Caliph AL-MUQTADIR decided that no-one was to practise medicine in Bagdad unless he was first examined by the physician SINAN IBN THABIT of Haaran.[7] But these requirements were not always insisted upon,[8] and there certainly was never any rigid system of control in the great era of Moslem medicine. In Christian Europe the licensing of physicians was first introduced by an order of the Norman King ROGER in the middle of the 12th century. It provided that no-one could practise medicine unless "he has presented himself before our officials and examiners in order to pass their judgment . . . and [was] found fit by the convention of the Salernitan masters".[9] A century later, this law was extended in the *Constitutiones Imperiales* issued by FREDERICK II, who supplied the medical school at Salerno with a complete syllabus to be covered before a licence would be granted.[10]

Although the system became more widely accepted in the following two centuries, the standard and value of medical degrees was generally low. We are informed that in Paris at the beginning of the 16th century they were often given to "common people who have not the slightest acquaintance with ARISTOTLE and are ignorant of even the first elements of grammar";[11] sometimes they were even sold for money. Consequently, some students refused to take any degree, and no diplomas can be traced of such celebrated doctors as J. SYLVIUS, VESALIUS, M. SERVET, J. THIBAULT and others.[12] A report of conditions in England at the same time declares that "the practice of physic was improperly supervised, and had fallen into the hands of smiths, weavers and women. Midwives were licensed by the same authorities".[13] These abuses led to the parliamentary statute of 1511 providing that "no person within the city of London . . . take upon him to . . . occupy as a physician or surgeon, except he be first examined, approved and admitted by the Bishop of London . . . sided by four doctors of physic, or persons expert in surgery . . . "[14] In 1540 the statute was followed by an Act which empowered the United Company of Barber Surgeons to impose fines on unlicensed practitioners in London.[15]

The reference to the Bishop of London illustrates an interesting and, in our context, significant phase in the history of medical licensure. For several centuries the right to confer medical degrees was exercised by the popes and their legates in many parts of Europe.[16] Already in 1310 the Synod of Treves had decreed: "Inasmuch as so many ignorant physicians have arisen, no-one shall henceforth practice or teach medicine and surgery without the permission of the bishop who shall examine the applicant both in respect to his knowledge and his morals".[17] Originally, this development no doubt grew out of the papal control over the seats of learning and the association, often to the point of identity, of the theological and medical professions in medieval times. But the granting of medical licences remained an ecclesiastical prerogative long after the profession and the schools of medicine had won their independence. An example of the retention by the bishops of what has been compared[18] to "the functions of the modern General Council" are the famous "Lambeth degrees."[19] Even after the Reformation the Archbishop of Canterbury retained the power, vested in him until 1534 as the pope's representative, to confer degrees in medicine. Not altogether accurate is the statement[20] that, following protests by the Surgeon's Company and the College of Physicians, no bishop's licences were granted in London after 1713. Officially the use of the Archbishop's prerogative was restricted only by the Medical Act of 1858[21] Since then the number of such "Lambeth degrees" was reduced, though one was still granted as late as 1880. The legal right to use an M.D. title conferred by the Archbishop continues to exist to the present day, provided the recipient is already on the Medical Register.[22]

Jewish law provided for the control of physicians since very early times. Already in the *Tosephta*[23] there is a reference to "an expert doctor who healed by permission of the [ecclesiastical] court". This reference is repeated in all the major codes, too (*Y.D., cccxxxvi.*1). Whether this sanction refers to a formal licence or registration of physicians cannot be established, nor do the sources shed any light on the conditions under which the "permission to heal" was granted. But it is evident that the rabbinical authorities were held responsible for ensuring the attainment of satisfactory standards by physicians and for the certification of their competence. In granting or withholding their sanction, the rabbis did not exercise an ecclesiastical right as much as a juridical prerogative vested in them as the administrators of civil as well as religious law. In the talmudic order of society they were charged with many similar supervisory duties.[24] The obligation of rabbinical courts "to set up [officers] appointed [to have control] over prices, so that everyone shall not make profits as he pleases" is still codified by KARO (*H.M., ccxxxi.*20). So is their duty to appoint inspectors of weights, measures and scales who shall prosecute any shopkeepers guilty of fraudulence (*ib.*, 2). It may be assumed that, in certifying the competence of physicians, too, the rabbis relied on the advice of special experts appointed for the purpose.

As late as the 19th century we still learn of a rabbinical ruling[25] against a Turkish ecclesiastical court which had wrongly certificated an unqualified doctor whose treatment had proved dangerous. The Jewish system, therefore, would appear to represent the oldest, and certainly the longest established, form of regular control over the practice of medicine. It gradually disappeared only after the licensing of physicians by the civil authorities came into general force. Already in the 18th century AZULAY[26] declared: "These days, when no person may practise medicine except by permission of the masters, anyone who engages in medicine is regarded as qualified [in Jewish law]". Later rabbis frequently confirmed the view that "all our physicians enjoy the status of 'competent doctors', because they are required to pass an examination before leading physicians appointed by the government".[27]

PHYSICIANS' LIABILITIES

While in general, then, provisions for medical licensure and supervision were few and far between before the 12th century, most ancient and medieval legislations set forth more or less elaborate laws on the physician's liability for damages. Some codes treated doctors with extraordinary harshness, others with great leniency. The first to codify the physician's responsibilities were the Babylonians.[28] According to the Code of HAMMURABI,[29] whose laws were rooted in the *lex talionis*, a doctor was liable to have his right arm removed if an operation he performed proved fatal. There were corresponding penalties of a retaliatory character for injuries sustained by free men in the course of their treatment. Persian law punished a surgeon whose patient died for "wilful murder", unless he had previously performed successful operations on three unbelievers.[30] In Egypt a physician could be put to death if he treated anyone in an unauthorised manner with fatal consequences.[31]

The earliest European legislations, outside Greece and Rome, were equally severe. At about the turn of the 5th century *C.E.*, an edict was issued under THEODORIC, King of the Ostrogoths, providing that, if a patient died through an operation, "the physician should be handed over to the relatives of the deceased to do what they pleased with him".[32] The Visigothic Code (5th-7th centuries) also followed the pattern set by the Code of HAMMURABI,[33] and so did some of the early Irish legislations, such as the Brehon laws.[34] Among the Greeks and Romans, on the other hand, the physicians won for themselves almost complete immunity from the law. The Greek law did not assign any legal responsibilities to doctors at all, even when the killing of their patients was premeditated.[35] The contemporaneous writer PHILEMON[36] therefore stated with justice that only the doctor had the right to kill but not to be killed. PLINY[37] reported similar conditions among the Romans, although the *Lex Cornelia*, as we have noted, had rendered a physician liable to arrest if he could be charged with fatal negligence.

During the Middle Ages the more severe laws generally prevailed. Where these did not operate effectively, the law of the mob would often wreak vengeance on the unsuccessful physician. We learn, for instance, that when a nobleman of Bologna was injured in 1250 no-one could be found to attend the case for fear of being lynched, should the treatment fail. Eventually, he was treated by a surgeon, but only after thirty friends had taken an oath that no harm would befall him.[38] In the 15th century an unsuccessful physician was still burnt to death by JOHN XXII; and when that Pope died, his friends flayed the surgeon who had failed to keep him alive.[39] A similar fate befell the first Jewish doctor in recorded Russian history, MESSER LEON of Venice, whom IVAN III took into his service; he was publicly beheaded in 1490 after the Grand Duke's son failed to respond to his treatment and died.[40] These conditions naturally helped to discourage the practice and progress of surgery for a long time.[41]

The medico-legal system of Judaism was, in the view of a modern historian,[42] from the beginning further advanced than the Babylonian. Jewish law sought to steer a middle course between the complete exoneration of the physician, leading to recklessness, and his subjection to such rigorous penal sanctions as would shy away students from medical careers or stifle enterprising methods of treatment. On the whole, the distinction between physicians and ordinary people causing physical harm to their fellow-men is greater in the case of injuries than if death ensues. In the former event, the doctor is placed into the same privileged category as a father or a teacher chastising a child, or a court official administering corporal punishment, with injurious effects. Like them, the physician—provided he is authorised by the court — is liable to pay damages for injuries inflicted in error only if he exceeded the proper bounds within which the operation should have been confined.[43] The *Tosephta*[44] —the original source of all these regulations—explains that this concession was enacted "for the sake of the social order", that is, as commentary[45] has it, "because, although a human being is always liable to [pay] full indemnity [even for damage done unwittingly], he is exonerated [in this case], so that doctors shall be found to heal". The physician is, however, still held to account before the Heavenly tribunal. But if the physician caused an injury deliberately, or acted without the court's permission however competent his skill, he can be sued for damages.[46] These regulations are still recorded in the *Shulhan 'Arukh*[47] (*Y.D., cccxxxvi*.1). Only in one instance is the authorised physician not exempted from legal liability for errors leading to injuries: If the patient was the doctor's own non-Jewish slave,[48] and he sustained a material injury in the course of his treatment, he must be granted his freedom under the biblical law of manumission (*Ex. xxi*.26-27), even though the master had performed the operation for his benefit (*Y.D., cclxvii*.36).

In contrast to the infliction of injuries, the death of a patient does not entitle the doctor responsible to the same privilege as is enjoyed by a father or a teacher who accidentally killed a child whilst beating it. While the latter are completely acquitted,[49] "[a physician] who killed [his patient], and realised that he was in error, is exiled [to the cities of refuge[50]]" (*Y.D., cccxxxvi*.1)—suffering the biblical penalty applicable to any "manslayer that killeth any person through error" (*Nu., xxxv*.11 *ff.*; and *Deut., xix*.3 *ff.*). The *Tosephta*,[51] on which this law, too, is based, again stipulates that the physician must have acted with the court's permission. It also mentions, as a parallel case, "one who dismembers an embryo in the mother's womb and killed [her]". The physician, then, is legally distinguished from an ordinary murderer in so far as his action, though deliberate in itself, is not held to contain the element of "guile"[52] (*Ex. xxi*.14). Nor is he guilty unless he became subsequently aware of his mistake. Otherwise, as NACHMANIDES[53] points out, he is free from all liability, just as a judge must pay compensation for a false award only if he afterwards recognised his error.[54] But if the doctor's treatment was correct, though unsuccessful, it is assumed that "the Creator desired [the patient's] death [in any case]".[55]

According to SOLOMON LURIA,[56] the doctor's guilt is also conditional on death resulting immediately from the abortive operation, to exclude the contribution of other factors to the fatal outcome.

The physician's liability may also compromise his status in a purely ritual respect. A priest who has slain a human being, even unwittingly, is disqualified from bestowing "the priestly benediction" (*Nu. vi*.24 *ff.*) upon the congregation by "the raising of hands"[57] (*O.H.*, *cxxviii*.35). Special reasons[58] account for the exclusion from this rule of a priest who circumcised an infant with fatal results (*ib.*, 36). But it may be assumed that a doctor of priestly descent to whom such an accident occurred is debarred from the performance of this rite, though the problem is, surprisingly, altogether ignored in the codes as well as in all the classic responsa.[59]

The regulations detailed in this chapter did not, it appears, find much practical application in Jewish life. Indeed, it is remarkable how rarely questions or disputes on the liability of doctors were referred to rabbinic judgment. For it is significant that these medico-legal subjects were treated only in the *Tosephta* and the codes, not in the Talmud proper or in the great responsa works—the two literary stores which usually reflect most faithfully the social conditions and problems of their time. An important reason for the absence of law-suits on these issues may be the reluctance to litigate against physicians owing to the high respect and confidence which they always enjoyed in Jewish society.[60]

CHAPTER EIGHTEEN

THE PHYSICIAN — 3

HIS PROFESSIONAL CHARGES

Physicians were no doubt the first—and, for very long, the only—occupational group of men whose right to, or even scale of, remuneration for their services was fixed by law. Already in the Code of HAMMURABI[1] we find a list of medical charges varying according to the success and the severity of the operation and to the patient's status as a freeman or a slave. The ancient Indian doctors, like other learned men, were free from taxes and other charges. While their services were generally rewarded by presents, their claims of payment were not small.[2] Similar conditions obtained in Egypt where physicians were often, moreover, maintained at the public expense as officials of the temple or the community. But they were expected to give free treatment to the poor as well as to soldiers and travellers. Some doctors, however, also practised privately by individual contract.[3] Greece, too, knew of a communal health service at quite an early period, though wealthy patients probably showed their recognition by gifts.[4]

But gradually this system gave way to the individual employment and payment of physicians. In Hippocratic times they were regarded as paid craftsmen; as such they were subject to the same aristocratic prejudice as any manual labourer—a fact which somewhat impeded medical progress.[5] The conditions are also illustrated by PLATO's complaint that the mass of the population had no medical service, since they could not afford to pay for any. As a result most people continued to have recourse to the healing shrines where the fees were small by comparison.[6] Yet, a Hippocratic writer[7] recommended doctors to take their patients' circumstances into account and to treat the stranger and the poor gratis. In Rome, as in most ancient societies, the payment of physicians in advance was the rule.[8] The majority of them were poor and often unable to support themselves. But a few received fabulous fees, and PLINY[9] speaks with particular bitterness of the avaricious demands made by the Greek doctors in Rome.[10] The Emperor AUGUSTUS granted physicians immunity from taxation and other burdens, and similar privileges were conferred on them by VESPASIAN and HADRIAN.[11] The Justinian Code[12] marked a return to the Hippocratic ideals in laying down that the public physician "shall choose rather to do honest service for the poorest than to be disgracefully subservient to the rich".

Christian theologians concerned themselves with medical fees only insofar as they affected the treatment of the poor, as an act of charity, or the practice of medicine by priests who, in cases of disputes, had to submit to the *jus canonicum*.[13] Later the interest of the Church was further limited by the close association of healing with the monasteries. These provided a sufficient living for clerical practitioners[14] in much the same way as the Church supports her medical missionaries today. But the Church did not seek to prescribe the professional charges of lay physicians or to challenge their right to a financial reward. Nor were their scales of remuneration fixed by civil statutes until comparatively modern times. Consequently, the material standards of physicians varied greatly. In some places the income of medieval doctors was often considerable, since their number was relatively small, and even practitioners not enjoying great renown made a good living.[15] In Elizabethan England, on the other hand, the medical fees were rather meager; but the surgeons were fairly well paid, whilst the apothecaries fared best of all.[16] The earliest American medical legislation (17th century) was, like the Code of HAMMURABI, again mainly concerned with the question of fees,[17] but in Europe family doctors often lived on gifts until the end of the 19th century.[18]

In Jewish law and practice the physician's title to payment was recognised from the beginning. Already the Bible decrees that, if a man inflicts an injury on his neighbour, "he shall cause him to be thoroughly healed" (*Ex. xxi*.19) —an obvious reference to the defrayment of medical expenses, as assumed in the *Septuagint*, the *Targum* and the *Vulgate* as well as by JOSEPHUS,[19] all rendering the phrase by: "he shall pay the doctor's fee".[20] In the Talmud[21] the indemnity for healing expenses is listed among the five items of compensation due by law to an injured party, and wide currency was enjoyed by the adage "a doctor for nothing is worth nothing"[22]—a proverb strikingly similar to the line attributed to the School of Salerno: " . . . *si quae detur gratis, nil affert utilitatis* . . . ".[23] This truism may also have inspired the 10th century medical writer ISAAC ISRAELI to declare in his *Aphorisms*: "The more thou demandest for thy service . . . , the greater will [it] appear in the eyes of the people. Thine art will be looked upon as insignificant by those whom thou treatest for nothing".[24]

At the same time, the Talmud naturally commends the ideal of free treatment for the poor. It holds up the example of "ABBA, the Bleeder, [who] had a box placed outside his office where his fees were to be deposited. Whoever had money put it in, but those who had none could come in without feeling embarrassed. When he saw a person who was in no position to pay, he would offer him some money, saying to him: 'Go, strengthen thyself [after the bleeding operation]' ".[25] This ideal was reiterated by Jewish medical authors at all times. ASAF JUDAEUS abjured his pupils: "Do not close thy heart to mercy toward the poor and the needy",[26] and he wrote a special chapter on medicine for the poor, comprising remedies which required no outlay.[27] ISAAC ISRAELI, his general attitude to fees notwithstanding, exhorted the physician: "Make it thy special concern to visit and treat poor and needy patients, for in no way canst thou find more meritorious service".[28] In the 16th century AMATUS LUSITANUS swore that he had "not been desireful for the remuneration for medical services and [that he had] treated many without accepting any fee, but with nonetheless care".[29] A century later JACOB ZAHALON of Rome urged that doctors "should not accept a fee from the poor nor from relatives and close friends".[30]

Only in the case of communal appointments were doctors not always expected to attend the poor without payment. The Portuguese-Jewish Congregation in Hamburg, for example, decided in 1666 not to accept the offer by a physician to treat the poor gratis as an act of charity, because "it is not fitting to engage someone without salary; for the payment will force the doctor to be in time when called in by a patient".[31] Yet in Poland, during the 17th and 18th centuries, physicians employed by the community or its sick-visitation societies were generally required to attend the poor gratuitously and to pay regular visits to the communal hospital; but in return they also enjoyed special privileges, including their exemption from many taxes and sometimes even the grant of a free residence.[32]

Jewish law introduced a further element into the ethical considerations regarding the physician's fees. According to a ruling by NACHMANIDES[33] recorded in the *Tur*[34] and the *Shulhan 'Arukh* (*Y.D.*, *cccxxxvi*.2), "[the physician] may accept payment only for loss of time and for his trouble, but not for instruction, since it is a matter of the decrease of his body [*i.e.* the health of one's neighbour] concerning which Scripture says: 'Thou shalt restore it to him'[35] (*Deut. xxii*.2), and we maintain in the fulfilment of religious precepts [the rule] 'Just as I [*i.e.* God acts] gratuitously, so shall you [render religious duties] gratuitously';[36] hence it is forbidden [to receive] payment for [one's medical] knowledge or instruction". This limitation, though already found in the *Sepher Hasidim*[37] and other early writings,[38] is not mentioned by MAIMONIDES. Doctors are thus placed into the same category as religious teachers (*Y.D., ccxlvi.5*), judges[39] (*H.M., ix.5*) and rabbis (*Y.D., ccxlvi.21*, gloss) who must not accept a reward for their professional services, though they may claim compensation for the interruption of their ordinary occupation during the time spent on their religious work.

This rule presupposed, and encouraged, the exercise of rabbinical and educational functions on a non-professional basis—a system which survived in some Jewish communities until the 15th century.[40] But it is doubtful whether, even before the professionalisation of the learned pursuits, Jewish physicians, too, actually practised their craft in harmony with this principle of honorary service. The frequent combination of the rabbinical and medical professions in the Middle Ages—with the income from the latter enabling the former occupation to be carried out without payment— would rather suggest that in practice the opposition was limited to the gainful pursuit of religion only. Evidently the legal fiction—of accepting payment not for services rendered, but for "interrupted labour" or simply for general subsistence, whereby the rabbis eventually justified the professionalisation of their calling[41] (*ib.*)— had always been applied to medical practitioners.[42]

Nevertheless, the law may have been a factor in discouraging the charging of fees from individual patients and it may thus have promoted the early development of communal medicine instead. While the Talmud evidently knew of no public medical appointments as the Egyptians and Greeks did,[43] such arrangements were fairly popular in medieval times. In Spain Jewish physicians played a prominent role in this system of "socialised medicine",[44] and elsewhere, too, many Jewish communities included a staff of surgeons, physicians, nurses and midwives among their salaried servants.[45] Even religio-legal sources take account of these conditions. A 13th century Spanish scholar[46] mentions doctors in the group of professionals paid by the community; as such they were not required, for instance, to replace an article lent to, or deposited with, them if it was lost or stolen whilst they were engaged on their work. This concession is also codified, though only communal blood-letters are specified in this category (*H.M.*, *cccvi.*12). Communally appointed barbers, but again no physicians, are further mentioned among the public officials who may be dismissed without notice if found guilty of neglect (*H.M.*, *cccvi.*8).

Notwithstanding the restriction on medical charges, it is evident that Jewish law tolerated the paid treatment of patients by private contract even in theory. In fact, NACHMANIDES[47]—again followed by KARO—maintains that the patient is liable to honour an agreement reached with his physician, even if it stipulated the payment of an excessive fee, for the very reason that the latter "sold him his expert knowledge which is beyond price" (*Y.D.*, *cccxxxvi.*3). Reference is also made without scruples to places where "it is the custom to give a reward to the physician", though the alternative practice of engaging a doctor without payment is mentioned at the same time (*Y.D.*, *ccxxi.*4). Moreover, the Talmud and the codes legislate at considerable length on legal claims in respect of sickness benefits and medical expenses, including the liability to the payment of doctors' bills. Thus, the law determines the husband's responsibility for medical expenses incurred by his wife on account of sickness (*E.H.*, *lxix.*2; and *lxxix.*1 and 3) or injuries (*E.H.*, *lxxxiii.*1), even if she turned insane[48] (*E.H.*, *lxx.*4); the obligation of heirs to defray the cost of medical attendance on the deceased (*H.M.*, *cviii.*1, gloss) and his widow (*E.H.*, *lxxix.*2); the division of medical costs among business partners if one of them fell ill (*H.M.*, *clxxvii.*2 and 3); and, above all, the compensation due to victims of violence and the basis on which the doctor's and other healing charges are to be assessed (*H.M.*, *cdxx.*3-23).

In contrast to the views on the physician's right to charge professional fees, the decisions on the treatment of the poor were more liberal in practice than in theory. Although, as we have seen, Jewish physicians were always prepared to attend insolvent patients without payment, there was no specific law requiring them to do so. Indeed, a ruling on this issue was sought only in the 19th century, when a rabbi[49] decided that, if a doctor refused to visit a patient who could not afford to pay his fee, the religious court could compel the doctor to give his services free of charge. The judgment was based on a similar verdict pronounced by AD-RETH[50] six centuries earlier, but the offender then was a circumciser, not a physician. ISSERLES codified the decision thus: "If the father does not know how to circumcise, and there is a circumciser who does not wish to perform the operation except for payment, it is [proper] to rebuke him, for that is not the way of ABRAHAM's seed; on the contrary, circumcisers regard it as an honour to be permitted to carry out that rite.[51] But if he persists in his refusal, and the father has no means to pay his fee, [the child] is considered as if it has no father and the obligation to circumcise it then rests with the court; hence, in the absence of another [competent person] who would perform the act, they can force the circumciser [to do so]" (*Y.D.*, *cclxi.*1, gloss). According to JACOB EMDEN,[52] it would then be lawful even to deceive the official by assuring him of his recompense without paying it to him afterwards. The medical practitioner who fails to treat the poor when he is in a position to do so may not have been subjected to quite the same pressure, but it was to such a doctor that the opprobium "To hell with the best of the physicians" was mainly applied.[53]

PAYMENT FOR SERVICES ON THE SABBATH

A question not dealt with in the codes concerns the right to be remunerated for medical services rendered on the Sabbath or other holy days. The problem arises from the law, clearly laid down in the Talmud[54] and the codes (*O.H.*, *cccvi.*4), that it is forbidden to pay wages to a hired labourer in respect of work done on the Sabbath, unless the payment covers a period of employment of which the Sabbath is an unspecified part.[55] As far as it affects medical attendance, the question was first raised in the 15th century by the German rabbis JACOB WEIL[56] and ISRAEL BRUNA[57] who permitted a midwife to receive payment for assisting a Jewess on the Sabbath on the grounds that her liability to be called at any time might technically be regarded as an employment for a period within which the Sabbath is absorbed and that, moreover, the fear that she might not be paid could lead to her withdrawal or negligence. Since the 19th century doctors were granted a similar concession in several responsa.[58] These referred to BRUNA's arguments and decision as a valid precedent; but, while one of them suggested it would be better to pay physicians either for a complete cure or at least on a weekly basis,[59] another held that professional services on the Sabbath could be charged for only if they had been engaged on the previous day and if no specified sum was mentioned as the fee.[60] Some rabbis, however, opposed the collection of any fees for distinct work done on the Sabbath, since the argument of negligence was not applicable to conscientious doctors.[61] This opinion was already advanced by JACOB ZAHALON[62] who urged that the physician "should not accept a fee for his services on holy days and Sabbaths", though he added: "Others permit this to be done by including it in the general charge for the weekdays". MOSES SCHREIBER[63] advised that fees from non-Jewish patients for Sabbath attendances should be given to charity, as one ought not to derive a personal benefit from them. A later authority, incidentally, ruled that physicians could legitimately charge a fee for viewing the dead and issuing a death certificate, even though it was unlawful to make a profit from the dead.[64]

PRICE OF MEDICINES

Jewish law also concerns itself with the price of medicines. Directly the Talmud[65] refers to this only by relating of a sage who offered the medicines he possessed free to all who wished to have some. But it also mentions two related issues[66] from which the following important inference was drawn: "He who has drugs, and his sick neighbour requires them, is forbidden to raise their price above the proper level. Furthermore, even if they agreed on a high price because of the need of the hour—for the drugs could only be found in his hand—he may only claim their [actual] value" (*Y.D., cccxxxvi.3*). In this respect, therefore, the charges of apothecaries are controlled more strictly than those of physicians who, as we have observed, may legally claim the payment of any fee, however excessive, if it had been agreed upon previously (*ib.*). Hence, when the 16th century Algerian talmudist ABRAHAM IBN TUVVAH[67] was asked whether a patient was required to honour his promise to pay a physician an unduly high sum for both the treatment and the medicines he had received, the reply was that the undertaking had to be carried out only in regard to the treatment, since the doctor "had sold his wisdom which is beyond measure". The rabbi added, however, that this ruling was subject to the patient's prior agreement to pay such a high fee; otherwise the doctor could merely claim compensation for his trouble and loss of time. But DAVID IBN ZIMRA,[68] also of the 16th century, ruled in similar circumstances that, notwithstanding any prior accord, payments above the usual rates could be claimed neither for medicines nor for professional services, if no other equally competent doctor was available; for "in that case the duty to heal. . . devolves upon him alone, and if he fails to discharge it, he transgresses a religious precept". Perhaps these rulings were not altogether unrelated to the advice of ZAHALON[69] a century later: "The physician should not sell the drugs himself, but the patient should send to the druggist. . .".

The legally enforced limitation of profits on the sale of pharmaceutical products is of particular interest when one remembers the exorbitant prices for drugs often charged by apothecaries, especially in 17th century England. Their unscrupulous exploitation of disease was immortalised by the century's leading poets, ALEXANDER POPE and Dr. GARTH. The latter, for instance, wrote bitterly:

"Thrice happy were these golden days of old,
When dear as Burgundy, ptisans were sold,
When patients chose to die with better will,
Than live to pay the 'pothecaries' bill".[70]

No less strikingly in contrast with the Jewish legislation against overcharges were the earliest professional rules drawn up by the apothecaries themselves. The "Code of Ethics" promulgated by the Philadelphia College of Pharmacy in 1848—the first pharmaceutical code ever issued—decreed that "no apothecary should intentionally undersell his neighbour with a view to his injury".[71] But there was no law to protect the customers from injury by fixing a maximum price for the apothecary's wares. A few years later the newly-founded American Pharmaceutical Association embodied a similar provision in the second article of its Ethical Code,[72] but the clause was eventually omitted in the revised code of 1922.[73]

CHAPTER NINETEEN

THE PHYSICIAN—4

THE ADMISSION OF HIS EVIDENCE

The administration of Jewish law, owing to its wide ram-ifications in every sphere of human activity, often pre-supposes a thorough knowledge of facts and circumstances which can be established only by competent experts. Accurate data bearing on medicine in particular may frequently de-termine religious decisions in virtually all branches of the Jewish law codes. Medical factors must be considered in the application of Judaism's civil and criminal laws, and of many other social as well as purely ritual regulations. Indeed, the resultant association of rabbinical and medical functions is so close that the members of the *Sanhedrin*, or Supreme Court, were required, according to MAIMONIDES,[1] to include a knowledge of medicine among their academic qualifications, so that—as a commentator[2] explains—they would be able, for example, to identify deadly poisons in murder trials or to distinguish between natural and magic cures.[3]

But since in practice the rabbis could hardly be expected to combine medical studies with their rabbinical training, they were compelled to seek opinions of physicians as a basis for many of their own rulings. The question therefore arose whether, and to what extent, such medical evidence could be utilised for the solution of religious problems. This question, treated technically under the heading of "the doctors' trust-worthiness", has exercised the minds of Jewish legislators in almost all ages, and its consideration occupies an important position in rabbinic literature.[4] A religious medical writer in Israel has recently suggested that the legal concept of "the doctors' trustworthiness" was created to emphasise "the moral responsibility of the Jewish physician in medical issues which border on the territory of religious principles. . ."[5]

The value of the moral factor cannot be gainsaid, but it must not obscure the purely legal aspect as the primary element in the shaping of this concept. The talmudic sages already recognised that the Jewish laws of evidence were not always completely rational and that the mere establishment or corroboration of the truth was not in itself their sole *rationale*. Some of them were regarded simply as "scriptural decrees", transcending the norms of logic and utility. Thus, Jewish jurisprudence refuses to accept the joint testimony of closely related persons—a provision explained in the Talmud[6] and the codes in these significant terms: "That the *Torah* disqualified the evidence of relatives is not due to the presumption that they have a friendly bias one towards the other. . . : even MOSES and AARON [however unimpeachable their integrity] are not qualified to act as witnesses one for [or with] the other; it is [therefore] only a scriptural decree" (*H.M.*, *xxxiii*.10.). This conclusion is further confirmed by the clause that proselytes, even if they are twin-brothers, may yet give evidence for each other, since they are legally regarded as "new-born" from the moment of their conversion to Judaism (*ib.*, 11; and *Y.D.*, *cclxix*.10). Conversely, as MAIMONIDES[7] is at pains to stress, "we are commanded to decide the law on the evidence of two qualified witnesses, and although it is possible that they testify falsely, we assume their fitness once they are [legally] qualified. Regarding such matters it is stated: 'The secret things belong unto the Lord our God, but the things that are revealed belong unto us' (*Deut. xxix*.28)."

A further important consideration must be borne in mind to appreciate the attitude to the admission of witnesses peculiar to Judaism. The evidence, to be valid, has to be submitted by eye-witnesses whose account of the facts must be complete (*H.M.*, *xxx*.13) and based on their personal verification.[8] Circumstantial evidence[9] or statements founded on mere knowledge or assessments are never admitted in capital cases,[10] and even in civil litigations such collateral or indirect evidence is at best accepted only in exceptional circumstances (*ib.*, 14; and *xc.*16). The sanction to rely on evidence in religious issues, too, is qualified by numerous conditions (*Y.D.*, *cxxvii.*3, gloss), particularly when offered by non-Jews (*Y.D.*, *xcviii.*1 and gloss; and *cccxiii.*2, gloss) or Jews whose own loyalty to the laws affected by their testimony is not beyond all doubt (*Y.D.*, *cxix.*1 *ff.*). All these general principles combine to form the essential background to the subject under discussion in this chapter.

The religious problem of "the doctors' trustworthiness" can arise in a variety of circumstances. Thus we have already seen in previous chapters that, while any physician's opinion is unreservedly accepted if given to certify the need for violating religious observances in the face of danger to life,[12] some rabbis hold that medical evidence regarding the onset of death[13] and the risk of infection when sucking the circumcision wound[14] may not be admitted if it conflicts with the rules laid down in Jewish law. But the real problem which has engaged so much attention in rabbinic literature concerns the validity of the physician's evidence when it affets mainly ritual decisions, especially in connection with the complex laws of menstrual uncleanliness.

The Talmud records no discussion on the problem itself, but it mentions several instances of religious and legal judgments based on medical evidence.[15] In some cases, as we shall indicate, the talmudic view was still accepted without reservation in the codes; in others they already introduced some limitations on "the doctors' trustworthiness".[16] In the administration of justice, for example, competent estimates, presumably by physicians, were sought to assess such data as the likely duration of an injured person's recuperation[17] (*H.M.*, *cdxx.*18), an offender's ability to survive the rigours of corporal punishment,[18] and whether the blow sustained by a person who ultimately succumbed to his injuries was directly responsible for his death.[19] In the latter two cases the medical verdict may clearly be of immediate consequence to the convict's life. Again, a midwife was relied upon to identify the first-born son in the event of a twin-birth[20] (*H.M., cclxxvii.*12). A healer's claim to be competent in the use of amulets was also accepted[21] (*O.H., ccci.*26). But regarding the establishment of the cause of death (to determine the validity of a conditional bill of divorce[22]) only the Talmud[23] was prepared to trust medical opinion; KARO shared the fear of ADRETH[24] that an unscrupulous and interested party might extort a statement favourable to himself from the doctor (*E.H., cxlv.*9), while ISSERLES categorically stated that in the view of some authorities "one must not rely at the present time on physicians' estimates [in such cases]"[25] (*ib.*, gloss). Yet he agreed to advise women to consult physicians on the effects of a hair lotion on allowing the proper contact between the body and the water at a ritual immersion[26] (*Y.D., cxcix.*2, gloss).

The Talmud also relates several specific cases in which physicians were consulted and their statements accepted in religious matters. Special experts were engaged to determine whether blemishes in first-born animals were transitory or permanent (warranting their slaughter and consumption by the owner).[27] On two occasions religious decisions were made on the strength of statements made by "THUDOS, the Physician", probably on alumnus of the Alexandrian school of medicine.[28] His declaration that in Alexandria the wombs of all pigs and cows were removed prior to their exportation (to prevent competitive breeding abroad) was used to prove that animals whose uterus was missing could live and were, therefore, ritually fit.[29] Again, he had identified some human bones placed before him as belonging to different skeletons and thus solved a problem regarding the laws of priestly defilement.[30]

Of particular importance are the talmudic accounts[31] of certain substances aborted by two women on the evidence of which the rabbis were asked to decide whether the women were ritually impure; the rabbis, in turn, submitted the exhibits to "the doctors" whose analysis of these unusual discharges, followed by a practical test,[32] determined the rabbinical verdict. But it is not clear whether the test was applied by the physicians to reach their conclusions, or suggested by the rabbis to confirm the diagnosis by independent means. KARO,[33] as well as several earlier authorities,[34] evidently accepted the former interpretation; hence, he was prepared to admit certain gynecological evidence, provided it was submitted by a Jewish doctor[35] (*Y.D., clxxxvi.*8). But ISSERLES,[36] in common with other dissenting scholars,[37] held that the medical opinion was accepted only because the rabbis corroborated it by their test.[38]

This controversy helped to furnish the basis for the many arguments and dissertations on the subject in nearly all subsequent responsa works of which only a brief summary can here be given. On several issues opinions varied widely. While MOSES SCHREIBER[39]—one of the most copious writers in this field—would accept the general facts established by medical research but not necessarily an individual diagnosis made by a doctor, another rabbi[40] subscribed to almost the reverse view. A third authority[41] admitted the reliability of medical evidence only in respect of cures and medicines, but not in regard to the cause of pathological symptoms. Underlying the growing hesitation to acknowledge medical findings as absolute was the belief that the standards of medical science had declined since the times of the Talmud—a belief to which ISSERLES, as we have seen, already gave emphatic expression.[42] Yet, more recent scholars agreed that with the use of instruments, especially the "uterine mirror", the results of medical examinations could be relied upon more readily.[43] It was, however, advisable that any medical problem affecting a religious decision should be submitted to the physician by a rabbi,[44] and that a questioner should not accept the physician's judgment for practical religious purposes until he had consulted rabbinical opinion, too.[45] The doctor whose advice was sought should himself be a God-fearing and observant Jew, and conscious of the gravity of the religious issues to be resolved through him. Consequently, the evidence of a conscientious non-Jewish practitioner might be accepted with greater assurance than that of a non-practising Jew,[46] while the statements of either would be regarded as less reliable than the findings of a trustworthy Jewish midwife.[47]

The reluctance of the rabbis to base their judgments on the physicians' opinions certainly did not imply that any aspersion was cast on the importance of their work, or indeed on the value of medical research even in the determination of some religious principles. The rabbis, in their responsa, often urged their questioners to consult doctors and to hear their views.[48] Frequently rabbinic decisions were justified or supported by quotations from medical sources. LAMPRONTI[49] cited the writings of HIPPOCRATES, "the head of the physicians", in a halachic context, and some original rulings in the code of MAIMONIDES were attributed to "his medical erudition"[50] and to "his greatness in medicine and the natural sciences".[51]Some of the rabbis' hygienic and dietary enactments, too, were assumed to be based on the health rules established by "the physicians".[52] Even in regard to the interpretation of biblical laws, the rabbis often relied on the counsel of medical experts, and there is a collection[53] of several instances from the responsa showing that the rabbinical authors sought and accepted technical guidance on medico-religious questions from physicians,[54] midwives[55] and even from the medical faculties of various universities.[56]

CHAPTER TWENTY

THE PHYSICIAN—5

PRIESTS AS PHYSICIANS

In ancient history the practice of medicine was, probably in its very origin, an integral part of the priest's ministrations. To him and his craft resorted those broken in body and spirit alike. Priestly medicine, which had grown into a highly organised system especially in Babylonia and Egypt, continued to flourish even in Greece, with its many shrines and cults, long after the rise of rational therapy.[1] We have previously often noted how close the personal association between religion and medicine remained throughout the Middle Ages,[2] and it may be characteristic that the only pope whom DANTE met in Paradise was JOHN XXI of the 13th century who had been the physician PETRUS HISPANUS.[3] After a comparatively brief break in this relationship, the present tendency is once again to seek a closer alliance between man's spiritual and physical mentors. "One of the most striking results of the modern developments of our knowledge concerning the influence of mental factors in disease", declared RIVERS[4] in his *Fitzpatrick Lecture* of 1923, "is that they are bringing back medicine in some measure to that co-operation with religion which existed in the early stages of human progress". In the same *Lecture* he also stated: "A striking feature of the last twenty years in this country is the frequent combination of priest and physician in one person, while in America a regular system of collaboration... has come into being in what is known as the Emmanuel movement".[5]

On the whole, the initiative and urge in this association

has come from within religion no less than from without. But, while in practice Judaism and Christianity have both encouraged the ministry's professional devotion to medicine, the Church was the more pronounced in her championship of this alliance as a matter of policy, if not of doctrine. "Monastic medicine", the ecclesiastical control of medical schools, the papal and "Lambeth degrees" of medicine, the "Ministry of Healing" and the medical work of the missionaries are all more or less distinct expressions of this attitude. In Judaism the conscious promotion of such an ideal is less in evidence. A common notion to the contrary notwithstanding, the Bible did not charge priests with medical duties,[6] and no provision in rabbinic Judaism sought to induce its ecclesiastics to practice the healing art. Nevertheless, the combination of the two professions was extremely popular among the Jews, as we have often pointed out.[7] In effect, then, the fusion of the two vocations represents a feature common to both religions, even though the respective causes leading to this development were very dissimilar.[8]

BAN ON PRIESTLY PHYSICIANS

In view of this long-established medico-theological relationship, it may appear extraordinary that opposition to the pursuit of medicine by priests is found in both Jewish and Christian teachings. But the motives, extent and practical effects of this opposition show only the most superficial resemblance. Christianity desired to divorce the priesthood from medicine because it regarded the two callings as fundamentally incompatible. In Judaism the objection to priestly physicians arose merely from an incidental aspect of medical work which might offend against the laws of priestly defilement.

Since the 12th century many Church councils and papal decretals have repeatedly forbidden clerics to engage in medicine and, particularly, in surgery.[9] In 1243 the Dominican Order even forbade medical treatises to be brought into the monasteries.[10] The very frequency with which this ban was reiterated in successive centuries seems to indicate that it was never completely obeyed.[11] Exemptions, too, were freely granted, often for political reasons.[12] But the ban remains in force to the present day.[13]

A variety of reasons were advanced for the interdict. Probably most prominent among these was the view expressed at the Council of Tours, held by ALEXANDER III in 1163, "that the devil, to seduce the priesthood from the duties of the altar, involved them in mundane occupations which, under the plea of humanity, exposed them to constant and perilous temptations."[14] The fear that the pursuit of medicine led the clergy to neglect their religious tasks is also mentioned as a principal factor by DIEPGEN,[15] GARRISON[16] and WALSH.[17] Some historians consider the edicts to be due to "the innate fear of rationalism" and to the fact "that the medical monks had become gluttenous and lascivious".[18] The aim to prevent clerics from treating wo--men is also acknowledged by PUSCHMANN[19] and GARRISON.[20] Other reasons suggested include the possibility of causing a patient's death[21] and especially the traditional "abhorrence of bloodshed" by the Church.[22]

In Jewish sources none of these motives are in any way related to the restrictions on the priestly exercise of medical functions. In any event, since in post-exilic times the Jewish priesthood was completely divorced from the ecclesiastical status it had enjoyed in the Temple cultus, the limitations are applicable only to Jews who trace their descent to AARON. The disability, therefore, strictly concerns laymen (in the professional sense); rabbis and other religious officials are altogether unaffected, unless they happen to be of priestly stock. The problem of such priests acting as physicians arises simply from the Biblical law (*Lev. xxi.*1, *et pass.*), which is still valid, forbidding the male descendants of AARON to defile themselves by contact with a human corpse, either by direct touch or by sharing a common roof with it.[23] This law is, of course, bound to affect the practice of medicine only insofar as it involves dealing with the dying or the dead in the course of one's medical studies or professional work. But there exists no objection in principle to priestly physicians; in fact, for the performance of circumcisions, priests were often preferred to others.[24]

Doctors of priestly lineage, by reason of the special restrictions imposed on them (to be detailed presently), naturally faced a number of religious problems not shared by other Jewish physicians. But there never was any formal ban on priests taking up medicine. Indeed, these problems were evidently raised only in comparatively late times. In the talmudic era, some of the most outstanding rabbi-physicians —including R. YISHMAEL[25] and SAMUEL whom we have mentioned several times—were of priestly descent.[26] So were a very considerable number of medical rabbis throughout the Middle Ages.[27] Yet none of them ever expressed the slightest scruples at the combination of the priesthood with medicine; nor did they even mention the special difficulties which might be expected to result from it.[28] Only from the 18th century onwards does the number of priests joining the medical profession appear, in fact, to fall short of their normal proportion to the rest of the Jewish population.[29] This phenomenon certainly reflects the growing misgivings with which the choice of a medical career by students of priestly descent came to be viewed.

PRIESTLY PHYSICIANS AND THE DEAD

In the codes and their principal commentaries there is still no reference to the problems affecting priestly physicians. It was only in more recent times that these difficulties were treated in rabbinic writings. The first question to be dealt with concerned the right of such doctors to visit patients during the final phase of life. Some authorities refer in this context to the precedent created by the Prophet

ELIJAH, himself a member of the priesthood, when he re-vived the dead child by physical contact[30] (I Kings *xvii*.17 *ff*.). Most rabbis rejected the view that KARO's ruling—forbidding priests to enter a house containing a dying per-son (*Y.D., ccclxx*.I)—applied to physicians, too. They re-lied on the amendment by ISSERLES—which legally per-mits priests to enter such a house but advises them to adopt the stricter view (*ib.*, gloss)—to sanction medical visits in these circumstances, at least if no other physician is avail-able to replace his priestly colleague.[31]

Far less favourable is the attitude taken towards the right of medical students who are priests to engage in anatomical dissections on human cadavers. One or two modern scholars are inclined to permit the practice, particularly if only non-Jewish bodies are used.[32] They base their leniency on a view attributed to ABRAHAM IBN DAUD[33] according to which the biblical ban on ritual defilement no longer binds priests in post-exilic times. But most authorities[34] oppose this view and strongly object to priests indulging in anatomical ex-aminations, even though a priestly student ignoring this ban may be considered merely an "unwitting sinner".[35] On the other hand, MOSES SCHREIBER[36] permits priests to take up medicine (provided their training involves no contact with the dead) even if, on being qualified, they may be re-quired to attend patients on their deathbed. But they may not defile themselves for the issuance of death certificates, unless the dead would otherwise remain unburied. A doctor defying these laws loses his priestly privileges until he undertakes to avoid contact with corpses in future.[37]

Recent responsa also give a variety of rulings on related problems. In particular, questions have often been raised in regard to the entry of priests into hospitals which may be presumed to house dead bodies from time to time. One res-ponsum permits priestly male nurses to work in such hos-pitals if necessary for their livelihood or in the interest of the sick.[38] Another allows priestly ministers of religion to accept a hospital chaplaincy for the visitation of the sick and the recitation of the confession prayer with the dying.[39] Ordinary priests, too, may visit hospitals, except if they definitely know Jewish corpses to be there at the time; but they are advised to enquire beforehand.[40] Similarly, priestly patients may go to hospital for urgent treatment, unless this can be procured with equal effect at home (notwithstanding any additional expenditure).[41] If a sick priest is in a building in which a death has occurred and he cannot be moved, the relatives of the deceased can be compelled to remove the body from it, since the laws of defilement take precedence over the respect due to the dead.[42] The fact that an amputated limb is also a source of defilement[43] (*Y.D.*, *ccclxix*.1) may well impose certain disabilities on surgeons of priestly stock. It may also be mentioned that a Roumanian rabbi forbade a boy of a priestly family to attend a school which contained a human skeleton.[44]

APPENDIX

ARTIFICIAL INSEMINATION

Procedures to bring about conception by artificial aids are of fairly recent origin. Legend has it that such methods were employed on horses as early as the 14th century.[1] But the first scientific research on artificial insemination in domestic animals was not carried out until late in the 18th century.[2] Experiments on human beings followed very soon afterwards, but no successful case was reported until 1866 when the first test-tube baby appeared in the United States.[3] Since then rapid and enormous advances have been made in this field. In Britain artificial insemination is not practised on a very large scale,[4] but in America there are today many thousands of human beings who were conceived as well as born in a clinic and whose fathers' identity is known only to God and the physician.[5] Accurate statistics cannot, for obvious reasons, be procured, and the incidence of such births usually becomes public knowledge only when it is by chance involved in some law-suit years later.

The legal position relating to artificial human insemination is still rather obscure and undefined. There does not appear to be any explicit legislation on the subject, either in Europe or in America. We can be guided only by a few, isolated judgments given in some celebrated court-cases. Thus the Supreme Court in Ontario (Canada) ruled in 1921 that artificial insemination with donated semen (A.I.D.) constituted adultery.[7] A similar conclusion is apparently indicated by Lord DUNEDIN's judgment in a British case which occurred in 1924,[8] but at least until 1947 no Amerian court had decided the issue.[9] In 1945 the then British

Minister of Health (Mr. WILLINK) told Parliament that he was advised "that it would be a breach of the law to register as legitimate a birth that occurred as a result of this operation when the husband was not in fact the father of the child".[10] As the law stands, therefore, there is little doubt that A.I.D. involves both the wife and the donor in an act of adultery and renders the child born in this way illegitimate.[11] On the other hand, A.I.H. (*i.e.* if the husband's semen is used) does not legally affect the marriage at all, and the resultant child enjoys the same status as that born after normal intercourse.[12]

The first Roman Catholic pronouncement on this problem was made in a Holy Office decree of 1897.[13] This has been followed by innumerable discussions and rulings in the many books and periodicals on Catholic moral philosophy and medical ethics. These make it clear that A.I.D. is definitely immoral, "because it is a violation of the natural law which limits the right to generate to married people, and which demands that right to be exercised personally and not by proxy".[14] In regard to A.I.H., however, Catholic opinions vary. But the margin of difference is being narrowed by a tendency among Catholic theologians in recent years to favour a stricter view which considers every form of artificial insemination as intrinsically unlawful except "assisted insemination in the wide sense", *i.e.* if it is applied after normal intercourse between husband and wife as an aid to the natural process, for instance by forcing the semen through artificial means into the wife's tract which it should have entered through the natural act, but was unable to enter owing to some physical impediment.[15] But there is practical unanimity among Catholic moralists that the husband may not procure the semen, either for medical examination in cases of suspected infertility or for artificial insemination into his wife, by any method which involves masturbation or other forms of *coitus interruptus*.[16]

The Protestant attitude is far less final and more flexible. In an official Report of the Church of England in 1948, all but one of the 13 commission members agreed that A.I.D. involved a breach of the marriage, was wrong in principle and contrary to Christian standards.[17] They recommended that, in view of the evils involved, early consideration should be given to the framing of legislation to make the practice a criminal offence. Regarding A.I.H. all members with again one exception agreed that even masturbation by the husband would be justifiable, if there was no other practicable alternative to bring about the successful insemination of the wife.[18]

For nearly thirty years now the problem has also been treated extensively in rabbinical quarters. Since Jewish law is based entirely on ancient authority and precedent, its treatment of such an altogether novel subject as artificial insemination may well serve as a classic example for the rabbinic method of applying old principles to new circumstances.

The first precedent found by the rabbis in this case represents a remarkable anticipation of one of the main factors involved in artificial insemination, some 1700 years before scientific research made its application in all but accidental cases possible. This occurs in a talmudic discussion[19] on whether a high priest is permitted to marry a virgin who is pregnant, notwithstanding the biblical insistence on her absolute virginity.[20] The answer given is in the affirmative, and the circumstances of her pregnancy are explained as due to an impregnation through water in which she had bathed and which was previously fertilized by a male. The possibility of such generation *sine concubito* was not apparently known to the Greeks or other nations of antiquity, and Jewish literature is certainly the first to refer to this recognition in a legal context.[21]

A second important precedent is contained in a late Midrash which is repeated in several medieval works, both historical and legal. It mentions the belief that BEN SIRAH was conceived in this way, the father having been the Prophet Jeremiah, and the mother, according to some sources, the Prophet's own daughter.[22] This Midrash, incidentally, is also quoted as "a legend of the rabbis" by the famous 16th century Marrano physician AMATUS LUSITANUS to clear a nun from the suspicion of fornication after a miscarriage.[23]

This Midrash has been utilized by various medieval authorities to establish the important principle that a man whose semen accidentally fertilized the female ovum by indirect contact through water is to be regarded as the legal father of the child so produced and is, in fact, considered as having fulfilled the religious duty of procreation in respect of that child.[24] Moreover, the early 18th century rabbi-physician ISAAC LAMPRONTI[25] proves from the account of BEN SIRAH's conception that such a child is not a *Mamzer*,[26] even if its father and mother would have committed an incestuous act had they had normal relations with each other. These rulings, though disputed by some authorities,[27] are of course of the greatest significance for our subject of A.I.D.

A further legal precedent to our problem is first mentioned by the 13th century glossator PERETZ BEN ELIJAH of Corbeil.[28] He rules that a woman must be careful with the use of linen on which a man other than her husband had lain, lest she become pregnant and the resultant child, not knowing the identity of the true father, marry the latter's daughter, *i.e.* his own sister. Yet he agrees that this offspring would not be regarded as born of an adulterous union, though the father is not the mother's husband. This ruling, which is also repeated by various later rabbis,[29] once again vindicates the principle that the relationship between father and child is not necessarily dependent on physical intercourse between the parents, and that, on the other hand, the legal consequences of incest render a child illegitimate only if the forbidden union between the parents was natural.

But there are scholars who do not agree with these rulings, or indeed with the literal interpretation of the talmudic passage and the traditional account of BEN SIRAH's conception. Thus JUDAH ROZANES,[30] the 18th century commentator of the code of MAIMONIDES, doubts if an impregnation through water can altogether be effected. Several eminent rabbis, even to the present century, have shared this view.[31] The historicity of BEN SIRAH's birth through a conception *sine concubito* has likewise been challenged centuries ago, for example, by DAVID GANS in his chonicle first published in 1592.[32] But the rather bold refusal of ROZANES and others to accept the literal meaning of a passage in the Talmud has been heatedly contested by such scholars as HAYIM J. D. AZULAY[33] and JONATHAN EYBESCHUETZ[34] in, respectively, the first and the second half of the 18th century.

The essential principles governing the Jewish legal attitude to A.I.D. have thus been laid down in the classics of Jewish law long ago. The considerations involved, though complex, may appear to warrant rather liberal conclusions on the legitimacy of the practice. Nevertheless, in the growing number of modern responsa on the subject, A.I.D. is unanimously and utterly condemned. The first to deal with the problem was probably the responsum in reply to an enquiry from Budapest dated 1930. Disregarding the earlier arguments on an accidental impregnation through water as irrelevant and resorting directly to a Biblical reference,[35] the author looks on A.I.D. as plain adultery and on the children so produced as *Mamzerim*.[36] But this extreme view found only isolated echoes in later responsa,[37] and the consensus of rabbinic opinion decidedly rejected both conclusions.

If Jewish law nevertheless opposes A.I.D. without reservation as utterly evil, it is mainly for moral reasons, not because of the intrinsic illegality of the act itself. The principal motives for the revulsion against the practice is the fear of the abuses to which its legalisation would lead, however great the benefits may be in individual cases. By reducing human generation to stud-farming methods, A.I.D. severs the link between the procreation of children and marriage, indispensable to the maintenance of the family as the most basic and sacred unit of human society. It would enable women to satisfy their craving for children without the necessity to have homes or husbands. It would pave the way to a disastrous increase of promiscuity, as a wife, guilty of adultery, could always claim that a pregnancy which her husband did not, or was unable to, cause was brought about by A.I.D., when in fact she had adulterous relations with another man. Altogether, the generation of children would become arbitrary and mechanical, robbed of those mystic and intimately human qualities which make man a partner with God in the creative propagation of the race.[38]

The practice would inevitably result in legal complications, too. Since only the mother, her husband and the physician are likely to know that the putative father is not, in fact, the child's progenitor at all, the mother—on the death of her husband—might be unlawfully freed from the levirate bond with his brother[39] on the false assumption that the deceased husband left a child. On the same assumption the child might be regarded as the legal heir to an inheritance which by law was due to someone else, or be deprived of an inheritance (from the donor) it could lawfully claim. The uncertainty about such children's paternity could quite conceivably lead to incestuous marriages;[40] for this reason they might have to be subjected to the severe marriage restrictions applicable to semi-foundlings.[41] The mother, while carrying or nursing a child begotten by a stranger, may also be debarred from conjugal relations with her husband during that period.[42] The whole procedure is therefore execrated as "an act of hideousness and an abomination of Egypt" in the unqualified verdict of all Jewish authorities.[43]

On A.I.H., however, rabbinic opinions are rather more favorable. The problem has often been discussed, especially in relation to the question whether a husband may produce a sample of his semen for medical testing. This, too, hinges largely around the controversy (already referred to) on whether a man who begot a child *sine concubito* has thereby fulfilled his duty of procreation. Otherwise the act would be condemned as "the bringing forth of semen for no purpose" which is strongly condemned in Jewish law (*E.H.*, *xxiii*.1-3). Yet there are some who hold that masturbation in such circumstances is unlawful even if the duty of procreation may thereby be fulfilled.[44] Others refute this view, holding that such an act performed for the sole purpose of making the eventual birth of a child possible can never be regarded as an offence, whether the precept of procreation is thereby technically carried out or not.[45] Although the majority view favours the more lenient attitude, sanction for such operations is granted only in extreme cases and with considerable reluctance;[46] furthermore, it is usually subject to the insemination not being made during the wife's period of impurity.[47]

From Israel has come very recently the welcome news of experiments which may eventually reduce, or altogether eliminate, the need for A.I.D. as an answer to sterile marriages when these are caused by a deficiency in the husband's semen. It appears now possible to use a donor's seminal plasma, completely freed from its sperm cells by a centrifugation process, and then resuspending the husband's spermatozoa in it to increase their motility and effectiveness on insemination into his wife.[48] If this method is indeed absolutely foolproof, and there is no possibility whatever of the donor's contribution producing any genetic traits in the offspring, the purely accessory function of the non-generative part of the donated seminal fluid may be regarded legally as being in the same category as blood-transfusions or skin-grafts transferred from one person to another. The procedure would then have to be adjudged like any other form of A.I.H.

NOTES

Foreword

[1] In addition to the authors cited in the present work who have treated the problems of medical ethics, among recent authors mention should be made of: W. Riese, Professor at the Medical College of Virginia, *La Pensée Morale en Médecine*, Paris, 1954; Professor P. M. Schuhl, *Le Merveilleux, la Pensée et l'Action*, Paris, 1952; Professor Pierre Mauriac, "Médecins et Philosophes" in *Histoire de la Médecine Francaise*, Paris, 1954; Professor H. Baruk and M. Bachet, *Le Test Tsedek, le Jugement Moral et la Délinquance*, Paris, 1950.

[2] *Cp.* Rashi *Ex.* XV, 26 and the commentaries of Ba'aleh Tosaphoth (*Da'at Zekenim*), and Nachmanides, on Ex. XV. 26; Issac Aboab in *Sefer Menorath Hamaor*, III, Chapter 183; *Sefer Hahinnukh*, 73; Isaac Arama, *Akeda*, Chapter 60. *Cp.* also M. M. Kasher, *Encyclopedia of the Pentateuch*, Tome XIV, pages 175 and 296.

[3] *Cp.* Dr. M. Grunwald, *Die Hygiene der Juden*, Dresden, 1911; H. Goslar, *Hygiene und Judentum*, Dresden, 1930. Many monographs treating special subjects have appeared in the reviews and periodicals cited in the bibliography at the end of this book.

[4] In antiquity, Jewish medical science already possessed a profound knowledge of anatomy. *Cp.* the article "Anatomy" in *The Medical and Health Thesaurus* (*'Otzar Ha-refu'ah Veha-bri'uth*, Tel Aviv, 1955) by Dr. A. Goldstein and Dr. M. Schechter. This knowledge was essentially based upon the dissection of animals and a highly developed empirical medicine. As concerns the latter, the illustrious Rabbi J. Karelitz (*Hazon 'Isch*) presents an extremely instructive chapter in his posthumous work, *'Emunah Bitahon*, Chapter V (Jerusalem, 1954).

[5] Pages 65–67.

[6] *Hilkhoth De'oth*, Chapter III and IV. See also *infra*, Chapter VII, page 93 *ff*.

[7] On the theories concerning psycho-physical relations, *cp.* C. Sommer, *Leib und Seele in Ihren Verhaltnis Zueinander*, Berlin, 1920.

[8] b'*Arakhin* 15b.

[9] *Deut*, Chapter XXVIII.

[10] *La Pensée Morale*, page 34. It must, however, be noted that, in general, modern medicine does not recognize the principle of interdependence. In his book, *La Désorganisation de la Personalité* (Paris, 1952), Professor H. Baruk presents a historical analysis of the dualist doctrine and defends on scientific grounds the "synthesis of the unity" (page 755).

[11] It is especially in the etiology of nervous and mental disease that the problem of a moral cause confronts the contemporary doctor. *Cp.* the capital work of Dr. Baruk, *Psychiatrie Morale Experimentale, Individuelle et Sociale; Haines et Reactions de Culpabilité* (Paris, 2nd edition, 1950). The same author has demonstrated in his book, *Le Désorganisation de la Personalité* (Paris, 1952), the importance of the prin-

ciple of the unity of the human personality in the domain of psycho-therapy.

12 *Cp. The Soul in Physical Life and its Relation to the Body*, in W. Hirsch's *Rabbinic Psychology* (London, 1947); and Rabbi S. Schabmar, *Torath Hanefesh*, Jassy, 1938, 2 vol.

13 *Cp.* Dr. Joseph Carlebach, "Das Religions-Gesetz als Grundlage", in *Hygiene und Judentum*, Dresden, 1930.

14 *'Iggereth Ha-Mussar*; and *Guide of the Perplexed*, III, 27.

15 *Shemoneh Perakim*. Translated into English by Joseph J. Gorfinkel, *The Eight Chapters of Maimonides on Ethics*, N. Y., 1942; translated into French by J. Wolf, *Les Huit Chapitres de M.*, Paris, 1937; *Hilkhoth De'oth*, Chapter I–III. Cp. Dr. A. Litvak, *Les Conceptions de Maimonides sur l'âme et leur Comparaison avec celles de notre temps*, in *Révue d'Histoire de la Médecine hébraique*, No. 1. Cp. also S. Horovitz, *Die Psychologie bei den jüdischen Religionsphilosophen des Mittelalters von Saadia bis Maimuni*, Breslau, 1912.

16 *Hanhogath Ha-Bri'uth*. See also *infra* page 120 *f*.

17 *Cp.* Dr. Muntner, "The Impact of Maimonides upon Medieval Writers in the Field of Medicine", in the *Hebrew Medical Journal*, Vol. II, (New York, 1954), pages 134–160. *Cp.* the article, "Refuah Ve-Dath", in *The Medical and Health Thesaurus*, *op. cit.*

18 *Ib. art.* "Psycho-Somatica".

19 E. Weiss and O. S. English in *Psycho-somatic Medicine* (New York, 1952); cited in P. Chauchard, *La Médecine psychosomatique*, page 72 (Paris, 1955), which includes the entire bibliography.

20 *Infra* page 147 *f*.

21 *Infra* page 163 *ff*.

22 *Infra* page 186 *ff*.

23 *Infra* page 168 *f*.

24 *Cp. Khuzari*, III, 49.

Introduction

1 On the significance of this phrase, see Preuss, *p*. 23.

2 Osler, *Evolution*, *p*. 43. On the long history of this cult, see E. T. Withington, "The Aescepiadae and the Priests of Asclepius", in *Studies in the History and Method of Science*, ed. C. Singer, 1921, part *ii*, *p*. 204 *ff*.

3 Harnack (*Medizinisches*, *p*. 96) calls Christianity a "medical religion." The historical reasons for this development are also discussed by Castiglioni, *History*, *p*. 242 *ff*.; and Sigerist, *Civilisation*, *p*. 138.

4 "Hippocrates is almost alone among Greek authors to be described as 'the saint' in Hebrew sources" (M. Steinschneider, *Die hebraeischen Uebersetzungen des Mittelalters*, 1893, *p*. 657 *f*.). Isaac Israeli, for instance, usually calls Hippocrates "the pious"; see Jacob Guttmann, *Die philosophischen Lehren des Isaak ben Salomon Israeli*, 1911, *p*. 11 (note 6).

5 In early Christian temples the face of Christ was often modelled on Hippocrates and on the traditional portrayal of Aesculapius, whose images became objects of worship and veneration; see Castiglioni, *loc. cit.* Cf. also Mary A. Hamilton, *Incubation, or the Cure of Disease in Pagan Temples and Christian Churches*, 1906.

6 These Christian saints, long associated with the healing art, were

twin brothers (beheaded in 303); see Hamilton, *op. cit., p. 119 ff. Cf.* also
Sigerist, *Civilisation*, p. 141 *f*. But Harnack (*Medizinisches*, **p.** 13) suggests that perhaps they never actually existed, although their veneration
must already have begun in the 4th century, when they achieved for
the Christians what Aesculapius accomplished at an earlier age. Later
other saints were associated with the cures for particular diseases; see
Hamilton, *op. cit.*, p. 128 *ff.*; D. Riesman, *Medicine in Modern Society*,
1939, p. 93. and especially Henry Sayles Francis, "Traditional Representation of Medicine and Healing in the Christian Hierarchy", in *Bulletin
of the Medical Library Association, vol. xxxii* (1944), p. 332 *ff*.

[7] This relic of the medieval belief in the healing power of every great
religious personality has survived to the present day; *cf*. E. Worcester
and S. McComb, *Body, Mind and Spirit*, 1931, p. 348 *f*.

[8] Sigerist, *Medicine*, p. 24.

[9] C. Singer, in *Oxford Classical Dictionary*, 1949, *art.* "Medicine", p. 549.

[10] See Allbutt, *Greek Medicine*, p. 19.

[11] See C. Capellmann, *Pastoral-Medizin*, 1904, p. 88 *ff*. According to
Diepgen (*Die Theologie, p.* 56 *f.*), the theological teachings of the
Church in the Middle Ages mainly concerned three fields of medical
interest: the prescription of extra-matrimonial sex-relationships, the in-
ordinate consumption of alcohol, and the transgression of the fast-com-
mands.

[12] So especially Hugo Magnus, *Religion und Medizin in ihren gegenseitigen Beziehungen*, 1902; P. Diepgen, *Die Theologie und der aerztliche Stand*, 1922; and W. H. R. Rivers, *Medicine, Magic and Religion*,
1924. Much useful material, though polemically and sometimes tenden-
tiously presented, is also furnished by A. D. White, *A History of the
Warfare of Science with Theology in Christendom*, 1896. Of particular
value for the Greek period is the study by L. Edelstein, "Greek Medicine
in Relation to Religion and Magic", in *Bulletin of the Institute of the
History of Medicine, vol. v* (1937), p. 201 *ff*.

[13] See M. Neuburger, "Doctrine of Healing Power of Nature throughout the Course of Time", in *Journal of the American Institute of Homeopathy, vol. xxv* (1932), *pp.* 861 *ff.*, 1011 *ff.*, 1167 *ff.*, 1320 *ff.* and 1425 *ff*.

[14] Surveyed most comprehensively by H. E. Sigerist, "The History of
Medical Licensure", in *Journal of the American Medical Association, vol.
xiv* (1935), p. 1057 *ff*.

[15] The ancient history of castration has been reviewed by Savas Nittis,
"The Hippocratic Oath in Reference to Lithotomy", in *Bulletin of the
History of Medicine, vol. vii* (1937), p. 723 *ff.*; this article includes data
on the attitude of the early Church (*p.* 727 *f.*). A more detailed study
on this subject, with special attention to the evolution of the religious
views on castration, has been made by A. P. Cawadias, "Male Eunuchism",
in *Proceedings of the Royal Society of Medicine, vol. xxxix* (1946), p.
502 *ff*. For further sources, see *infra, chpt.* XIII.

[16] The best historical study on this subject is by N. E. Himes, "Medical
History of Contraception", in *New England Journal of Medicine, vol. ccx*
(1934), p. 576 *ff*. (This article has been separately reprinted and en-
larged.) Much material on birth-control, particularly among primitive
races, is to be found in Ploss and Bartels, *Woman*.

[17] An exhaustive survey of the attitude to abortion in antiquity has been
made by R. Huehnel, "Der kuenstliche Abortus im Altertum", in *Sudhoff's Archiv fuer die Geschichte der Medizin, vol. xxix* (1936), p. 224 *ff*.
The subject is treated briefly in all standard works on medical history,
and at considerable length in the second volume of Ploss and Bartels,

Woman. For the history of the penal legislation in abortion, see Ebinger and Kimming, *Ursprung und Entwickelungsgeschichte der Bestrafung der Fruchtabtreibung,* 1910; and S. B. Burk, "The Development of the Law of the Criminal Abortion", in *Medical Times, vol. lvii* (1929), *p.* 153 *ff.*

18 The history of anatomical dissection is fairly fully treated in all general works on medical history, and especially in C. Singer's *The Evolution of Anatomy,* 1925. For the history of the practice in ancient times, see L. Edelstein, "Die Geschichte der Sektion in der Antike", in *Quellen und Studien zur Geschichte der Naturwissenschaften und der Medizin, vol. iii* (1932), *p.* 50 *ff.* A useful survey of later developments can be found in E. B. Krumharr's "History of Autopsia and its Relation to the Development of Modern Medicine", *Report of the Com. of Necropsies of the American Hospital Association Bulletin, no. clxiii* (1938).

19 This is a very wide and complex field whose varied aspects have been the theme of numerous historical works. The whole range has been thoroughly treated by Thorndike, *Magic*; Singer, *From Magic to Science,* 1928; and Rivers, *op. cit.*

20 I. S. Kahana, "Medicine in Halachic Literature after the Compilation of the Talmud", in *Sinai, vol. xiv* (1950), *pp.* 62 *ff.* and 221 *ff.* The author states that, to his knowledge, "there exists not one book on the subject" (*p.* 62).

21 H. J. Zimmels, *Magicians, Theologians and Doctors; Studies in Folk-Medicine and Folk-lore as Reflected in the Rabbinical Responsa* (12th–19th centuries), 1952. This work supplements the rabbinic sources treated in our study in respect to several subjects in the field of Jewish medical ethics; but it does not deal with therapeutical sterilisation, certain eugenic regulations, euthanasia, the licensing of physicians by religious authorities, contraception, non-Jews as physicians and patients, and male doctors and attendants for women.

22 J. Preuss, *Biblisch-Talmudische Medizin,* 1911.

23 So B. Condronchus, *De Christiana, ac tuta medendi ratione, etc.,* Ferrariae, 1591.

24 So H. Bardi, *Medicus politico catholicus, seu medicinae sacrae tum cognoscendae, tum faciundae idea,* Genevae, 1644.

25 So *Medicina Theologica, etc.,* Lisboa, 1794.

26 So especially C. Capellmann, *Pastoral-Medizin,* 1878; and A. O'Malley and J. J. Walsh, *Essays in Pastoral Medicine,* 1906. Medical ethics also features prominently in the many Catholic compendia of moral theology, such as Petr. Scavini, *Theologia moralis universa,* Paris, 1859; and Gury, *Compendium Theologiae Moralis,* Rome, 1874. A fuller list of works on this subject has been compiled by Capellmann in the bibliography at the end of his book.

27 For 19th-century examples, see De Valenti, *Medicina Clerica, oder Handbuch der Pastoral-Medizin fuer Seelsorger, Paedagogen und Aerzte,* Leipzig, 1831; E. Bottacchiari, *Manuali medico ad uso dei parrochi di campagna e delle famiglie,* Foligno, 1887; and J. Tillie, *Manuel de médecine, à l'usage du clergé parroissial, suivi des soins à donner dans les cas urgents,* Saint-Omer, 1891. More recent works in this rubric are, for instance: A. E. Sanford, *Pastoral Medicine, A Handbook for the Catholic Clergy,* New York, 1904; A. Klarman, *The Crux of Pastoral Medicine,* Ratisborn, 1912; J. Fletcher, *Notes for Catholic Nurses,* 1912; I. Antonelli, *Medicina Pastoralis in usum confessariorum et curiarum ecclesiasticarum,* Rome, 1920; P. A. Finney, *Moral Problems in Hospital Practice,* 1935; and A. Bonnar, *The Catholic Doctor,* 1948.

28 E. g., *The Linacre Quarterly,* A *Journal of the Philosophy and Ethics*

of Medical Practice; and *Hospital Progress* (both published in the United States). Since 1935 there has appeared a French quarterly publication, *Cahiers Laennec*, sponsored by an organisation similar to the American Catholic Physicians' Guilds. G. Kelly considers this "the best current contribution in the field of medical ethics" (in *Theological Studies, vol. x* [March 1949], *p.* 80 [note 25]).

29 On this Code and its revision, see G. Kelly, *Medico-Moral Problems,* 1950, part *i*, *p.* 1 *ff*.

30 Published by "The Catholic Hospital Association of the United States and Canada" at St. Louis. It has been prepared "for the guidance and benefit of Catholic Hospitals in those Dioceses which do not now have official Codes of Medical and Hospital Ethics" (Foreword). An introductory note further states that "these directives concern all patients in this hospital, regardless of religion, and they must be observed by all physicians, nurses, and others who work in the hospital" (*p.* 3).

31 "To the authors of the *Shulhan 'Arukh*", writes David Hoffmann (*Der Schulchan Aruch,* 1894, *p.* 140) in a comment which equally applies to other Jewish codes, "the principal criterion for the codification of laws was their mention in the Talmud, even if such laws can be applied nowadays only seldom or not at all". See also Hamburger, *RE, Suppl. iv* (1897), *p.* 104.

32 Of the seventy-odd groups and types of ailments and physical complaints specified less than half a dozen are not mentioned in the Talmud.

33 A larger, but still small, percentage of the approximately forty cures and treatments mentioned is not of talmudic origin.

34 The code refers to about twenty drugs and medicinal articles of food; less than a quarter of these do not originally occur in the Talmud.

35 Thus Sylvius averred, following the anatomical findings of Vesalius which differed materially from the teachings of Galen accepted as infallible for nearly a millenium and a half, that the human femur (described as curved by Galen) became straightened out by the adoption of cylindrical nether garments, and that "in ancient times the robust chests of heroes might very well have had more bones (Galen had listed eight bones in the sternum) than our degenerate day can boast"; see F. J. Cole, *A History of Comparative Anatomy,* 1944, *p.* 46. Even so bold a critic as Paracelsus defended his advocacy of new medical treatments on the grounds that conditions had altered with the times: "Therefore, no physician can be content to say I only require books composed 2,000 years ago. There are no longer the same causes" (*Works,* 1589, *vol. ii, p.* 168); see Rudolf Euken, *Beitraege zur Einfuehrung in die Geschichte der Philosophie,* 1906, *p.* 35 (in chapter: "Paracelsus' Lehren von der Entwickelung").

36 It was calculated that Achitophel begot Eliam (2 *Sam. xxiii.*34), and that the latter begot Bathsheba (*ib., ix.*3), at the age of eight years (b*Sanhedrin* 69b).

37 b*Sanhedrin* 69b; see also *Melo Haro'im, a. l.*

38 b*Yevamoth* 64b.

39 Tosaphoth, *Mo'ed Katan* 11b. Ya'ir Bacharach (r*Havath Ya'ir, no.*234) explains that talmudic medicines can no longer be applied because (a) the names of herbs, etc. cannot be identified with certainty, (b) their dosage and usage are not specified, and (c) human nature has changed, as recognised by Tosaphoth. *Cf.* also Azulay's commentary on *Sepher Hasidim, no.* 477.

40 So r*RIVaSH, no.* 447; r*RaSHBaSH, no.* 513; and r*TaSHBeTZ,* part *ii, no.* 101; see Zimmels, *p.* 60. These decisions are in opposition to the Talmud (b*Niddah* 38b).

41 So Tosaphoth, 'Avodah Zarah 24b; against the Talmud (ib.).

42 So Tosaphoth, 'Avodah Zarah 35a (bottom), and Yoma 77b; see also supra, p.xlix f.

43 So Tosaphoth, loc. cit.; and Yam shel Shelomo, Hullin, viii.12.

44 Ib. According to the Talmud (bYoma 77b), such danger was to be overcome by observing specially enacted precautions, e. g., the washing of hands before they touch the face in the morning.

45 Israel Isserlein, rTerumath Hadeshen, no. 271; against the Talmud (bBekhoroth 20b).

46 The Talmud (mTa'anith, iii.4) provided for the proclamation of special fasts in times of pestilence, but "nowadays" lack of food during such epidemics may prove dangerous; see M.A., dlxxvi.2, quoting Azulay (Birkei Yoseph) in the name of Isaac Luria.

47 Regarding the omission by Maimonides of the talmudic enactment, for health reasons, against roasting meat and fish together, Moses Schreiber (rHatham Sopher, Y.D., no. 101) observes: "Maimonides tested the matter by investigation and found that conditions had changed...". Epstein (A.H., O.H., clxxiii.2) advances a similar argument to explain why Maimonides does not mention the law of washing hands before eating cheese after meat. For further examples of such efforts to reconcile apparent contradictions between talmudic law and later findings of medical science, see rHatham Sopher, E.H., no. 19; and M.B., cccxxxi.31.

48 Tosaphoth, Yoma 77b.

49 Yam shel Shelomo, loc. cit.

50 bShabbath 129a, b. See also note 75 below.

51 Keseph Mishneh, Hil. De'oth, iv.18.

52 Quoted by B. Lewin, "Zur Charakteristik und Biographie des R. Scherira Gaon", in JJLG, vol. viii (1910), p. 335; citing Tachkemoni, Jahrbuch, ed. B. Lewin, Bern, 1910, p. 41.

53 See Browne, Arabian Medicine, p. 13.

54 Likkutei MaHaRIL, Amsterdam, 1730, p. 90. This view is also quoted with approval in Novellae of R. Akivah Eger, on Y.D., cccxxxvi.1.

55 Quotation in Kovetz 'al Yad, on Hil. De'oth, iv.8; see also Sedei Hemed, s. v. "Resh", no. 54; and D.T., cxvi.44.

56 Yam shel Shelomo, loc. cit. See also Likkutei MaHaRIL, loc. cit.

57 The sources cited in note 54 above stipulate that the ban does not include the recitation of the magic formula which the Talmud (bShabbath 67a) prescribes against a bone stuck in the throat, because its efficacy "has been tested". Even Galen praised the usefulness of a similar incantation against the same complaint; see quotation by Alexander of Tralles, ed. Puschmann, ii, p. 474. For further details, see Preuss, pp. 166 and 244.

58 E.g., Likkutei MaHaRIL does not refer to any ban; nor is it to be found in any code.

59 mShabbath, xix.3.

60 bShabbath 134b.

61 Hil. Shabbath, ii.14. But elsewhere (Hil. Milah, ii.8) Maimonides sanctions the practice only in places where it is customary to provide such baths.

62 Tur, O.H., cccxxxi.

63 Beth Yoseph, O.H., cccxxxi. But Isserles (Darkei Mosheh, a.l.) questions this decision, though he suggests that the water should be heated by a non-Jew. See Preuss, p. 283.

64 b'Avodah Zarah 30a, b.

65 Hil. Rotze'ah, xi.6.

66 Tur, Y.D., cxvi.

67 See note 42 above. The repeal of this law required no formal revocation, because the original decree was only made on the assumption that

open drinks were in danger of being poisoned by snakes; see Tosaphoth, *loc. cit.*, and *Levush, Y.D., cxvi.*1. This argument is also accepted by Hezekiah Silva (*Peri Hadash, a.l.*) and Elijah of Vilna (*Bi'ur HaGRA, a.l.*). Some authorities, however, are in doubt regarding such abrogation; see *P.T., a.l.,* 16. Solomon Ganzfried again incorporated the original law in his abridged code, *Kitzur Shulchan Aruch, xxxiii.*5.

68 See note 40 above.

69 *Cf.* Loew, *Lebensalter, p.* 48 *ff.*

70 *M.A., clxxix.*8. Karo (*O.H., clxxix.*6) still recorded the talmudic view (b*Berakhoth* 40a) that such an admixture of food and drinks was necessary to avoid bad oral smells and, at night, also the danger of "choking" (diphtheria?); see Preuss, *p.* 179.

71 *M.A., clxxiii.*1. The law requiring such rinsing of hands, codified in *O.H., clxxiii.*2, is based on the Talmud (b*Pesahim* 76b).

72 "There are several items, mentioned as dangerous in the Talmud due to the 'evil spirit', which are no longer harmful in our days" (*M.A., loc. cit.*).

73 *M.A., dlxxvi.*2. See note 46 above.

74 The Talmud (b*Ta'anith* 5b) prohibits conversations during meals, including even the uttering of the wish "health!" after a sneeze (j*Berakhoth, vi.*6) "lest the windpipe come before the gullet thus causing danger", *i.e.* lest the food produce choking by entering the trachea. This law is still retained by Karo (*O.H., clxx.*1); but its operation has now lapsed—according to Joshua Falk (*Perishah, a.l.*) because we no longer eat in a reclining position, and according to some later views (*A.H., a.l.,* 2; and *S.T., a.l.,* 1) because of the principle derived from "The Lord preserveth the simple". The former explanation seems to be supported by the talmudic rule that drinking whilst lying on one's back is likewise dangerous (b*Pesahim* 108a; see Preuss, *p.* 104)—showing that the position causes the danger.

75 Certain days, particularly the eve of festivals, were considered bad for blood-letting in the Talmud (b*Shabbath* 129b) and, in greater variety, by a tradition ascribed to Judah the Pious (see *TaZ, Y.D., cxvi.*6). These restrictions were later relaxed; see *Levush, a.l.,* 5; and *M.B., cdlxviii.*38.

76 According to the Talmud (b*Yevamoth* 72a), circumcisions and venesections should not be performed on cloudy days or days when a southerly wind blows; yet, "nowadays" this is often disregarded as "the Lord preserveth the simple". Hence RITVA (*Novellae a.l.*), in his teacher's name, permits the postponement of a circumcision if the due day is cloudy; for the operator need not rely on the divine protection of "the simple". But Luria (*Yam shel Shelomo, Yevamoth, viii.*4) opposes this view, as none are more "simple" than the present generation "who, in some mysterious way, are always saved from danger". See also J. L. Unterman, *Shevet Miyehudah,* 1955, *p.* 57 *ff.*

77 For the application of this phrase to justify a concession not sanctioned in the Talmud, see note 74 above.

78 The Talmud employs this argument in four cases, *viz.*, to vindicate those who ignore (i) the astrological indications against blood-letting (b*Shabbath* 129b; *cf.* note 75 above), (ii) the contraceptive precautions to be taken by minor, pregnant or lactating women (b*Yevamoth* 12b), (iii) the climatic indications against circumcision and blood-letting (b*Yevamoth* 72a; see note 76 above), and (iv) the danger of poisoning by snakes when eating grapes or figs at night (b'*Avodah Zarah* 30b; *cf.* also j*Terumoth, viii.*3).

79 See, *e.g.,* r*Hatham Sopher, E.H., nos.* 17 and 18; and r*MaHaRaM*

*Shik, Y.D., no.*244. *Cf.* Loew, *Lebensalter, p.*52; and Zimmels, *p.*8. Thus, the regulations regarding the ritual fitness of animals, though based on the assumption that the disqualifying symptoms of disease listed by the rabbis indicate that the vitality of animals so affected is reduced to a maximum of twelve months (m*Hullin, iii.*1; and b*Hullin* 54a), cannot be altered even if—in the words of Maimonides (*Hil. Shehitah, x.*13)—"it will appear, according to the teachings of medicine in our hands, that some of them [*i.e.* such animals] will not die [within the expected time]". This view is also shared by other early authorities. Adreth (r*RaSHBA, no.*89) even maintains that an animal showing any of the pathological indications enumerated by Sinaitic tradition in the Talmud is bound to die within a year, and he explains any apparent exception as due to some mistake in the diagnosis or to "a miracle". *Cf.* also *SHaKH, lvii.*48. Isaac ben Shesheth (r*RIVaSH, no.*447), too, confirms the ruling of Maimonides, adding sarcastically: "If you will base your judgments concerning issues of ritual fitness on the evidence of medical scholars, you will receive a great reward from the butchers...". *Cf. Yam shel Shelomo, Hullin, iii.*80; and *Y.D., lvii.*18, gloss.

80 The belief in the decline of man, though in complete contrast to the theory of progressive evolution, is very widespread. The Talmud expressed this attitude in the saying: "If the former generations were sons of angels, we are sons of man; if they were sons of man, we are like asses" (b*Shabbath* 112b; j*Demay, i.*3; and j*Shekalim, v.*1). *Cf.* the reduction in human longevity, *supra. p.*6.

81 *Novellae of RaMBaN,* on *Niddah, iii* (beginning). A similar view was put forward in the 18th century by Jacob Poppers (r*Shav Ya'akov, no.*40). See *D.T., clxxxiii.*6.

82 See b*Niddah* 57b; and *Y.D., cxc.*1.

83 So r*Teshurath Shay, no.*457; see *D.T., loc. cit.*

84 *Birkei Yoseph, E.H., i.*7; in the name of Jonah the Pious.

85 b*Yevamoth* 62b; and b*Sanhedrin* 76b. The usual age of marriage was, however, eighteen years; see m'*Avoth, v.*26. See also *E.H., i.*3.

86 Loew (*Lebensalter, p.*380 [note 165]), giving numerous illustrations from Tosaphoth and elsewhere, mentions Amram Gaon (see *Tur, O.H., cclxxxviii*) as the oldest authority for this rule.

87 He applies the rule especially in regard to tests to determine the pathological condition of suspect animals; see, *e.g.,* glosses in *Y.D., lv.*10; *lvii.*18; and *lviii.*6. *Cf.* also glosses in *Y.D., xviii.*6; *xci.*5; *cxcvi.*13; and *E.H., cxlv.*9 where the rule is employed to deny our competence to carry out tests for the determination of other religious issues.

88 So Maimonides, *Hil. Shabbath, ii.*15; and *Tur, O.H., cccxxx.*

89 b'*Arakhin* 7a; see Preuss, *p.*490 *ff.*

90 *M.A., a.l.,* 11.

9,1 It is evident that the law was not, in fact, acted upon since the time of the Geonim; see Chayim Benevisti, *Keneseth Hagedolah, O.H., cccxxx* (citing *Teshuvath Hage'onim* [*ed.* Mantua], *no.*248); and Azulay, *Birkei Yoseph, O.H., cccxxx.*2. But there is no proof for Loew's assumption (*Gesammelte Schriften, vol.iii, p.*392) that the law was never implemented, not even during the talmudic era.

92 The view that the law lapsed because of the declining competence to ascertain the precise moment of death is first encountered in the 15th century work '*Issur Vehetter* (ascribed to Jonah Gerondi, Ferrara, 1955, *cap.lix, no.*11); see Isserles, *Darkei Mosheh, O.H., cccxxx*; and Zimmels, *pp.*69 and 213 (note 87). Loew (*op. cit., p.*393) wrongly indentifies this work with the 14th century *Issur Vehetter* by Isaac ben Meir of Dueren;

but elsewhere (*Lebensalter, p.71*) he speaks of the amendment as dating from the 16th century. It is noteworthy that Isserles, though he embodied the opinion in the *Shulhan 'Arukh*, still envisaged the successful outcome of such an operation in his responsa (r*ReMA, no.40*). At the turn of the 17th century, however, the noted medical writer R. Tobias Cohen (*Ma'asei Tuvi'ah*, Venice, 1707, *p.*138a *f.*) confirmed that the performance of a post-mortem caesarian section was a "strange and unimaginable" operation and that it was not carried out on Jewish women; see Loew, *Gesammelte Schriften, loc. cit.* Yet the original law still enabled Cohen's contemporary Jacob Reischer (r*Shevuth Ya'akov*, part *i*, *nos.*1 and 13) to rule that a Jew, who had hastened to open the belly of a woman on the Sabbath in order to remove her child immediately after she had been accidentally decapitated, required no atonement for his act, since the mother's death was certain; see Loew, *op. cit., p.*394. Cf. also *infra, pp.* 127 and 130 *ff.*

93 b*Yevamoth* 80b.
94 *M.A., cccxxx.*6.

Chapter One

1 Sigerist, *Civilisation, p.*68 *ff.*
2 Thus, fasting for the recovery from illness is mentioned together with fasting for the relief from other misfortunes (*O.H., dlxix.*1). Revealing, too, is the formula to be used on greeting the sick on the Sabbath: "It is Sabbath [to-day] when one does not lament, and healing will be speedy in coming" (*O.H., cclxxxvii.*1; and *Y.D., cccxxxv.*6).
3 This belief is clearly taught in the Talmud: "The sick person does not rise from his illness until all his sins are forgiven him" (b*Nedarim* 41a). The codes, too, presume a relationship between sickness and atonement when advising people to encourage the patient's confession with these words: "As a reward for your confession of sins you shall live" (*Y.D., cccxxxviii.*1). On the moral value of suffering in general, *cf. O.H., ccxxii.*3.
4 The Talmud (b*Shabbath* 12b) bases this on the verse: "The Lord support him upon the bed of illness" (Psalms *xli.*4). See also Rashi, *Gen.* xlvii.31.
5 This view is only faintly apparent in the Talmud. It records the individual opinion of R. Acha, permitting the practice of medicine only "because people were already accustomed to it" (b*Berakhoth* 60a); see Preuss, *p.*25; and Krauss, *vol.i, p.* 9. The Karaites, following their founder's (Anan ben David) strong opposition to the use of medicines (see A. Harkavy, in *Likkutei Kadmoniyoth*, Petersburg, 1903, *vol.ii, p.*148), held that "God alone should be sought as physician and no human medicine should be resorted to" (Friedenwald, *p.*9). For the only other Jewish sect in which this attitude reappeared, though as a completely isolated phenomenon and evidently as a personal belief, see *infra, p.* .
6 See *infra, p.*8 *f.*
7 A late midrashic source relates that when R. Yishmael and R. Akivah once prescribed some medicine to a sick person consulting them, a farmer who accompanied them asked why they had interfered in a matter of no concern to them; as God had smitten, they—by offering a cure—had transgressed His will. Whereupon the rabbis replied that he—by cultivating

the soil—likewise interferred in a matter that did not belong to him. To his further argument that the fruits he would eat were the produce of his own labour, they retorted: "Fool! From your own work, do you not understand that... even as the plant, if not weeded, fertilized and ploughed, does not grow..., so is the body of man. The fertilizer is the medicine, and the farmer is the physician" (*Midrash Samuel, iv.*1; and *Midrash Temurah*; see J. D. Eisenstein, *'Otzar Midrashim*, 1928, *p.*580 *f.*); see Preuss, *p.*29. To a similar category may belong the argument advanced in some earlier sources that most illnesses were not, in fact, caused by God at all, but by human carelessness; hence it could not be wrong to cure them. Thus, several teachers held that only 1% of all diseases were caused "by the hand of Heaven", the remainder being due to common colds or, according to another opinion, to negligence; see *Lev. Rabbah, xvi.*8. On the significance of this view, see W. Ebstein, *Die Medizin im Neuen Testament und im Talmud*, 1903, *p.*191. The Talmud expressly exempts colds, and possibly all diseases (*cf.* Tosaphoth, *B. Bathra* 144b), from the rule that "everything is in the hands of Heaven" (b*Kethuboth* 30a). This implies a recognition that the operation of the *fatum* may be limited (*cf.* Rashi and Tosaphoth, *a.l.*). But *cf.* also Tosaphoth, *Niddah* 16b, where diseases generally are included among the experiences "determined by Heaven". For the view expressed in the codes, *cf. infra*, *p.*31.

8 Explaining that the rabbis approved of King Hezekiah's action in hiding the *"Book of Medicines"* (m*Pesahim, iv.*9) solely because it contained astrological and other forbidden prescriptions, Maimonides (*Mishnah Commentary, a.l.*) rejects the view (*cf.* Rashi, *Pesahim* 56a) that Hezekiah's action was intended to restore people's faith in prayer by destroying their reliance on human cures: "How could one attribute such folly (argues Maimonides) to Hezekiah...? According to this worthless and corrupt opinion, any person who is hungry and goes for bread and eats it, though he will doubtless be healed from that grave illness (the illness of hunger), would have to be considered as lacking in faith and reliance on his God...". Maimonides thus justifies the healing of disease on purely rational grounds; his system does not, therefore, require any biblical sanction for the practice of medicine.

9 b*Berakhoth* 60a; and b*B. Kamma* 85a; in the name of the School of R. Yishmael.

10 *Tur, Y.D., cccxxxvi.*

11 So, *e.g.*, John of Baldus (in MS at the Laurentian Library in Florence) and other writings of the 15th century; see L. Thorndike, *Science and Thought in the 15th Century*, 1930, *p.*50 (and note). Early Christians also quoted this passage to reconcile ancient medicine with their faith; see Diepgen, *Die Theologie, p.*8; Sigerist, *Medicine, p.*18; and Loren M. McKinney, "Medical Ethics and Etiquette in the Early Middle Ages", in *Bulletin of the History of Medicine, vol.xxvi* (1952), *p.*5.

12 See Cumston, *An Introduction, p.*187.

13 Rashi, *B. Kamma* 85a.

14 Tosaphoth, *B. Kamma* 85a.

15 *Novellae of RaSHBA*, on *B. Kamma* 85a.

16 *Torath Ha'adam, Sha'ar Sakkanah*; quoted by Karo, *Beth Yoseph, Y.D., cccxxxvi.* See OY, *vol.x, p.*8.

17 *Tur, loc. cit.*

18 Pardo, *Hasdei David*, Livorno, 1776; see Preuss, *p.*30.

19 Zimmels, *p.*7.

20 See, *e.g.*, *MaHaRaTZ Chajes*, on *B. Kamma* 85a.

21 See J. Epstein, *Torah Temimah*, on *Ex. xxi.*19 (*no.*145); *cf.* r*TaSHBeTZ*, part *iii, no.*82, for a similar explanation.

22 On *Nedarim, iv.*4; *cf. MaHaRaTZ Chajes,* on *B. Kamma* 81b. Maimonides describes the duty to heal as a religious precept (without, however, citing the biblical source) also in *Hil. Nedarim, vi.*8. Friedenwald
(*p.*14) is therefore wrong in stating that Maimonides does not refer to
any biblical warrant for the view that "one who is ill has not only the
right but also duty to seek medical aid". See also note 8 above.

23 b*B. Kamma* 81b; and b*Sanhedrin* 73b. *Cf. Siphri,* on *Deut. xxii.*2. On
the proper care of the human body as a religious duty, see also *Lev.
Rabbah, xxxiv.*3.

24 *Torah Ha'adam, loc. cit.*; based on a similar reasoning in b*Sanhedrin*
84b.

25 Arama, *'Akedath Yitzhak, Sha'ar xxvi* (*ed.* Frankfurt a/Oder, 1785,
*p.*57a).

26 See *Deut. xxii.*8. *Cf.* also Rashi's significant comments on this passage.

27 *Cf.* "There is nothing in the world regarding which God did not issue
a religious command to Israel; if one goes out to plough the field, one
must not plough with an ox and an ass together, if. . ." (*Midrash Yelam-
denu, Shelakh*); *cf.* also r*TaSHBeTZ,* part *i, no.*140. This rabbinic dictum
illustrates the tendency to find a biblical mandate for every legitimate
human action. On the subordination of all activities to the revealed will
of God, *cf.* also *O.H., ccxxxi.*

28 So, *e.g.,* Krauss, *vol.i, p.*264; and Zimmels, *p.*170 (note 45).

29 See note 5 above. *Cf.* also Zimmels, *p.*6 *f.*

30 The ancient Egyptians also differentiated, as did primitive peoples, between wounds inflicted by man (which were treated by rational means)
and conditions arising from proper diseases (dealt with by spells and
incantations); see Stern, *Society, p.*4.

31 Tosaphoth, *B. Kamma* 85a.

32 Ibn Ezra, on *Ex. xxi.*19. *Cf.* also his commentary on *Ex. xv.*26; and
*xxiii.*25. He cites *Job v.*18 and 2 *Chron. xvi.*12 in support of his view.

33 Bachyah, on *Ex.xxi.*19 (*ed.* Amsterdam, 1726, *p.*109b).

34 Eybeschuetz, *Kerethi Upelethi, Y.D., clxxxviii.*5.

35 Nachmanides, on *Lev. xxvi.*11. *Cf.* Zimmels, *p.*171 (notes 46–50).

36 *'Akedath Yitzhak, loc. cit.*

37 See particularly W. Hofmann, "Zur Bewertung des Arztes und der
Medizin in der juedischen Auffassung", in *Jeschurun, vol.iv* (1917),
*p.*394 *ff.*

38 Ibn Ezra even composed a medical work (*Medical Experiences*); see
Friedenwald, *p.*619 *f.* On Nachmanides, see *Seder Hadoroth,* Karlsruhe,
1769, *p.*131a.

39 *Cf.* Bachyah ibn Pekudah, *Hovoth Halevavoth. Sha'ar Habittahon,
chpt.iv.*

40 See Zimmels, *p.*6 f.

41 See D. Margalith, "La Médecine et la Mouvement Hassidique", in
Révue, vol.xv (1952), *p.*212.

42 Azulay, *Birkei Yoseph, Y.D., cccxxxvi.*2.

43 See Cumston, *An Introduction, p.*208.

44 See Campbell, *Arabian Medicine, vol.i, p.*59; and Garrison, *Introduction, p.*138.

45 See M. Meyerhof, "Science and Medicine", in *Legacy of Islam,* 1931,
*p.*337.

46 See Meyerhof, *loc. cit.*

47 Campbell, *op. cit., p.*43.

48 *Ib., p.*93 *ff.* The memory of Hippocrates, too, was dishonoured by
medieval Christians because he refuted the intervention of a punishing

deity in physical suffering and denounced recourse to penances and abjurations for its appeasement (*On Epilepsy*, ed. Kuehn, *vol.i, p.561*); see E. Haas, "Hippocrates und die indische Medizin des Mittelalters", in *ZDMG, vol.xxxi* (1877), *p.656.*

⁴⁹ Diepgen, *Die Theologie*, p.2, where the references in the following six notes are given.

⁵⁰ *Gratian Decretals*, ed. Friedberg, *vol.i, p.541.*

⁵¹ *Ib., p.399.*

⁵² *Ib.*

⁵³ *Ib., p.909.*

⁵⁴ Aquinas, *Opera, vol.xii, p.422.*

⁵⁵ Antonius, *tit.vii, cap.i,* §1. A monastic MS of the 8th century (Bamberg Cathedral), too, declared: "Therefore [following the quotation of Ecclesiasticus; cf. note 11 above] he who does not seek medicine in time of necessity deserves the name stupid and imprudent... God wishes to be honoured by His miracles performed through man...". For this and further proofs of the legality of healing in early medieval MSS, see McKinney, *op. cit., pp.5* and 9 *f.*

⁵⁶ Allbutt, *Greek Medicine*, p.402.

⁵⁷ Puschmann, *Medical Education*, p.136.

⁵⁸ Osler, *Evolution*, p.84 *ff.*

⁵⁹ Singer, *Evolution*, p.63 *ff.*

⁶⁰ See E. S. Cowles, *Religion and Medicine in the Church, Report for the Joint Commission on Christian Healing*, 1925, *p.14; cf.* Haggard, *Devils*, p.271 *f.* For further details, and examples of "holy men" who were "eminent for filthiness", see White, *Warfare, vol.ii, p.69 ff.*; and Lecky, *European Morals, vol.ii, p.117 f.*

⁶¹ See Preuss, *p.28*; citing Luther, *Tischreden*, ed. Irmischer, *no.1411*; and Sam Maresius, *an possit et debeat homo Christianus in suis morbis medicum adhibere*, Groning., 1656.

⁶² See *OY, vol.x, p.8.*

⁶³ See H. Magnus, *Religion und Medizin in ihren gegenseitigen Beziehungen*, 1902, *p.39 ff.*

⁶⁴ For a graphic description of the physician's work in the 16th century, see H. W. Haggard, *The Doctor in History*, 1935, *p.200 ff.*

⁶⁵ On the influence of Christianity in the maintenance of the medical authority of the ancients throughout the Middle Ages, see Magnus, *op. cit., p.41 ff.* Neuburger (*History, vol.i, p.273*) states: "... never have the doctrines of one man exercised so long, unbroken and tyrannical a power over the minds of others as did those of Galen". Avicenna legislated in medical matters with such absolute authority that he called his chief work *The Canon*, with the idea that it should constitute an immutable law; see Castiglioni, *History, p.272.* Throughout the 16th century, his works, together with those of Hippocrates and Galen, still served as the standard text-books in all European universities; at Montpellier and Louvain they remained in general use until 1650; see D. Campbell, "The Medical Curriculum of the Universities of Europe in the Sixteenth Century", in *Science, Medicine and History*, ed. E. A. Underwood, 1953, *vol.i, p.359 f.*; and Z. Muntner, "Persian Medicine and Its Relation to Jewish and Other Medical Science", in *The Hebrew Medical Journal, vol.xxv* (1952), *p.196. Cf.* Puschmann, *Medical Education*, p.295 *ff.*

⁶⁶ See Magnus, *op. cit., p.41 ff.*

⁶⁷ See P. Diepgen, "Die Bedeutung des Mittelalters fuer den Fortschritt in der Medizin", in *Essays*, ed. Singer and Sigerist, *p.119.*

⁶⁸ A practical example of particular relevance may be the alleged papal

intervention in the first experiments on human blood-transfusion in 1675. According to several scholars, this led to the complete suspension of such experiments until early in the 19th century; see Castiglioni, *History*, p.553; and L. M. Zimmermann and K. M. Howell, "History of Blood-Transfusions", in *Annals of Medical History*, vol.iv (1932), p.419.

69 The use of untried medicines is also discountenanced in Jewish sources. But this ban is expressly restricted to articles otherwise prohibited on religious grounds. Thus, only "known [*i.e.* tried] medicines" may contain ritually forbidden substances and be consumed, if necessary (*Y.D.*, clv.3, gloss). On the definition of "known medicines", see J. L. Unterman, *Shevet Miyehudah*, 1956, p.15. Apart from this limitation, the administration of doubtful remedies in a desperate gamble to save life is, in fact, encouraged, and several authorities expressly permit giving a patient a possibly effective drug even at the grave risk of hastening his death if it proves fatal; see Jacob Reischer, rShevuth Ya'akov, part *iii*, no.75; Jacob Ettlinger, rBinyan Tziyon, no.111; Abraham Danzig, *Binath 'Adam*, on *Hokhmath 'Adam*, lxxxviii, no. 93; Solomon Eger, *Gilyon MaHaRSHA*, on *Y.D.*, clv.v. See also *D.T.*, clv.2; and Zimmels, p.181 (note 109).

70 For further illustrations, see *infra*, p.103 *f.*

71 Lecky, *European Morals*, vol.i, p.356.

72 Castiglioni, *History*, p.242 *ff.*

73 See *JE*, vol.x, p.69 *ff.* Josephus, too, regarded diseases, especially the plague, as punishments sent by God; see M. Neuburger, *Die Medizin im Fl. Josephus*, 1919, p.15 *f.*

74 rMaHaRIL, no.35.

75 bB. *Kamma* 60b; see *MaHaRSHA*, a.l.; and Preuss, p.174. Cf. *Torah Temimah*, on *Deut.* xxxii.25 (no.75). For other biblical and talmudic parallels, see Bi'ur HaGRA, *Y.D.*, cxvi.16.

76 *Yam shel Shelomo*, B. *Kamma*, vi.26; see Zimmels, p.103.

77 Horowitz, *Shenei Luhoth Haberith*, *Sha'ar Ha'othiyoth*, ed. Fuerth, 1764, p.63b.

78 Y. M. Epstein, *Kitzur SHeLaH*, ed. Fuerth, p. 10 b.

79 *M.A.*, dlxxvi.3.

80 Bachyah, on *Nu.* xvi.21 (ed. Amsterdam, 1726, p.197b).

81 Nachmanides, on *Gen.* xix.17. That plagues were "due to changes in the air" is also mentioned by Isserles (*O.H.*, dlxxvi.5, gloss). This widespread belief persisted into the 19th century; see Haggard, *op. cit.*, p.169.

82 The association of Lot's experiences with the duty to flee from places contaminated by pestilence—Bachyah's remarks are quoted by Akivah Eger in his *Novellae* on Isserles's ruling—also suggests that this duty may be morally rationalised by the desire to prevent people who survive a divine visitation from seeing the destruction of its victims.

83 rRaSHBaSH, no.195; see *P.T.*, *Y.D.*, cxvi.8; and Zimmels, p.101 *f.*

84 See Preuss, p.173.

85 See White, *Warfare*, vol.ii, p.60.

86 H. T. Buckle, *History of Civilisation in England*, 1857, vol.ii, p.593.

87 *Tiph'ereth Yisra'el*, 'Avoth, iii.1. See also other sources cited by Zimmels, p.233 (note 142). Some time before the publication of Jenner's discovery (1798), a Jewish author in London defended the religious lawfulness of the earlier practice of variolation, introduced into England from Constantinople at about 1720; see Abraham ben Solomon, 'Aleh Teruphah, London, 1785. The dissertation also appeared in Ha—Me'asseph, Koenigsberg, 1785, p.5 *ff.* See also Zimmels, p.108.

88 B. J. Stern, *Should We Be Vaccinated? A Survey of the Controversy*,

1927. The spirit of the times is well typified in the little tract by E. Massey, *A Sermon Against the Dangerous and Sinful Practice of Innoculation*, 1722.

89 White, *Warfare, vol.ii, p.55 ff.*

90 Tagliacozzi's attempts to restore the loss of noses and lips were considered a "presumptious interference with the rights of the Creator"; after his death, following much agitation, his corpse was exhumed and re-interred in unconsecrated ground at the instance of the Bologna clergy; see Puschmann, *Medical Education, p.305.* Following the ban by the Church, rhinoplasty remained unknown until reintroduced by Offenbach in 1822; see Castiglioni, *History, p.473.*

91 See Sigerist, *Civilisation, p.78;* quoting A. Vorberg, *Zur Geschichte der persoenlichen Syphilisverhuetung,* 1911, *p.21.*

92 See H. L. Gordon, *Sir James Young Simpson and Chloroform,* 1879, *p.123 ff.* For further details, see *infra, p.103.*

93 See Sigerist, *loc. cit.* For these and similar examples of religious opposition to medical innovations there is probably no parallel in Jewish sources, much as they abound with discussions on the various ritual problems arising from the advance of medical science. The only medical operations which have encountered serious opposition by many rabbis are anatomical dissection (see *infra,* chapter XII), organic kerastoplasty with transplants removed from the dead (for some details, see Grunwald, *Kol Bo, p.45 ff.;* and J. L. Unterman, *Shevet Miyehudah,* 1955, *p.313 ff.*), and artificial insemination, especially with donated semen (see I. Jakobovits, "Artificial Insemination, Birth-Control and Abortion", in *The Hebrew Medical Journal, vol.xxvi* [1953], *p.180 ff.*). But these objections were due entirely to considerations of the inviolable dignity attaching to dead as well as living human beings; the question of defeating the designs of Providence was not in any way related with these issues.

94 D. Martin Luther, *Werke,* ed. Weimar, 1901, *vol.xxiii, p.323 ff.;* see Zimmels, *p.103 f.;* and Preuss, *p.173 f.*

95 See note 8 above.

96 See *supra, p.4.*

97 See *supra, p.11.*

98 This divergence of views touches on the problem (considered *infra, p.96 ff.*) regarding the extent to which one may, or must, endanger one's life to save that of another.

99 See Preuss, p.174.

100 See Galen, *ed.* Kuehn, *vol.xv, p.309. Cf.* also the Hippocratic counsel: "Prayer indeed is good, but while calling on the gods, man should himself lend a hand" (*Oevres Complètes d'Hippocrate,* ed. Littré, *vol.iv, p.642;* cited by Sigerist, *Medicine, p.14*).

101 See M. Neuburger, "Zur Geschichte des Problems der Naturheilkraft", in *Essays,* ed. Singer and Sigerist, *p.333.* See also E. F. Podach, "Ursprung und Bedeutung des Spruches 'Ich behandelte ihn, und Gott heilte ihn' (A. Paré, 1575)," in *Medizinische* (Stuttgart), *vol.xxxvi* (1955), *pp.1279 ff.* and 1352 *ff.*

102 See Cumston, *An Introduction, p.24.*

103 See F. Hartmann, *The Life... of Paracelsus,* 1896, *p.227.* See also R. Euken, *Beitraege zur Einfuehrung in die Geschichte der Philosophie,* 1906, *p.31.*

104 In the bibliographical essays contained in the first volume of his *The Jews and Medicine,* 1944. See following notes.

105 See Friedenwald, *p.27.*

106 *Ib., p.* 315.
107 *Ib., p.*273 *ff.*, where an English translation of the prayer is reproduced in full. For the original Hebrew version, with a French rendering and introduction, see I. Simon, "La Prière des Médecins de Jacob Zahalon", in *Révue, no.*25 (1955), *p.*38 *ff.*
108 This is to be found in the Appendix to the *Sepher Hahayim* (Amsterdam, 1703) by Simon Frankfurther of Schwerin-an-der-Warthe; it was republished by Leiser Landshuth (b. 1817 at Lissa) in his *Seder Bikkur Holim* (Berlin, 1867); see L. Lewin, "Juedische Aerzte in Grosspolen", in *JJLG, vol.ix* (1911), *p.*413; and Friedenwald, *p.*27. Landshuth's work for long enjoyed much popularity; see *JL, vol.iii, p.*973.
109 See Friedenwald, *p.*27 *ff.* LaWall (*Pharmacy, p.*112 *f.*), however, accepts the Maimonidean origin of the prayer. He regards it as ranking with the Oath of Hippocrates and as "a great factor in the development of medical and pharmaceutical ethics". See also I. Simon, "Le Serment Médicale d'Asaph", in *Révue, no.*9 (1951), *p.*41 *f.*
110 See, *e.g., Matth. viii.*13; *ix.*2, 22 and 29; and *xv.*28.
111 See, *e.g.,* 1 *Cor. xii.*
112 Augustine, *De Civitate Dei, xxii.*8.3; see *ERE, vol.v, p.*698 *f.*
113 Castiglioni, *History, p.*348.
114 See Castiglioni, *History, p.*385. See also *supra,* Introduction (note 6).
115 E. T. Withington, "The Asclepiadae and the Priests of Asclepius", in *Studies in the History and Method of Science,* ed. C. Singer, 1921, *vol. ii, p.*205.
116 See Sigerist, *Civilisation, p.*141.
117 For a comparison of the cult of prayer and pilgrimage by the sick which has grown up at Lourdes since 1858 with the scenes witnessed in the Aesculapian temples during the first centuries of our era, see E. Worcester and S. McComb, *Body, Mind and Spirit, p.*348 *f.*
118 See the exhaustive report on present-day religious healing movements and practices by W. Oursler, *The Healing Power of Faith,* 1958.
119 J. J. Walsh, *The Popes and Science,* 1912, *p.*199 *ff.*
120 Even from the papal throne has been occupied by physicians. On the medical pope John XXI (13th century), see D. Riesman, "A Physician in the Papal Chair", in *Annals of the History of Medicine, vol.v* (1923), *p.*291 *ff.* Garrison (*Introduction, p.*169) claims that Pope Paul II, too, was a physician. There was also an Archbishop of Canterbury skilled in medicine; see White, *Warfare, vol.ii, p.*36. Harnack (*Medizinisches, p.*96) mentions some sixteen physicians, among them bishops, who reached distinction in the early stage of Christianity; see J. J. Walsh, *The Catholic Church and Healing,* 1928, *p.*15 *ff.* It has also been suggested that the author of the third Gospel and the Acts of the Apostles was "well acquainted with the language of the Greek medical schools" (W. K. Hobart, *The Medical Language of St. Luke,* 1882), and that Luke himself was probably a physician (Sigerist, *Medicine, p.*15).
121 Walsh, *op. cit., p.*107. The book bears the *imprimatur* of the Archbishop of New York.
122 See M. Meyerhof, *L'Oevre Médicale de Maimonide;* cited by Friedenwald, *p.*197.
123 See Osler, *Evolution, p.*101.
124 Castiglioni, "The Contribution", in *The Jews, p.*1024 *f.*
125 See Singer, *Prayer-Book, pp.* 47, 94d and f; see also *p.*101.
126 See *ib., p.*47 (note).
127 The formula, as originally mentioned in the Talmud (b*Berakhoth* 60a), is to be recited by him "who goes in for a blood-letting", but it was

later applied to other medical operations, too (*M.A., ccxxx.*6). *Cf.* also the prayer which the 6th century physician Aetius of Amida, when applying certain ointments, asked the patient to say: "May the God of Abraham, of Isaac and of Jacob give virtue to this medication" (see Cumston, *An Introduction, p.*188).

[128] See Singer, *Prayer-Book, p.*69.

[129] Fasting for the sick is mentioned in early talmudic literature; see t*Ta'anith, iii.*2. It is also assumed in *Midrash Rabbah,* on *Eccl. v.*6. *Cf.* the custom to fast on Wednesdays against the incidence of diphtheria among children; see Rashi, on *Gen. i.*14. Josephus adds to prayer and fasting (*Antiquities, vii.*7.4) the offering of special sacrifices to procure healing (*ib., iii.*9.4), though such custom cannot be found in the Bible or Talmud; see M. Neuburger, *Die Medizin im Fl. Josephus,* 1919, *p.*16; and Preuss, *p.*24.

[130] *Cf. Nu. x.*9.

[131] See Preuss, *pp.*179 and 182; and *OY, vol.ii, p.*150 *f.*

[132] See *supra,* Introduction (note 46).

[133] Lewin, *loc. cit.* For further sources on such prayers, see Zimmels, *p.*232 (note 121).

[134] The belief that the righteous can "annul a divine decree", based on *Ps. cxlv.*19, is strongly upheld in the Talmud (b*Mo'ed Katan* 16b; and b*Shabbath* 63a); *cf.* also Edels, *MaHaRSHA,* on *Yevamoth* 64a. See *JE, vol.x, p.*169, for further details. On whether one may even desecrate the Sabbath to ask for such intervention (by sending a telegram to a famous saint), see J. L. Unterman, *Shevet Miyehudah,* 1955, *p.*50 *f.*

[135] Puschmann, *Medical Education, p.*151; and Magnus, *op. cit., p.*33 *ff.*

[136] "Because one thereby becomes another person on whom that fate is not decreed" (*Levush, Y.D., cccxxxv.*10); see also *MaHaRSHA,* on *Rosh Hashanah* 16b, citing *SeMAG,* Positive Commandment *no.*16. On the origin and usages of this custom in the Talmud (b*Baba Bathra* 116a) and rabbinic literature, see Loew, *Lebensalter, p.*107 *ff.*; and Zimmels, *p.*143.

[137] For a critical discussion of this law and its origin in the Talmud (b*Sanhedrin* 101a), see Loew, *Gesammelte Schriften, vol.ii, p.*86.

[138] As will be seen in the following chapters, this principle is often applied in Jewish law; see also Kahana, in *Sinai, vol.xiv* (1950), *p.*239; and Zimmels, *p.*36 *f.*

[139] *Hil. 'Avodah Zarah, xi.*12; so also *TaZ, Y.D., clxxix.*8. See also A. A Neuman, *The Jews in Spain,* 1948, *vol.ii, p.*109.

[140] Joshua Falk adequately sums up these laws and their spirit when he explains that recitations from the Bible over sick people are prohibited if they are regarded as taking the place of rational cures; but if such readings are meant to procure the "reward of good deeds and faith", they are obviously commendable (*Perishah, Y.D., clxxix.*17). The universality of this outlook among Jews is attested by its adoption even in the *Zohar,* "the mystics' Bible". Its therapy—in the judgment of its medical historian, K. Preis ("Die Medizin im Sohar", in *MWGJ, vol.lxxii* [1928], *p.*183)— is remarkably rational, forbidding the use of mystic and divine names for healing purposes; see *Zohar, ed.* Amsterdam, 1800, *vol.iii, p.*296a.

[141] See Isak Unna, "Christian Science", in *Jeschurun, vol.*ii (1015), *p.*583 *ff.*; and B. Drachman, "The So-called 'Science' Movements and their Relation to Judaism", in *Essays Presented to J. H. Hertz,* 1943, *p.*131 *ff.* Drachman also mentions a "Jewish Science" movement;; founded by Rabbi Morris Lichtenstein in New York in 1922, it taught (in contrast to its Christian counterpart) "that all help and healing are of God but that medical science is a divine gift and should not be rejected" (*p.*142 *f.*).

142 So Puschmann, *Medical Education*, p.27; and Castiglioni, *History*, p.77.

143 Singer, "Judaism", in *The Jews*, p.1065.

144 Indeed, the talmudic studies and outlook of Jewish physicians in the Middle Ages may have been an important contributory factor in their services to medicine. Analysing their phenomenal devotion to the healing art, L. Wallerstein ("Behind the Pioneer Role of Jews in Medicine", in *Commentary, vol.xix* [March, 1955], p.245) declares: "Particularly in the five hundred years between the 10th and the 16th centuries, Jewish physicians attained universally recognised eminence in three characteristic pursuits: the translation of medical works from Greek to Arabic, and later from Arabic to Hebrew, the composition of original medical treatises, and the practice of medicine at noble courts... A key factor in understanding this remarkable phenomenon is that these men were not only distinguished physicians, but Rabbinic scholars and leaders of the Jewish community. This cultural element, possibly indeed the key to the whole story, has not been understood by non-Jewish medical historians. The tendency, rather, has been to attribute the historical Jewish role in medicine to a congenital national aptitude". C. Roth ("The Qualification of Jewish Physicians in the Middle Ages", in *Speculum, vol.xxviii* [October, 1953], p.835) also recognises that "to some extent, of course, they [*i.e.* the Jewish medieval doctors] got their medical knowledge from books; all the more so perhaps since the Jew's Talmudic training and interests gave him a peculiar devotion to book-lore". Significant, too, is the remark by Neuman (*op. cit.* p.106) that among the rabbi-physicians in medieval Spain "the opposition to, rather than the defence of, the fantastic notions of astrology was based on biblical and talmudic authority".

Chapter Two

1 See Sigerist, *Medicine*, p.9, where numerous references to magical elements are shown to occur in the *Ebers, Hearst, Brugsch* (*Maior* and *Minor*) and *Berlin papyri*.

2 *ERE, vol.viii*, p.267.

3 See Sigerist, *Civilisation*, p.138; and *ERE, vol.vi*, p.540 ff.

4 See Osler, *Evolution*, p.54; and Sigerist, *Medicine*, p.14.

5 So Preuss, p.166; and Thorndike, *Magic, vol.i*, p.172 ff.; against the claim of other scholars that there are in Galen's voluminous works "no recommendations of charms and magical procedures of any kind"; so F. J. Payne, *English Medicine*, 1904, p.95 f.; and Stern, *Society*, p.8.

6 See Payne, *op. cit.*, p.102 f.

7 Preuss, p.4.

8 Singer, "Judaism", in *The Jews*, p.1044. But it may be open to doubt whether this is altogether due to lack of scientific interest "by those whose lives were passed within the talmudic universe of discourse".

9 *Zohar, ed.* Amsterdam, 1800, *vol.iii*, p.299a; see K. Preis, "Die Medizin im Sohar", in *MGWJ, vol.lxxii* (1928), p.184; *cf.* p.179. But the identity of the physician mentioned in the *Zohar* with the famous doctor at Trajan's court has been in doubt; see R. Eisler, "Zur Terminologie und Geschichte der juedischen Alchemie", in *MGWJ, vol.lxx* (1926), p.197 f.

10 G. A. Wherli, "Das Wesen der Volksmedizin", in *Essays, ed.* Singer and Sigerist, p.369 ff.

[11] Puschmann, *Medical Education*, p.33; quoting *Vendidad*, *vii*.118–121.

[12] See *Oxford English Dictionary*, *vol.ii*, p.251, *s.v.* "Chaldean".

[13] See G. Maspero, *The Dawn of Civilisation. Egypt and Chaldea*, ed. A. H. Sayce, 1910, p.780 *ff*.; and Castiglioni, *History*, p.39 *ff*.

[14] Sigerist, *Civilisation*, p.132; see also Sigerist, *Medicine*, p.2 *ff*.

[15] See Osler, *Evolution*, p.119 *ff*.

[16] See Rashdall, *Universities*, *vol.i*, p.242 *f*.

[17] For these and other sources on the importance of astrology for me-dieval doctors, see Zimmels, p.15 *f*. Among Jewish medieval thinkers, only Maimonides opposed astrology as a base superstition (especially in "*Letter to the Men of Marseilles*"); but it was generally agreed that faith in God could overcome the stars' influence on human destiny; see *JE*, *vol.ii*, p.244 *f*.; and A. A. Neuman, *The Jews in Spain*, 1948, *vol.ii*, p.104 *ff*. The importance of physicians knowing astronomy was also stressed by the classic medical writers of earlier times, such as Hippocrates, Galen and Abulcasis; see M. Steinschneider, *Die Hebraeischen Uebersetzungen des Mittelalters*, 1893, p.742. The association of medicine with astronomy may likewise be indicated by the surname "*Yarchinai*" ("of the moon", *i.e.* versed in lunar science) added to the names of the physicians Samuel and Asaf, as suggested by S. Muntner, "The Antiquity of Asaph the Physician", in *Bulletin of the History of Medicine*, *vol.xxv* (1951), p.109.

[18] See H. W. Haggard, *The Doctor in History*, 1935, p.173; and *Oxford English Dictionary*, *vol.v*, p.271.

[19] See LaWall, *Pharmacy*, p.81.

[20] J. G. Frazer, *Psyche's Task; a Discourse Concerning the Influence of Superstition on the Growth of Institutions*, 1913, p.4.

[21] In Jewish law, the main provisions on superstitious cures are, signi-ficantly, featured under the heading of "Laws on Idolatry".

[22] For examples, see Matth. *iv*.24; *viii*.28 *ff*.; *Mark v*.2 *ff*.; *Luke viii*.27 *ff*.; *xiii*.32; and Acts *x*.38.

[23] See Friedenwald, p.104.

[24] See Haggard, *Devils*, p.298.

[25] See White, *Warfare*, *vol.ii*, p.27 *ff*. A long list of references to the belief in the power of magic by the Church Fathers is also given in *ERE*, *vol.xviii*, p.277. See also E. Worcester and S. McComb, *Body, Mind and Spirit*, 1931, p.346 *f*.

[26] See Zimmels, p.82, where Jewish sources referring to similar incubuses are also cited. *Cf. infra*, p.37.

[27] White, *Warfare*, *vol.ii*, p.75 *f*.

[28] See LaWall, *Pharmacy*, p.89.

[29] See Payne, *op. cit.*, p.112 *f*.; quoting Maitland, *The Dark Ages*, 1841, p.150.

[30] See Osler, *Evolution*, p.119 *ff*.

[31] The first specialised study of the subject is G. Brecher's *Transcen-dentale Magie und magische Heilarten im Talmud*, 1850. Another useful work in this field is L. Blau's *Das altjuedische Zauberwesen*, 1898. See also *JE*, *vol.iv*, p.516 *ff*.

[32] See *JE*, *vol.i*, p.547. Chajes already pointed out that the supernatural element was much more in evidence in the Babylonian than the Palesti-nian Tamud; see Z. H. Chajes, *The Student's Guide through the Talmud*, ed. J. Schachter, 1952, p.233 *f*.

[33] M. Guedemann, *Geschichte des Erziehungswesens und der Cultur der Juden in Frankreich und Deutschland*, 1880, p.199 *ff*.

[34] Guedemann, *op. cit.*, p.219.

[35] Guedemann, *op. cit.*, p.217 *f*.; see also Zimmels, p.80 *ff*. and notes.

36 Guedemann, *op. cit.*, *p*.222. See also Neuman, *op. cit.*, *vol.ii*, *p*.112.

37 See L. Rabinowitz, *The Social Life of the Jews of Northern France in the XII—XIV Centuries*, 1938, *p*.204 *ff*.

38 See Friedenwald, *pp*.365 and 383; citing Amatus, *Centuria* I, *Cur*.34.

39 Friedenwald (*p*.428 *ff*.) attributes the advanced views on witchcraft held by Amatus Lusitanus, Andres a Laguna (1499—1542) and Montaigne (1533—1592) to the influence of Maimonides, Isaac Abarvanel (1437—1508) and Levi ben Garson (1288—1344).

40 Ibn Ezra, on *Lev. xvii*.7; *cf.* also Nachmanides, *a.l.* See JE, *vol.iv*, *p*.519.

41 I. Abrahams, *Jewish Life in the Middle Ages*, 1932, *p*.391 (note 4).

42 *Ib.*, *p*.312.

43 Maimonides, *Mishnah Commentary*, on 'Avodah Zarah, iv.7; and *Hil.* 'Avodah Zarah, xi.16. *Cf.* also his *Guide to the Perplexed*, part *i*, *chpt*.61.

44 See Loew, *Gesammelte Schriften*, *vol.i*, *p*.328 *f*. See also H. S. Lewis, "Maimonides on Superstition", in *JQR*, *vol.xvii* (1905), *p*.485 *ff.*; I. Weiss, *Dor Dor Vedarshav*, 1924, *vol.iii*, *p*.223; and *JE*, *vol.ix*, *p*.85. Maimonides's refusal to accept the literal interpretation of the talmudic references to demons and magic was strongly attacked by Elijah of Vilna (*Bi'ur HaGRA*, *Y.D.*, *clxxix*.13) and Z. H. Chajes (*loc. cit.*). *Cf.* also Nachmanides, on *Deut. xviii*.9.

45 In fact, the strictures of Elijah of Vilna on Maimonides (see preceding note) were occasioned by Karo's repetition of Maimonides's critical views. *Cf.* note 107 below.

46 b*Horiyoth* 13b.

47 See *OY*, *vol.iv*, *p*.230 *f*.

48 See J. Goldziher, "Muhammedanischer Aberglaube ueber Gedaechtniskraft und Vergesslichkeit mit Parallelen aus der juedischen Litteratur", in *Berliner Festschrift*, ed. A. Freimann and M. Hildesheimer, 1903, *p*.131 *ff*. Such systems of mnemonics have retained their popularity to the present day; see, *e.g.*, D. Feldmann, *Kitzur Shulhan 'Arukh*, 1933, *p*.228 *ff*.

49 According to Maimonides, this contingency also includes him "who ate food well-known to be injurious" (*Mishnah Commentary*, on *B. Bathra*, *ix*.4).

50 *Tur*, *Y.D.*, *cccxxxv*. The actual wording is based on the Talmud (*Semahoth*).

51 b*Mo'ed Katan* 15a. Maimonides (*Hil. 'Avel*, *v*.18) still codified the law in its original form. The fear of arousing the suspicion of sorcery as one of the reasons for the abrogation of the custom is first mentioned by the Franco-German authorities Tosaphoth (*Mo'ed Katan* 21a), Asheri (*Mo'ed Katan*, *iii*.78) and his son Jacob (*Tur*, *Y.D.*, *ccclxxxvii*).

52 Zimmels, *p*.88 *f.*, and notes. See also Neuman, *op. cit.*, *p*.111.

53 Guedemann, *op. cit.*, *p*.224. But *cf.* note 51 above.

54 See Zimmels, *p*.221 (note 90). The question is not treated in the codes.

55 So Samuel Halevi, r*Nahalath Shiv'ah*, *no*.76, where earlier authorities for this view are cited and discussed. See also note 73 below.

56 See SHaH, *Y.D.*, *clxxix*.1; and Jacob Ettlinger, r*Binyan Tziyon*, *no*.67.

57 See *Beth Yoseph*, *Y.D.*, *clxxix*; and Solomon Luria, r*MaHaRSHaL*, *no*.3.

58 See Zimmels, *p*.193 (notes 186 *ff*.). *Cf.* also *supra*, *p*.30.

59 See Zimmels, *p*.35.

60 See *JE*, *vol.i*, *p*.529 *f.*, *s.v.* "Amorites".

60a *Cf.* the statement that the belief in eclipses as bad omens belonged to non-Jews only (*Mekhilta*, on *Ex. xii*.2; based on *Ter. x*.2).

61 t*Shabbath*, vii and viii.

[62] b*Shabbath* 67a; and b*Hullin* 77b.

[63] For the uses of these amulets, see commentaries on m*Shabbath*, *vi.*10 and b*Shabbath* 67a. L. Blau (*JE*, *vol.i*, *p.*547) wrongly states that the Talmud "forbade the use of all such remedies as being 'heathen practice' ".

[64] See *Beth Yoseph*, *loc. cit.* For a summary of these views, see Hamburger, *RE*, Supplement *ii* (1891), *p.*82 *f.*

[65] r*RaSHBA*, *nos.*167, 413 and 825.

[66] Asheri, *Shabbath*, *vi.*19. *Cf.* also *Kitzur Piskei HaROSH*, *a.l.*

[67] Rashi, *Shabbath* 67a.

[68] There would otherwise be a contradiction between this view of Rashi and that he expresses on another passage (*Hullin* 77b), where he permits the recitation of a charm-formula over a wound; see J. Z. Jalisch, *Melo Haro'im*, on *Shabbath* 67a.

[69] Following *RaN*, on *Shabbath* 67a.

[70] So originally *RaN*, *loc. cit.*, in the name of R. Jonah. *Cf. supra*, chpt.I (note 69).

[71] Maimonides, *Mishnah Commentary*, on *Yoma*, *viii.*6; and *Guide of the Perplexed*, part *iii*, chpt.37. *Cf.* also Thorndike, *Magic*, *vol.ii*, *p.*209.

[72] See *supra*, chpt.I (note 138). The Roman physician Soranus (though he, too, rejected charms and the like) permitted their use for women in childbirth, since "this soothes them and does no harm"; see Payne, *op. cit.*, *p.*96.

[73] See r*Nahalath Shiv'ah*, *loc. cit. Cf.* the view of R. Samuel of Meseritz (1625–1691): "The people should be permitted to retain the means of divining the fate of a sick person; for real magic existed only at the time when it was originally prohibited. To-day there is none" (cited by L. Lewin, in *JJLG*, *vol.ix* [1911], *p.*414). Earlier MaHaRaM ibn Haviv (*Kunteres Yom Kippur*, on *Yoma* 83) also regarded only such astrological and magic cures as forbidden as have emerged from the heathen cult of the Emorites, whereas supernatural methods proved effective by physicians might be employed; see *D.T.*, *clxxix.*7. *Cf.* also the statement by I. Hagiz, in *Etz Hahayim*, quoted by Epstein, *Torah Temimah*, on *Deut. xviii.*11 (*no.*64).

[74] See *D.T.*, *clxxix.*24; citing commentary on *Sepher Hasidim*.

[75] *SHaH*, *clv.*7.

[76] See *Beth Yoseph*, *Y.D.*, *clxxix*; and *SHaH*, *a.l.*, 8.

[77] See *supra*, *p.*22.

[78] See Preuss, *p.*167 *f.*; Krauss, *vol.i*, *p.*204; and *JE*, *vol.i*, *p.*546 *ff.*, *s.v.* "Amulets".

[79] See *supra*, *p.*33.

[80] b*Shabbath* 65a; see Preuss, *p.*192.

[81] So Falk, *Perishah*, *O.H.*, *ccci.*35. But this measure may also well have been prompted by perfectly rational considerations.

[82] This is first mentioned in b*Shabbath* 66b. A similar talisman is also described by Pliny (*Nat. Hist.*, *xxxvi.*39.3). It was probably a hollow stone containing a small pebble making a sound like a clapper in a bell, no doubt a representation of the fruit in the mother's womb. On the properties of this stone (often identified with *aetitis*), with ancient and medieval parallels, see Loew, *Lebensalter*, *p.*63; Guedemann, *op. cit.*, *p.*214; Preuss, *p.*446 *f.*; and Krauss, *vol.ii*, *pp.*4 and 425.

[82a] For a similar distinction between preventive and healing incantations, see *supra*, *p.*22.

[83] The Talmud (b*Shabbath* 53b) explains that man has a guardian angel and thus a chance of recovery from diseases fatal to animals. Hence, his luck helps some amulets to be effective, which is not always the case with animals; see *M.B.*, *cccv.*60.

84 Generally, sacred writings may be rescued without question (*O.H.,* *cccxxxiv.*12).

85 See sources cited in note 44 above. Maimonides omits the reference to demons in the rulings given here.

86 Meir ben Gedaliyah, r*MaHaRaM* of Lublin, *no.*116. *Cf.* Innocent's bull, *supra,* p.28.

87 *Zohar,* quoted by Karo, *Beth Yoseph, Y.D., clxxix.*

88 So expressly Karo, *loc. cit.*

89 See Zimmels, *p.*86 *f.* and notes, *a.l.*

90 Karo, *loc. cit.*

91 Hebrew "קְשֻׁב מְרֹורִי" (*Deut. xxxii.*24); the expression is demonologically interpreted by the *Targum* and Rashi, *a.l.* See also *JE, vol.iv, p.*516.

92 See Jaffe, *Levush, Y.D., ccclviii.*3.

93 This law is omitted by Maimonides; see *Lehem Hishneh, Hil. Shevithath 'Asor, iii.*2.

94 Maimonides (*Hil. Rotze'ah, xii.*5) explains this law as due to the fear lest something harmful fall unnoticed into the food.

95 According to the Talmud (b*Hullin* 105b), the washing of hands after meals was to protect the eyes from hurt through contact with salty hands, but with the disappearance of the harmful sea-salt, the enactment was later revoked (Tosaphoth, *Berakhoth* 53b; and *O.H., clxxxi.*10). The reference to "the evil spirit" resting on water so used, though mentioned in the Talmud (b*Hullin* 105b), is omitted by Maimonides (*Hil. Berakhoth, vi.*16).

96 Maimonides, *Hil. Gerushin, ii.*14; and *Mishnah Commentary,* on *Shabbath, ii.*5, where he identifies "the evil spirit" with "melancholy". *Cf.* also his *Guide of the Perplexed,* part *i, chpt.*7.

97 See, *e.g.,* Epstein, *A.H., O.H., ccxxxviii.*17, who regards a person possessed of "the evil spirit" as suffering from a dangerous disease which may lead to suicide.

98 Similar attempts to rationalise classic references to "possessed people" are found in Christian sources, too. Preuss (*p.*360) recalls that Th. Bartholin, in a 17th century dissertation on the subject, "first dared to describe the demoniacs of the New Testament as epileptics and lunatics". Writing on "Angels and Demons", an official Anglican report recently stated: "For many of the phenomena recorded in the Gospels it is no doubt true that an alternative interpretation, based upon medical or psychological considerations, might in our time be suggested" (*Doctrine in the Church of England,* 1950, *p.*46).

99 *Cf.* Rashi, *Ta'anith* 22b. See also Karo, *Beth Yoseph, Y.D., ccxxviii.*

100 This belief is of medieval origin, but is not mentioned by Guedemann, *loc. cit.*

101 For literature on the subject, see *JE, vol.v, p.*280, *s.v.* "Evil Eye".

102 This charm, mentioned in the Talmud (b*Shabbath* 57b), probably contained balsam (so Jastrow, *Dcitionary, p.*436), though Rashi (*a.l.*) and the codes appear to interpret the word used for "balsam" (קִימֹוף) as "sudden death" or "plucking" of the evil eye (so also Kohut, *Aruch Completum, vol.iii, p.*436).

103 b*B. Bathra* 126b. Maimonides (*Hil. Nahaloth, ii.*16) avoids mentioning the belief.

104 See *John ix.*6; and *Mark viii.*23.

105 Tacitus, *Hist., iv.*81. For this and further Roman sources, see Preuss, *p.*321. *Cf.* also the widespread belief in the virtue of *saliva jejuna* to cure eye-complaints, found in Pliny and even Galen; see Thorndike, *Magic, vol.i, pp.*82 and 174. See also *JE, vol.x, p.*651.

106 Guedemann (*op. cit., p.*215), referring to several Jewish and non-Jewish medieval sources for this occult remedy against head-ache, claims that this could also be found in the Talmud. But the passage (*Shabbath* 157b) on which the codes base this law deals with measuring for religious purposes in general, not with this particular practice which is unknown in the Talmud.

107 This practice, too, is not mentioned by Maimonides, though it is recorded several times in the Talmud and Midrash; see Preuss, *p.*463; and Krauss, *vol.ii, p.*8. But even the other codes omit reference to the many other magic customs and superstitions widely practiced in connection with child-birth; see Loew, *Lebensalter, p.*76 *f.*; Preuss, *p.*488; and *JE, vol.iv, p.*30 *f.*

108 On the origin of this medieval legend, see L. Ginzberg, *The Legends of the Jews,* 1939, *vol.vi, p.*22 (note 135). Another health token mentioned in the Talmud (j*Mo'ed Katan, iii.*7) and codified by Karo (*Y.D., cccxciv.*4) is the belief that all the family will be healed if a son is born during the year of mourning.

109 The source for this fear is to be found in the *Sepher Hasidim;* see *Darkei Mosheh, Y.D., xi.*2. The tradition is not mentioned in the earlier codes.

110 So *TaZ, a.l.,* 1, in the name of *BaH,* who bases his view on the Talmud (b*Nedarim* 40a).

111 See b*Shabbath* 129b. But in cases of danger, the operation was permitted even on the eve of Pentecost; see *M.B., a.l.,* 38. Cf. also *supra,* Introduction (notes 75 and 78).

112 See *supra,* Introduction (note 74). On the ancient origin and wide currency of the belief that sneezing often proved fatal, see Preuss, *p.*83 *ff.*; and *JE, vol.ii, p.*255 *f.*

113 These laws, first codified in the *Shulhan 'Arukh,* are based on stories related in the Talmud (b*Berakhoth* 18b; and b*Mo'ed Katan* 28a); see *Beth Yoseph* and *Darkei Mosheh, Y.D., clxxix.* In the 19th century, one rabbi (Jacob Ettlinger, r*Binyan Tziyon, no.*67) permitted a patient to be treated by "magnetising" (Mesmerism) because the forces thus invoked could be attributed to purely "natural phenomena still undiscovered by us", whilst another (Solomon Kluger, r*Tuv Ta'am Vada'ath,* 3rd *ed.,* part *ii, no.*48) strongly objected to participation in spiritualistic seances as plain sorcery; see *D.T., clxxix.*6. More recently, A. I. Kook (r*Da'ath Kohen, no.*69), too, was inclined to view spiritualism as compromising the true faith in God; see Zimmels, *p.*219 (note 53).

114 For numerous medical reports on such cases in recent times, see lists of articles in *Index Catalogue of the Library of the Surgeon-General's Office, U.S. Army,* Third Series, *vol.x* (1932), *p.*1021, *s.v.* "*Vagitus Uterinus*"; and Fourth Series, *vol.x* (1940), *p.*956, *s.v.* "Fetus, Respiration."

115 b*Niddah* 42b; see Preuss, *p.*445. The inference drawn by Guedemann (*op. cit., p.*216) to the contrary effect is wrong.

116 The *Shulhan 'Arukh* evidently held that the child's sounds could be heard in *exceptional* cases before the delivery of its head; for it declares the 8-day period to commence "from the day its head emerged *or* from the day it was heard to cry". Elsewhere, however, Karo (*Y.D., cxciv.*12) states expressly that "it is impossible to hear the child's voice if it did not bring out the head outside the birth-canal"; but *cf. P.T., a.l.,* 9. Maimonides, therefore, follows the Talmud more accurately in omitting the reference to the child's crying altogether and in dealing only with the emergence of the head as determining the birth-day (*Hil. Milah, i.*15). According to Isserles (*E.H., iv.*14, gloss), incidentally, it was possible

(CHAPTER II)

that an embryo aborted after less than five month's gestation could be heard to cry at birth before its death; see *He.M.*, *a.l.*, 13.

117 See Haggard, *Devils*, p.61; and McKenzie, *Infancy*, p.310 f. This belief was firmly held throughout antiquity and shared by Hippocrates and Galen; see Preuss, p.456. According to A. Stern (*Die Medizin im Talmud*, 1909, p.14), this notion was definitely of foreign origin; see Krauss, *vol.ii*, p.427 (note 26). In Jewish law, the idea that 8-months' babies could not live became so axiomatic that it was suggested that if such a child nevertheless survived, neither its puberty (b*Yevamoth* 80a; and *Novellae of RaSHBA*, *a.l.*) nor its viability (Rashi, *a.l.*) would be definitely established before reaching the age of twenty years; see Loew, *Lebensalter*, p.49 f.

118 So *TaZ*, *a.l.*, 8, based on the Talmud (b*Yevamoth* 80b; and b*Niddah* 38b); see Loew, *loc. cit.*; and Preuss, p.456. The same reasoning occurs to explain the circumstances of a pregnancy exceeding nine months (*E.H.*, *iv.*14).

119 This is among the original practices prohibited as "Emorite" customs (t*Shabbath*, *vii.*3). Other authorities, however, were prepared to permit the act completely (sor*MaHaRIL*, no.118); see Guedemann, *op. cit.*, p.209 (note 1).

120 See McKenzie, *Infancy*, p.109 ff. Garrison (*An Introduction*, p.274) remarks that C. F. Paulini's *Die heilsame Dreckapotheke* (published in 1696) is "a title which amply symbolises the tendency of many 17th century prescriptions". In fact, this tendency was not at all restricted to that period.

121 Galen, *ed.* Kuehn, xii.248, 284—285, and 290.

122 *Ib.*, 293; see Thorndike, *Magic*, *vol.i*, p.167 f.

123 See McKenzie, *loc. cit.*

124 See LaWall, *Pharmacy*, p.247 f.

125 Osler, *Evolution*, p.15.

126 H. L. Strack, *Der Blutaberglaube in der Menschheit*, 1892, p.83.

127 Preuss, p.509. Krauss (*vol.i*, p.257 ff.) enumerates 72 kinds of domestic and pharmacological medicines mentioned in the Talmud; only six items in this list belong to the "*Dreckapotheke*" (nos. 51—56).

128 E. A. W. Budge, *Syrian Anatomy, Pathology and Therapeutics;* or "*The Book of Medicines*", 1913, end of second volume.

129 We may here remark that the long and notorious popularity of uroscopy is hardly reflected in Jewish law; it refers only once to vessels used for the examination of urine (*O.H.*, xliii.9). On the history of this quaint department of medieval medicine, see D. Riesman, *The Story of Medicine in the Middle Ages*, 1935, p.328 ff. (in chapter on "Uroscopy").

130 See *SHaKH*, *a.l.*, 3. Cf. *D.T.*, cxvi.100.

131 Cf. *supra*, chpt.I (note 69).

132 *Levush*, *Y.D.*, cxvi.6.

133 See, *e.g.*, *A.H.*, *Y.D.*, lxxxi.10.

134 See Zimmels, p.126 ff.; and the few illustrations given by Guedemann, *op. cit.*, p.216.

135 See Preuss, p.140 (note 8).

136 Cf. the pointed observation by Guedemann (*op. cit.*, p.220 [note 4]): "Even in the darkest times, Judaism never went so far as to grant dogmatic recognition to the belief in sorcery, as happened in the Church which set up the doctrine: '*Haeresis est maxima, opera maleficarum non credere*' (*Malleus Malefic.*, iii, quaest.25)".

— 273 —

Chapter Three

[1] These words are omitted in the *Munich MS* of the Talmud.

[2] m*Sanhedrin, iv.*5.

[3] *Koran, v.*35; quoted by Cumston, *An Introduction, p.*187.

[4] b*Shabbath* 151b.

[5] *Sepher Hasidim, no.*724.

[6] *SHaKH, a.l.,* 1. This law is derived from the Talmud (b*Kethuboth* 17a).

[7] See Hamburger, *RE,* Supplement *ii, p.* 37.

[8] For numerous sources on the Karaite attitude, see Zimmels, *p.*172 (note 72).

[9] The Sabbath laws, due to their numerical and practical prominence, usually serve as a prototype to exemplify the setting aside of any religious precept for medical considerations; see Joseph Babad, *Minhath Hinnukh,* commandment *no.*32 (*ed.* Vilna, 1912, *vol.i, p.*103). *Cf.* also Moses Ribkes, *Be'er Hagolah, O.H., cccxxviii.*10 (*no.*100); and *P.T., Y.D., clv.*4.

[10] J. M. Tucatzinsky, "The Death Penalty according to the Torah in the Past and Present", in *Hatorah Vehamedinah, ed.* S. Israeli, 4th series, 1952, *p.*34 *f.* But the editor, in a footnote, has contested the validity of the deduction on technical grounds.

[11] b*B. Kamma* 26b and 27a. The argument there concerns the capital guilt of a person who beheads a child thrown from a roof by another person.

[12] b*Yoma* 85a and b. *Cf. Mekhilta,* on *Ex. xxxi.*13, where the same teachings are ascribed to a slightly varied group of authors.

[13] *Cf. Matth. xii.*8.

[14] *I.e.* Israel "shall keep the Sabbath" only on condition that they shall be able "to observe the Sabbath" in the future; see Malbim, *a.l.*; and Rashi, *Yoma* 85b. For another interpretation, see J. L. Unterman, *Shevet Miyehudah,* 1955, *p.*62 *ff.*

[15] The Talmud (*loc. cit.*) prefers this view to the other deductions because it proves more conclusively that the Sabbath may be profaned even if the resultant saving of life is in doubt. See also Unterman, *op. cit., p.* 5 *ff.*

[16] Atar, *'Or Hahayim,* on *Ex. xxxi.*16.

[17] See *Minhath Hinnukh, loc. cit.*

[18] See *M.B., cccxxix.*4.

[19] Maimonides, *Hil. Shabbath, ii.*3.

[20] So *M.B., loc. cit.*

[21] Me'iri, *Beth Habehirah,* on *Yoma* 85b. See also Chajes, r*MaHaRaTZ, no.*28. On the correspondence of this view with the Christian doctrine of confession, see *infra,* chapter XI (beginning).

[22] See *M.B., loc. cit.*

[23] See Adreth, r*RaSHBA, no.*689.

[24] So Asheri, *Yoma, viii.*14; and r*RoSH, no.*26, §5. He compares the suspension of the Sabbath laws for the sick with the abeyance of laws affecting the preparation of food on festivals for healthy people.

[25] So Nissim, *RaN,* on *Yoma* 83a.

[26] r*RaSHBA, loc. cit.*

[27] For detailed discussions on these arguments, see *Beth Yoseph, O.H., cccxxviii; Minhath Hinnukh, op. cit.* (*p.*102); *A.H., O.H., cccxxviii.*3–5; and Samuel Hacohen Borstein, *Minhath Shabbath,* 1905, *xcii.*1.

[28] *Cf.* the controversy on the extent to which the Sabbath laws may be disregarded for patients in danger; see *infra,* chapter V (beginning).

29 See *supra*, *p.6 f.*

30 For further details, see *infra*, *p.196 f.*

3,1 *TaZ*, *a.l.*, 21.

32 "Moreover, he who is asked is reprehensible" (*Tur*, *O.H.*, *cccxxviii*; based on *jYoma*, *viii*.5), "for he should have expounded the sanction in public" (*Beth Yoseph*, *a.l.*).

33 All other biblical festivals must be observed (in the Diaspora) on the original dates and on the days immediately following them (*O.H.*, *cdxcvi*.1).

34 So Adreth, *rRaSHBA*, *no.*175; see *Ba'er Hetev*, *O.H.*, *cccxviii*.1.

35 *M.A.*, *cciv*.21.

36 Responsum of Maimonides, quoted by Karo, *Beth Yoseph*, *O.H.*, *dcxviii*.

37 See *M.B.*, *dcxviii*.5.

38 "For they all aimed at accomplishing a meritorious deed, considering that whoever is zealous to [assist] the sick is praiseworthy" (Rashi, *Menahoth* 64a).

39 So Nachmanides, *Torath Ha'adam*, *Sha'ar Hasakkanah*; and David ibn Zimra, *rRaDBaZ*, part *iii*, *no.*885.

40 So *M.A.*, *cccxxviii*.6; *Ba'er Hetev*, *O.H.*, *cccxxviii*.1; and *P.T.*, *clv*.4. According to Moses Schick (*rMaHaRaM Shik*, *O.H.*, *no.*260) and Judah Assad (*rMaHaRYA*, *O.H.*, *no.*160), a seriously sick person eating unleavened bread and bitter herbs on Passover against medical advice must not recite any benediction over them, for this would be as contemptible as to say a blessing over forbidden foods when healthy.

41 *Nu. Rabbah*, *xxiii*.1; and *Tanhuma*, Ma'sei (beginning).

42 *Gen. Rabbah*, *lxxxii*.9. See also Elijah of Vilna, *Bi'ur HaGRa*, *Y.D.*, *clvii*.20.

43 Maimonides, *Hil. Yesodei Hatorah*, *v*.4.

44 See *SHaKH*, *clvii*.1. Karo himself comments on the ruling of Maimonides: "There are, however, many truly pious men who hold that, if one preferred death to transgression, it is accounted as a meritorious act for him" (*Keseph Mishneh*, *a.l.*). See Unterman, *op. cit.*, *p.*38 *ff.*

45 See *rRaDBaZ*, part *i*, *no.*67; quoted in *D.T.*, *clvii*.12.

46 *rRaDBaZ*, part *iii*, *no.*885; see Zimmels, *p.*9 *f.*

47 *bSanhedrin* 74a. For various sources on the date of this ordinance, see Zimmels, *p.*172 (note 76).

48 We here use the term 'incest" to denote any carnal relationship (including adultery) which is proscribed as immoral. See also *infra*, *p.*55 *f.*

49 Maimonides, *Hil. Yesodei Hatorah*, *v*.6. See Unterman, *op. cit.*, *pp.*24 *ff.* and 44 *ff.* The distinction is not incorporated in the later codes, probably because they are not usually concerned with penal considerations.

50 See *infra*, chapter XIV.

51 See H. L. Strack, *Der Blutaberglaube in der Menschheit*, 1892, *p.*36 *ff.*; and Preuss, *p.*168 *f.*

52 See M. Dworzecki, "Jetons l'anathème contre la science criminelle nazie", in *Révue*, *no.*1 (1948), *p.*60 *ff.*; and H. Baruk, "Les médecins allemands et l'experimentation médicalle criminelle", in *Révue*, *no.*7 (1950), *p.*7 *ff.*

53 *bYoma* 82b. This argument implies that the absolute ban on bloodshed operates only if one person seeks to save his life at the expense of another. Yet, as will be shown (see *infra*, chapter VII [end]), a man must not kill another even if a refusal would lead to the death of both. Hence, Karo (*Keseph Mishneh*, *Hil. Yesodei Hatorah*, *v*.5) assumes that the main basis of the law is not the "obvious argument" but an authentic tradition handed down to the rabbis.

54 Maimonides, *Hil. Yesodei Hatorah, v.*7.

55 For a complete list of the thus forbidden relationships, see *E.H., xv, xvi* and *xvii.*1.

56 The Roman Catholic Church, too, teaches that a virgin "may discontinue external positive resistance [to an attack on her virtue] for a very grave cause like danger of death" (J. McCarthy, in *Irish Ecclesiastical Record, vol.lv* [1940], *p.*636).

57 b*Sanhedrin* 75a.

58 Maimonides, *Hil. Yesodei Hatorah, v.*9. So also Karo, *Beth Yoseph, Y.D., clvii.* The ruling is not recorded in the *Shulhan 'Arukh*, but Shabbatai Cohen (*SHaKH, Y.D., clvii.*10) suggests that the inclusion of non-capital cases in Isserles's gloss refers to the circumstances envisaged in the decisions of the Talmud and Maimonides.

59 Maimonides, *Sepher Hamitzvoth*, Negative Commandments, *no.*353; and *Hil. 'Issurei Bi'ah, xxi.*1. But Nachmanides (*RaMBaN*, on *Sepher Hamitzvoth, loc. cit.*) regards any physical intimacy (other than actual cohabitation) as merely a rabbinical offence; see also *Maggid Mishnah, Hil. 'Issurei Bi'ah, xxi.*1. Cf. note 66 below.

60 H. L. Strack, *The Jew and Human Sacrifice*, transl. H. F. E. Blauchamp, 1909, *p.*95 *f.*; and particularly E. D. Baumann, "Antike Betrachtungen ueber Nutzen und Schaden des Koitus", in *Janus, vol.xliv* (1940), *p.*123 *ff.*

61 Pliny (*Nat. Hist., xxviii.*43), for instance, promised relief from epilepsy "*si virgo dextro pollice attigat*"; see Allbutt, *Greek Medicine, p.*36.

62 Maimonides, *Hil. De'oth, iii.*2. In the *Shulhan 'Arukh* (*O.H., ccxxxi.*1) the medical motive is omitted.

63 During this period (terminated only by immersion in a ritual bath at least twelve days after the onset of menstruation) a woman may not be in any physical contact with her husband (*Y.D., cxcv.*1 and 2).

64 The law is first mentioned by Israel Isserlein, r*Terumath Hadeshen, no.*252.

65 So Karo, *Beth Yoseph, Y.D., cxcv.* See also *SHaKH, a.l.*, 20.

66 So Nachmanides, r*RaMBaN, no.*127; see also note 59 above. Other authorities are cited by Isserles (*Y.D., cxcv.*16, gloss). See *SHaKH, loc. cit.*; and *Bi'ur HaGRA, a.l.*, 21.

67 This law is first recorded by Asheri, r*ROSH, no.*29, §3. It is held that a man is less capable of controlling his passions once aroused than a woman; hence when he is weak and confined to bed, physical contact between him and his wife is less likely to lead to conjugal intimacy than her being ill (*Beth Yoseph, Y.D., cxcv*).

68 See L. Ginzberg, *Ginzei Schechter*, 1928, *vol.*i, *p.*19.

69 See Daniel Tirni, '*Ikrei Dinim, xv.*3 (*ed.* Vilna, *Y.D.*, end of 2nd *vol., p.*14a). Zimmels (*p.*242 [note 89]) refers to another source (r*Shemesh Tzedakah, no.*29).

70 Found, *e.g.*, in Abukalsen, *ed.* Channing, *p.*371; see Preuss, *p.*169. For this reason Saladin refused to follow his Jewish doctor's advice; see E. Ashtor-Strauss, "Saladin and the Jews", in *HUCA, vol.xxvii* (1956), *p.*311 f.

71 See *supra, p.xxxiii.*

72 C. Capellmann, *Pastoral-Medizin*, 1878, *p.*99.

73 See Diepgen, *Die Theologie, p.*49 *ff.* For further illustrations on this attitude, see L. M. McKinney, "Medical Ethics... in the early Middle Ages", in *Bulletin of the History of Medicine, vol.xxvi* (1952), *p.*9 *f.*

74 Hefele, German *ed., vol.v, p.*1053; cited by Friedenwald, *p.*559.

75 Ambrosius, *Opera, vol.ii, p.*709; and *Gratian Decretals, d.v., cap.*21; cited by Diepgen, *loc. cit.*

76 See *infra, p.*121 *f.*

Chapter Four

1 *Cf. supra, p.xxxvi.* See also Kahana, in *Sinai, vol.xiv* (1950), *p.68.*

2 *Cf. supra, p.xxxvii ff.*

3 This applies even when the evidence against the Talmud is given by a non-Jewish physician, "for your eyes testify that changes have occurred in all these matters" (*rBesamim Rosh,* [ascribed to Asheri,] *no.59*). For references to further sources, including a ruling by Isaac Lampronti, in support of this view, see *D.T., cxvi.43.* Recently, this opinion was also confirmed by D. Feldmann (*Metzudath David,* on *Kitzur Shulhan 'Arukh, xcii* [end]); *cf.* Kahana, *op. cit., p.224 f.*

4 See *P.M., O.H., cccxxviii.2*; quoted by Kahana, *loc. cit.* These views are clearly shared by the codes, for, while enumerating the conditions regarded as dangerous by the Talmud in its Sabbath regulations, they rule categorically that "the Sabbath may be profaned for *all* diseases which the doctors declare to be dangerous" (*O.H., cccxxviii.10*). But *cf.* also *Minhath Shabbath, xcii.24* and *32.*

5 This division has been compared with the modern distinction between "*morbi internae et externae*" (B. Saltzberg, *Meshiv Kehalakhah, or On the Religious Duties of Physicians and Patients,* 1922, *p.36* [note 15]). For a similar distinction among the ancient Egyptians and in the religious philosophy of Ibn Ezra, see *supra, p.5.*

6 Hebrew: "אחזו דם", translated by Jastrow (*Dictionary, p.39*) as "an attack of congestion". The Talmud (*tBekhoroth, iii.17*) mentions this condition to indicate venesection only as an affliction of animals. Preuss (*pp.289* and *511*) calls it "*Blutandrang*".

7 Preuss (*p.208*) surmises that the talmudic definition of this complaint (*b'Avodah Zarah 28b*) refers to a kind of eczema.

8 Regarded in the Talmud (*b'Avodah Zarah 28a*) as "a herald of severe fever"; see Preuss, *p.223.*

9 See Preuss, *p.185.*

10 So suggested by Krauss, *vol.i, p.253.*

11 See Preuss, *p.310 f.*

12 Hebrew: "תחלת אוכלא". Jastrow (*Dictionary, p.25*) renders this (actually Aramaic) term simply by "an eye disease", or "itching". Preuss (*p.311*) is uncertain as to the exact meaning of the expression, but he cites Kohut (*Aruch Completum, vol.i, p.76*) who translates it as "cancer". Literally the word means "consumption", and according to the Talmud (*b'Avodah Zarah 28b*) this disease is dangerous only in its incipient stage.

13 For details on this illness (well known to several medical writers of antiquity), see Preuss, *p.209.* But Krauss (*vol.i, p.255*), opposing Preuss, believes that "*bulimus*", as used in the Talmud (*mYoma, viii.6*), probably refers not to the pathological, chronic feeling of hunger, but to the ravenous appetite experienced by healthy people after a protracted fast.

14 The Talmud (*mYoma, viii.5*) considers this as sufficiently dangerous to justify breaking the fast on the Day of Atonement only if manifested in pregnant women, but the *Shulhan 'Arukh*—following Asheri (*Yoma, viii.13*)—regards it as a possibly fatal disease in any person, with the difference that the demand for food by pregnant women must be satisfied even if their morbid desire is not accompanied by "a change in [the appearance of] the face".

15 Preuss (*p.442*) identifies this malady with the «κισσᾶν» of the ancient Greeks.

16 See *supra, chpt.I* (note 130).

17 See Preuss, *p.220.*

18 In ancient times, the deadly character in injuries caused by iron (as a septic agent) was widely feared; for talmudic and classical sources, see Preuss, *p.*219 *f.*

19 See Preuss, *p.*224 *f.*

20 See Preuss, *p.*225.

21 Leeches were regarded as poisonous in antiquity; see Preuss, *p.*230.

22 See Preuss, *pp.*294 and 297.

23 See *supra, p.*38.

24 The phrase used here is: ". . . one against whom an evil spirit breathed —[a condition] in which there is no danger".

25 This was a treatment for certain heart complaints; see Preuss, *pp.*205 and 671.

26 For details on these acts in the treatment of new-born children (already mentioned in *Ez. xvi.*4), see Preuss, *p.*467; and Krauss, *vol.ii, p.*8. Gumbiner (*M.A., a.l.,* 3), following Tosaphoth (*Shabbath* 129b [end]), regards these actions as necessary only to avoid undue pain; hence, he merely permits the transgression of rabbinic laws in this connection. But more recent halachists (so *A.H., a.l.,* 12; and *M.B., Bi'ur Halakhah, a.l.*) agree with the view of Maimonides (*Hil. Shabbath, ii.*14) that the failure to carry out these operations may be dangerous, so that they override even biblical precepts if necessary. *Cf.* also *supra, p.xlix.*

27 This act, also mentioned by Galen and Soranus, was considered indispensable; see Preuss, *p.*467. The custom was still practised among Turkish Jews in the 18th century; see Zimmels, *p.*74.

28 The Talmud (b*Shabbath* 128b) also records some opposition to this operation being performed on the Sabbath. For further sources, see Preuss, *p.*463 (note 2).

29 For details, see *infra,* chapter XV.

30 But the powder should not be compounded on the Sabbath in the ordinary manner; instead it should be ground with one's teeth (*O.H., cccxxxi.*7; and *Y.D., cclxvi.*3). If the powder was scattered or lost on the Sabbath *before* the circumcision, some rabbis (against the view of others) hold that the whole operation must be postponed to the next day, so that it should not necessitate violating the Sabbath by an action rendered essential only *post facto* (the danger not being acute at the time the mixture is prepared); see *SHaKH, a.l.,* 6; and J. L. Unterman, *Shevet Miyehudah,* 1955, *p.*32 *ff.*

31 See Preuss, *p.*66. 4

32 *Cf. infra,* chpt.VI (note 2).

33 For sources, see *D.T., clv.*15. *Cf.* also Zimmels, *p.*111 and notes. For numerous talmudic data on epilepsy, see Preuss, *p.*343 *ff.*

34 Thus, Solomon Luria (r*MaHaRSHaL, no.*3) opposes the view of R. Tam that the danger to an organ or a limb is in itself a sufficient cause for profaning the Sabbath; see also Asheri, *'Avodah Zarah, ii.*10. Karo (*loc. cit.*) inclines to the view that the danger does not warrant "any action which leans on a biblical prohibition", but he also records the more lenient rulings. See Unterman, *op. cit., p.*23 *ff.* Only serious injury to the eye was always regarded as dangerous condition (*cf. supra, p.*60), because "[an affection of] the eye-muscles is connected with the chamber of the heart (or mental faculties)" (b*'Avodah Zarah* 28b); see Preuss, *p.*80 *f.*

35 This is permitted by one authority (*M.B., Bi'ur Halakhah, cccxxix.*4), but doubted by another (Moses Chagiz, *Halakhoth Ketannoth,* part *ii, no.*38). See also *Minhath Hinnukh,* commandment *no.*32; and *Ba'er Hetev, O.H., cccxxviii.*40.

36 In one important source (r*Beth Ya'akov, no.*59) the breach of the Sabbath laws for the sake of dying persons is discountenanced, but the

consensus of rabbinic opinion agrees with Tosaphoth (*Yoma* 84b) that this is permitted; see Azulay, *Birkei Yoseph*, *O.H.*, *cccxxix*.4; Lampronti, *Pahad Yitzhak*, *s.v.* "*Holeh beshabbath*"; Chajes, r*MaHaRaTZ*, *no.*28; and Aeurbach, *Nahal Eshkol*, *xxxvi* (end), *no.*1. Cf. also *Minhath Hinnukh*, *loc. cit.*

37 While Joseph Te'umim (*P.M.*, '*Eshel 'Avraham*, *O.H.*, *cccxxix*.4) permits the violation of the Sabbath to save a person under sentence of death, another opinion disputes this (*M.B.*, *loc. cit.*).

38 Nachmanides (*Torath Ha'adam*, *Sha'ar Sakkanah*) forbids profaning the Sabbath for the protection of an unborn child's life, unless the process of parturition has set in or the mother is already dead (the child then being regarded as a separate being); see *Minhath Hinnukh*, commandment *no.*296; and *TE*, *vol.i*, *p.*75. But according to Nissim (*RaN*, on *Yoma* 82a) and Asheri (*Yoma*, *viii*.13), every danger to the foetus involves a risk of life to the mother as well, thus setting aside the Sabbath laws; *cf.* r*RaDBaZ*, part *i*, *no.*695; and r*Havath Ya'ir*, *no.*31. For a summary of these views, see *M.A.*, *cccxxx*.15; E. Landau, *Dagul Mervavah*, on *O.H.*, *dcxvii*.2; *P.M.*, *Mishbetzoth Zahav*, *O.H.*, *cccxxviii*.1; and Unterman, *op. cit.*, *p.*9 *ff.*

39 See *supra*, *p.xli*. Thus, Joseph Trani (r*MaHaRIT*, *no.*97) explains that this ruling permits the desecration of the Sabbath only because the child, after the mother's death, is no longer regarded as *pars ventri*; *cf.* preceding note.

40 See *supra*, *p.*40.

41 b*Pesahim* 21b; based on *Lev. xxv.*35.

42 The "stranger" here refers to any non-Jew who observes the "seven Noachidic commandments"; see D. Hoffmann, *Der Schulchan Aruch*, 1894, *p.*150 *ff.*; and M. Guttmann, *Das Judentum und seine Umwelt*, 1927, *p.*43 *ff.*

43 Maimonides, *Hil. 'Avodah Zarah*, *x.*2.

44 So, for instance, Nachmanides, *Sepher Hamitzvoth*, additions to positive commandments, *no.*16; and Adreth, r*RaSHBA*, *no.*120 (*ed.* Venice, 1545; in the later editions this responsum was excised by the censor; see A. A. Neumann, *The Jews in Spain*, 1948, *vol.ii*, *pp.*109 and 309 [note 93]).

45 See b*Yoma* 84b; and Tosaphoth, *a.l.* (85a [top]).

46 Me'iri, *Beth Habehirah*, on *Yoma* 84b; *cf.* also on 85a. See further quotation by Bezalel Ashkenazi, *Shittah Mekubbetzeth*, on *Baba Kamma* 38a.

47 The principal 17th century authorities dealing with this problem are: Joel Sirkes, r*Beth Hadash Hahadashoth*, Koretz, 1785, *no.*2; Gur Aryeh Halevy of Mantua, commentary on *O.H.*, *cccvii*; and Gershon Ashkenazi, r'*Avodath Hagershuni*, *no.*123. For extensive quotations from these and later sources, see Kahana, *op. cit.*, *p.*227 *ff.*

48 So, *e.g.*, Chayim Halberstam, r*Divrei Hayim*, part *ii*, *O.H.*, *no.*25 (see Zimmels, *p.*25). The main objection concerned biblically prohibited work, not rabbinical prohibitions, for the non-Jewish sick; see also *M.B.*, *cccxxx*.8. Halberstam (*loc. cit.*) mentions he had heard that the "Council of the Four Lands" (which functioned in Poland between the 16th and 18th centuries; see *JE*, *vol.iv*, *p.*304 *f.*) had sanctioned the treatment of non-Jews on the Sabbath, but he had seen no confirmation of such an enactment; see also Kahana, *op. cit.*, *p.*230.

49 So Nachmanides, cited by Bezalel Ashkenazi, *op. cit.*, on *Baba Kamma* 90a; and Gur Aryeh Halevy, *loc. cit.* Sirkes (*loc. cit.*) also advised doctors to resort to this expedient with certain reservations; see Kahana, *op. cit.*, *p.*227 *ff.*

[50] See especially Moses Schreiber, r*Hatham Sopher*, *Y.D.*, *no.*131; and his addenda to *H.M.*, *no.*194. See also *P.T.*, *Y.D.*, *cliv.*2; and Kahana, *op. cit.*, *p.*229.

[51] So Sirkes, *loc. cit.*, and most other authorities previously cited.

[52] So Israel Lipschuetz, *Tiph'ereth Yisrael*, on '*Avodah Zarah*, *ii.*1 (*no.*6), who refers to a concession by Maimonides (*Hil. Shemittah*, *i.*11) in similar circumstances; David Ungar, r*Yad Shalom*, *no.*57; and *Shibbolei David*, cited in *D.T.*, *cliv.*9. Professional and economic pressure also forced the Jewish authorities in Prague to sanction similar relaxations in medical practice; see Joab of Deutschkreuz, r*Imrei No'am*, *no.*8; quoted by Kahana, *op. cit.*, *p.*232. But such sanction could be given only for the violation of rabbinical Sabbath laws; see I. J. Weisz, r*Minhath Yitzhak*, *no.*53.

[53] For instance, when called upon to visit prominent citizens. So Gershon Ashkenazi, *loc. cit.*; and Meir Zvi Vitomir, r*ReMaTZ*, part *i*, *O.H.*, *no.*21; see Kahana, *op. cit.*, *p.*227 *ff.*

[54] So Joseph Te'umim, *P.M.*, *Mishbetzoth Zahav*, *O.H.*, *ccxxxviii.*6. But this view is opposed by M. J. Breisch, r*Helkath Ya'akov*, *no.*45.

[55] The Talmud (b*Yoma* 83a) regards this scriptural proof as necessary (although any doubt involving danger to life is in any case always resolved by suspending the law) to show that the patient's view is accepted even though the fear of death may lead him to exaggerate his needs; see Asheri, *Yoma*, *viii.*13; and Preuss, *p.*170.

[56] Even if the patient is himself a medical expert (*P.M.*, *Mishbetzoth Zahav*, *a.l.*, 2).

[57] So Joel Sirkes (*BaH*, *a.l.*) following Nachmanides; see *M.A.*, *a.l.*, 4.

[58] See *infra*, chapter XIX.

[59] So first Simon Duran, r*TaSHBeTZ*, part *iii*, *no.*271; followed by Jacob Poppers, r*Shav Ya'akov*, *nos.*41 and 42; Moses Schreiber, r*Hatham Sopher*, *E.H.*, part *ii*, *no.*82, and *Y.D.*, *no.*153; Moses Schick, r*MaHaRaM Shik*, *Y.D.*, *nos.*155 and 243; and A. I. Kook, r*Da'ath Kohen*, *no.*140. For further sources, see Kahana, *op. cit.*, *p.*64 *ff.*; and Zimmels, *p.*24 with corresponding notes.

Chapter Five

[1] This general rule, though always taken for granted, is not clearly codified except in relation to the Sabbath laws (*O.H.*, *cccxxvii.*2), the Fast of Atonement (*O.H.*, *dcxviii.*1) and the use of ritually forbidden substances (*Y.D.*, *clv.*3).

[2] So explicitly Vidal of Tolosa, *Maggid Mishnah*, *Hil. Shabbath*, *ii.*14; and evidently also Me'iri, *Beth Habehirah*, on *Yoma* (end); and Duran, r*TaSHBeTZ*, part *i*, *no.*54.

[3] See *M.A.*, *a.l.*, 4.

[4] As implied by his commentary on *Yoma* 84b.

[5] r*RaSHBA*, *no.*214.

[6] For a full summary and discussion of these views, see *M.B.*, *Bi'ur Halachah*, on *O.H.*, *cccxxviii.*4. Cf. also I. Abramsky, *Hazon Yehezkel*, on t*Shabbath*, *xvi.*12.

[7] By Elijah of Vilna, *Bi'ur HaGRA*, *Y.D.*, *clv.*24.

[8] See *supra*, *p.*47 *ff.*

[9] b*Yoma* 84b.

[10] Sabbath work so performed does not constitute a biblical offence and

is not therefore culpable. Regarding the attendance on women during childbirth on the Sabbath, even Karo rules that any essential act should preferably be performed in some unconventional manner (*O.H.*, *cccxxx.*1); in this case the sages insisted on greater stringency "seeing that the birth-pangs are natural and that not one out of a thousand women die in child-birth" (*M.A.*, *a.l.*, 3; citing *Maggid Mishnah*). See also note 34 below.

11 *RaN*, on *Yoma* 84b.

12 Asheri, *Yoma*, *viii.*14.

13 Tosaphoth, *Yoma* 84b.

14 Maimonides, *Mishnah Commentary*, on *Shabbath*, *xviii.*3; and *Hil. Shabbath*, *ii.*3.

15 So Jacob Molin, quoted by Joel Sirkes, *BaH*, *O.H.*, *dcxviii* (end). See also *A.H.*, *O.H.*, *cccxxviii.*7.

16 *TaZ*, *a.l.*, 5.

17 See other commentaries, *a.l.*

18 Cf. *M.B.*, *cccxxviii.*35.

19 See *supra*, *p.*60.

20 This practice is also mentioned by several non-Jewish writers of an-tiquity; cf. Lucian, *Works*, *vol.i*, 41–44; and Tertullian, *De anima, chpt. xxvi*. V. Aptowitzer (*JQR, vol.xv* [1924], *p.*70 [note 55]), discussing this custom, has pointed out that Loew (*Lebensalter*, *p.*379 [note 141]), by a "remarkable oversight", thought that, according to the Talmud (b*Yoma* 82b), *Biblical verses* were whispered into their ears.

21 That is, extinction by the hand of Heaven; see *Lev. xxiii.*29. A ca-pital offence against the Day of Atonement is committed only if the statutory volume of food or drink was consumed; the consumption of a lesser measure, while still biblically prohibited, is not culpable in the same way; see *O.H.*, *dcxii.*5.

22 "Because the sages established that, by [consuming] a smaller volume, one's mind is not set at ease" (b*Yoma* 79a and 80b); *i.e.* one does not gratify one's hunger to the extent of avoiding the self-affliction demanded by the law.

23 This calculation is made by Moses Schreiber (r*Hatham Sopher*, part *vi*, *no.*16); see *M.B.*, *dcxviii.*21. The period specified in the Talmud (b'*Eruvin* 83a) and the codes (*O.H.*, *dcxii.*4) is "as long as it takes to eat a piece [of bread], that is, the time taken to consume three or [ac-cording to others] four eggs".

24 In the codes, as in the talmudic source (b*Yoma* 83a), this law is mentioned in connection with him "who is seized by *'bulimus'*" (see *supra*, *p.*60).

25 As explained in b*Menahoth* 64a and b; see *M.B.*, *cccxxviii.*43.

26 It follows that, in performing other prohibited acts (such as cooking on the Sabbath), the volume involved should also be reduced to the minimum required by the patient; see *M.B.*, *cccxxviii.*44.

27 Cf. *supra*, *p.*48 f.

28 This law applies only to the blood of deer or fowl; see *Lev. xvii.*13.

29 According to Nissim (*RaN*, on *Hullin* 84a—the source of this law), this act must not be performed even if the shovelling of the soil would only involve a rabbinic offence, "since the sages wanted to provide an obvious indication [to remind people] that slaughtering is [normally] pro-hibited on that day; hence, they did not sanction except what is necessary for the sick"; see *TaZ*, *a.l.*, 13.

30 *I.e.*, if one of the houses in danger is occupied by sick people or by children who cannot escape (*M.A.*, *a.l.*, 1).

31 Cf. *supra*, *p.*35.

[32] This proviso is added by Maimonides (*Mishnah Commentary*, on *Shabbath*, ii.5). The law itself; though obvious as codified, is separately recorded, because it included in its earlier formulations some controversial contingencies; see *A.H., a.l.,* 2.

[33] *I.e.,* even from beyond the Sabbath limits, *viz.,* a distance of 2000 cubits (or medium steps) beyond the outer limit of the town or village in which one lives (see *O.H., cccxcvii f.*).

[34] This reason is given in the Talmud (b*Shabbath* 128b). But Gumbiner (*M.A., a.l.,* 2) questions the need for this argument, since the light may be required simply to enable the assistants to see what has to be done for the mother. Epstein (*A.H., a.l.,* 2) suggests that the affirmation of the entire law is due only to the distinction between ordinary cases of danger to life and the circumstances of childbirth. The latter is a natural process which is anticipated by the mother and which does not, therefore, usually cause her undue anxiety. Hence, the acts listed here are sanctioned only if the necessary services cannot be rendered in a more lawful manner (by making all possible preparations on the previous day and by doing all Sabbath work in an unconventional way), provided her mind is not distracted. Cf. also note 10 above.

[35] See *infra,* chapter VII (note 10).

[36] See *supra, p.*51.

[37] That is, without cooking and salting it (*SHaKH, a.l.,* 5). Both acts offend against the Sabbath laws.

[38] Cf. note 26 above. According to Isserles, this restriction applies even if a non-Jew was engaged to cook the food (*ib.,* gloss). But he admits that the ban on dishes prepared by non-Jews is then waived, so that such food is permissible as soon as the Sabbath has terminated (*Y.D., cxiii.*16, gloss).

[39] This condition is added by Karo, *Beth Yoseph, O.H., cccxxviii.*

[40] Any object completing its natural growth on the Sabbath must not be handled until after its termination (*O.H., cccxxii.*1 and 3).

[41] Epstein (*A.H., a.l.,* 14 and 15) questions the logic of the law, because he cannot discover any material difference between this case and that of meat from an animal (slaughtered on the Sabbath) whose growth also continues on that day. Gumbiner (*M.A., a.l.,* 8) and Elijah of Vilna (*Bi'ur HaGRA, a.l.*), too, doubt the validity of this ruling, though for a different reason; see *M.B., a.l.,* 16.

Chapter Six

[1] In the sources of rabbinic law, there is no search for an express "sanction" to justify the modification of religious rulings for the sake of moderately sick persons, as there is for those in danger (see *supra, p.*46). But since dangerous diseases warrant the setting aside of biblical laws, a "divine sanction" had to be sought. Other illnesses, however, can only compromise the operation of rabbinic laws. The authority for such suspension lies not in any "sanction", but in the assumption that "the rabbis did not enact their laws [to be effective] in cases of sickness" (*O.H., cccxxviii.*33; and *cccxvii.*1, gloss); see *M.B., cccxxviii.*50.

[2] The cold was always regarded as a particularly treacherous cause of serious illness. Indeed, some talmudic sages attributed 99% of all deaths to it; see *Lev. Rabbah, xvi.*8; and j*Shabbath, xiv.*3. Cf. Preuss, *p.*161.

[3] See *supra, p.*61.

4 See note 1 above.

5 See rRaSHBA *attributed to Nachmanides*, no.127, where the grada-
tion of different rabbinic enactments is analysed in relation to their violation for the sake of moderately sick persons. Hence, it is suggested that
in such cases only acts expressly sanctioned in the Talmud can be permitted; see *M.A., cccvii.*6.

6 For a comprehensive summary of these 39 principals and derivatives,
see Israel Lipschuetz, *"Kalkeleth Hashabbath"*, Introduction to his Mishnah
Commentary *Tiph'ereth Yisra'el*, on *Shabbath*. The different headings of
biblically prohibited work mentioned in the notes to this chapter are placed
in inverted commas to indicate that the acts so marked merely represent
typical characteristics of similarly creative (and therefore forbidden) activities.

7 Forbidden under the heading of "grinding"; see *"Kalkeleth Hashabbath"*, *op. cit.*, (*ed.* Romm, Vilna, 1911, *vol.iii, p.*3a, *no.*8).

8 While the ban is assumed in the Mishnah (*e.g.*, mShabbath, xiv.3, 4;
and *xxii.*6) and elsewhere (*e.g.*, bShabbath 109b, 110a and 147b), its
enactment is not recorded in the Talmud—a rather anomalous omission
in view of the many other rabbinic decrees of a simliar nature mentioned
in the Mishnah itself (*e.g.*, mShabbath, i.4 ff.). The anomaly has not apparently aroused any comment in later rabbinic writings.

9 *M.B., a.l.*, 1.

10 See Preuss, *p.*195; and Krauss, *vol.i, p.*240.

11 Unless it is afterwards swallowed or taken as an ordinary antepast
(*ib.*). Neither the mastich- nor the vinegar-cure against toothache is mentioned by Preuss, though both are found in the Talmud (tShabbath, *xii.*8;
and mShabbath, *xiv.*4).

12 See Preuss, *p.*197.

13 See Preuss, *p.*321.

14 Because such action makes it obvious that the ointment is applied for
purely medical reasons; see Rashi, *Shabbath* 108b.

15 Such ointment being too offensive to be used for cosmetic purposes,
it clearly serves medical ends only (*ib.*; and *M.B., a.l.*, 67). Preuss
(*p.*322), following the commentaries, identifies the substance with *saliva
jejuna*, the curative powers of which were particularly valued (see *supra,
chpt.*II [note 105]). He also cites modern views that such spittle con-
tains antiseptic properties. *Cf.* Krauss, *vol.i, p.*259.

16 This is forbidden to prevent the preparation of salves under the
heading of "scraping"; see *infra, p.*80.

17 See Preuss, *p.*322 *f.*; and Krauss, *vol.i, p.*260. Otherwise collyrium
prepared before the Sabbath may be used, as it appears merely like bathing the eye (*ib.*).

18 Possibly lumbago; see Preuss, *p.*355 *f.*

19 See Krauss, *vol.i, p.*236.

20 The Talmud (bShabbath 134b) merely distinguishes between new
and old rags. According to Maimonides (*Hil. Shabbath, xxi.*26) and Asheri
(*Shabbath, xix.*3), the latter must not be used because they heal. Rashi
(*a.l.*), however, on the contrary, forbids only the use of new rags (*i.e.*
material which has not been previously on a wound), as only this can
effect a cure. Karo's ruling synthesises both views. Preuss (*p.*277) follows
Rashi's interpretation.

21 But not if it fell on the ground (*ib.*), because one may be tempted
to smooth the poultice ("scraping") (*M.A., a.l.*, 26).

22 Provided the wound caused ill-effects on the whole body (*M.A.,
a.l.*, 29).

23 *Cf.* note 166 below.

24 On these talmudic treatments of wounds, see Preuss, *p.277 †.*

25 For the same reason, soap must not be used on the Sabbath (*O.H.,* *cccxxvi.*10, gloss). But *cf. M.A., a.l.,* 11; and "*Kalkeleth Hashabbath*", *op. cit., p.*3b, *no.*10.

26 Because such a mixture obviously serves medical ends; see Rashi, *Shabbath* 134b.

27 This does not necessarily look like a medical treatment; see Rashi, *loc. cit.*

28 The Talmud (*bShabbath* 148a) permits only "to restore a fractured bone". Hence, Gumbiner (*M.A., a.l.,* 51) contests the ruling given here, while Maimonides omits it altogether. Preuss (*p.*222) is in doubt whether the talmudic reference is to the setting of a fracture or to the restoration of a dislocated limb; *cf. A.H., a.l.,* 39.

29 See Preuss, *p.*222.

30 Because it may lead to heating the water (*M.A., a.l.,* 1). See also Preuss, *p.*638 *f.*

31 See Preuss, *pp.*512 and 626; and Krauss, *vol.i, p.*214 *ff.* On more recent rulings, see Kahana, in *Sinai, vol.xiv* (1950), *p.*79.

32 According to Maimonides (*Hil. Shabbath, xxi.*29), this is forbidden because it would conflict with the command to "call the Sabbath a delight" (*Is. lxviii.*13). But Rashi (*Shabbath* 109b) explains that the prohibition is due merely to the manifest demonstration of the medical motive.

33 On the prevalence of this reprehensible custom among the Romans and its denunciation in the Talmud (*bShabbath* 147b), see Preuss, *p.*507.

34 This law is first mentioned by Karo (*Beth Yoseph, O.H., cccxxviii* [end]).

35 Since that may easily lead to the administration of purgatives by mouth prohibited under the enactment against medicines (Maimonides, *Hil. Shabbath, xxi.*39).

36 Generally, the ban on medicines does not apply to remedies in which no material substances are used, because the possibility of compounding cannot then arise; see *M.B., cccvi.*36. The two last-mentioned cures are nevertheless prohibited, as they may lead to using alternative means involving the use of medicaments (*M.B., cccxxviii.*130).

37 But see preceding note.

38 See Preuss, *p.*320 *f.*

39 See Preuss, *p.*207. He suggests that this practice—originally mentioned in the Talmud (*bShabbath* 66b)—may have been a psychological stratagem to divert the patient's attention from his pain. The same law is mentioned again in another clause (*ib.,* 40) where the vessel is described as "a cup from which hot water has been poured, even if it was still filled with steam". The reference, therefore, is probably to an ordinary hot water bottle. To prevent the danger of being scalded, however, it was not permitted, even on weekdays, to put the receptacle on the abdomen whilst still containing hot water (*O.H., cccxxvi.*6). *Cf.* Preuss, *p.*510.

40 The purpose of this talmudic operation (*b'Avodah Zarah* 28b) is obscure. Rashi (*a.l.*) explains that "the tendons of the ears sometimes cause down and dislocate the jaws", the trouble being relieved by reversing the movement. Preuss (*p.*233) also thinks of a luxation of the jaw-bone, though he suggests that "the ears" are not those of the patient but the name of a special bandage originally called (in the nomenclature of the Greeks) "a hare with *ears*".

41 So Jastrow, *Dictionary, p.*30, following Rashi's second interpretation of the source in the Talmud (*b'Avodah Zarah* 29a). Preuss (*p.*245) is "altogether not clear" on it.

[42] This procedure to mitigate the intoxicating effects of wine is mentioned in the Talmud (b*Shabbath* 66b), but Preuss has evidently overlooked it.

[43] See *infra*, p.81. According to one view in the Talmud (b*Shabbath* 53b), the rabbinical ban is inapplicable, because "a man's excitement over the treatment of his animal is not so great as to lead him to [the forbidden] compounding of spices" (Alfasi, *a.l.*); see also *TaZ*, *O.H.*, *ccv*.2; and *M.A.*, *cccxxxii*.2.

[44] This law is first mentioned by Mordecai, *Shabbath*, *xiv*.384.

[45] In these circumstances the stick is considered as if it were a shoe, belonging to one's ordinary wearing apparel (Asheri, *Betza*, *iii*.5).

[46] This applies even to the festivals, because it is a "weekdaily habit" which disregards their sanctity; see Rashi, *Betza* 25a.

[47] It is remarkable that these artificial arms and legs, though already mentioned in the Mishnah (*Shabbath*, *vi*.8), were unknown to the classical physicians, including Hippocrates, Galen, Celsus and Oribasius; see Preuss, p.247. But Krauss (*vol.i*, p.183) is undecided on whether the appliance served, in fact, as an artificial limb or merely to support the stump. Rashi (*Shabbath* 65b) evidently also regarded the object mentioned in the Talmud as a cosmetic instrument to conceal the lost limb rather than as an aid to walking; see also Tosaphoth, *Shabbath* 65b (bottom).

[48] Because they may then easily be removed and carried separately (*M.B.*, *a.l.*, 56).

[49] In the rabbinic sources, artificial teeth are never mentioned as worn by men, and the reference to them in the Mishnah (*Shabbath*, *vi*.5) and the codes (*e.g.*, Maimonides, *Hil. Shabbath*, *xix*.7; and *Tur*, *O.H.*, *ccciii*) always occur under the heading of "female ornaments". Preuss (p.333) therefore surmises that such teeth may have been worn for cosmetic reasons only in antiquity. *Cf.* note 47 above.

[50] Karo's explanation that the suspected removal of the tooth may be prompted by its unsightly appearance is contested by Rashi (*Shabbath* 65a) and Maimonides (*Hil. Shabbath*, *xix*.7); they fear that she may, on the contrary, remove it in order to show it to her friends in the street.

[51] While the ban on medicines operates only if the treatment is applied for manifestly healing purposes, the prohibition of "carrying", by contrast, is relaxed if the object to be worn serves such ends, since it is then not technically regarded as a "burden". Hence the apparent contradiction in these two Sabbath laws.

[52] For other regulations on the use and replacement of bandages and plasters, see *supra*, p.75 f. On bandages, etc. in the Talmud, see Preuss, p.277 f.; and Krauss, *vol.i*, p.263.

[53] In the absence of any curative benefits, this is regarded as carrying a "burden" (*ib.*).

[54] Because this may evoke ridicule and induce the wearer to take it off (*ib.*).

[55] Because it cannot be classed as an ordinary clothing apparel, though it is normally worn in that condition; see b*Shabbath* 11b, and Rashi, *a.l.*; and Maimonides, *Hil. Shabbath*, *xix*.22. Preuss does not mention the appliance.

[56] It then counts as a kind of garment.

[57] See *supra*, p.36.

[58] See *supra*, pp. 36 and 39.

[59] But horses may not carry such cushions, since they do not suffer from the cold (*ib.*).

60 So Rashi, *Shabbath* 53a. But Krauss (*vol.ii, p.*126) suggests that, without the fodder basket, the old animals would grudge the young ones their food.

61 This appliance was made of metal (b*Shabbath* 59a) and served to shield the animal's feet from stones (so Rashi, *a.l.*; and on *Shabbath* 53a), or to prevent the animal from slipping (m*Parah, ii.*3); see Krauss, *vol.ii, p.*516 (note 907).

62 Forbidden as a derivative of "giving a stroke with the hammer" according to the reading and interpretation of Maimonides (*Hil. Shabbath, x.*17) followed here. The talmudic source (b*Shabbath* 107a), however, speaks of "opening the wound"; hence, Rashi (*a.l.*) places the offence under the heading of "building a door" or "mending a vessel". See also Krauss, *vol.i, p.*254.

63 In this case, it is considered that the main object of the operation is not the opening of the wound (aimed at by the doctors), but the discharge of its fluid contents; hence, the action is regarded as "work not required for its own sake" and thus sanctioned to avoid pain; see *M.A., a.l.,* 33; and *M.B., Bi'ur Halakhah, cccxvi.*7.

64 So as not to stain the material, "dyeing" being a principal act of work (*ib.*).

65 Any forcible expression of blood constitutes an offence as an "infliction of a wound"; see *M.A., a.l.,* 53.

66 This popular treatment is not found in the Talmud; it appears to be of medieval origin. Karo (*Beth Yoseph, a.l.*), though quoting the law in the name of some earlier authorities, himself critisises this use of the spider-web on the Sabbath because he attributes healing properties to it.

67 For it then loses the character of a "vessel" and may not, therefore, be used (being "מוקצא"); see *A.H., a.l.,* 28. This law, while based on the Talmud (m*Shabbath, xvii.*2), was first formulated by Me'iri; see Kahana, *op. cit., p.*74.

68 This is forbidden under the heading of "shearing"; even by hand a nail or shreds of skin may be removed only if the greater part had already been severed (*ib.*).

69 See *supra, p.*74.

70 See note 21 above.

71 On the talmudic use of this medicament, see Preuss, *pp.* 671 and 205; and Krauss, *vol.i, p.*118.

72 This is expressly included under the heading of "catching animals" (*ib.*).

73 These are prohibited within the category of "threshing" (*ib.*).

74 So Jastrow, *Dictionary, p.*259, translating "גונח". Literally, the word means "one who groans [from his heart]". The Talmud (b*Kethuboth* 60a; and b*B. Kamma* 80a) advises such a patient to drink naturally warm goat's milk; see Preuss, *p.*199; and Krauss, *vol.i, p.*253.

75 The milking of animals, too, is forbidden as a derivative of "threshing" (Maimonides, *Hil. Shabbath, viii.*10). *Cf. O.H., dv.*

76 As recorded in a contemporaneous work (r*Binyamin Ze'ev, no.*209); see Kahana, *op. cit., p.*70.

77 See *supra, p.*61.

78 See Preuss, *p.*468; and Krauss, *vol.ii, p.*8.

79 See preceding note.

80 This law derives from a rather obscure passage in the Talmud (b*Shabbath* 123a) and follows the interpretation of it offered by R. Tam (*Tosaphoth, a.l.*) and the 'Arukh (see Kohut, *Aruch Completum, vol.i, p.*164). Preuss (*p.*469) believes that the operation "is evidently the clean-

ing of the new-born child's mouth for the removal of phlegm, as demanded by all ancient accoucheurs". So also Jastrow, *Dictionary, p.* 89. But Krauss (*vol.ii, p.*431 [note 70]), following Rashi (*a.l.*), holds that the expression used ("אסובי ינוקא") refers to the "straightening of the position of the limbs dislocated by the birth".

81 This would be forbidden as an act of "threshing" (*M.B., a.l.,* 111). *Cf.* note 75 above.

82 For the medieval sources of these laws, see Karo, *Beth Yoseph, O.H., cccxxviii.*

83 According to the Talmud (b*Shabbath* 135a), excess milk in the mother's breasts may even endanger her life (see Rashi and Tosaphoth, *a.l.*).

84 This applies only if it is certain that the fruit is premature and inviable (*M.A., a.l.,* 16). *Cf. supra, pp.* 40 and 62.

85 Lest that will lead to "writing" (the bill of divorcement); see *M.B., a.l.,* 28.

86 *I.e.* so as to obviate the necessity of a levirate divorce which, according to biblical law (*Deut. xxv.*5 ff.), must be effected between the widow of a man who died without issue and his brother before she can be remarried. The concession granted in this case is designed to ease the patient's mind; see *M.B., a.l.,* 29.

87 Provided the document was written on the previous day (*TaZ, O.H., dxxiv.*2).

88 See *supra, p.*73 *f.*

89 Provided the pain affects the entire body (*M.A., a.l.,* 3). Although a sore attacking the teeth is regarded as a dangerous condition (see *supra, p.*60 *f.*), an aching tooth must not be removed on the Sabbath by a Jew, because the extraction involves a principal act of work (*M.A., loc. cit.; cf.* note 65 above) which can be sanctioned only if the pain is extremely strong (*A.H., a.l.,* 23). Moreover, the extraction itself is not a certain cure; on the contrary, the operation may sometimes lead to danger (*M.B., a.l.,* 10). For further rabbinical sources, see Kahana, *op. cit., p.*72 *f.*

90 See *supra, chpt.*V (note 33).

91 While the laws on the "Hebrew slave" have been in abeyance since the days of the first Temple (*Y.D., cclxvii.*14), those an the "Canaanite [*i.e.* non-Jewish] slave" are valid and still fully recorded in the *Shulhan 'Arukh* (*ib.,* 1–85); see *JE, vol.xi, p.*403 *ff.*; and Krauss, *vol.ii, p.*83 *ff.* Such slaves must submit to circumcision, ritual immersion and the religious laws applicable to Jewish women (*ib.,* 1 *ff.*). Hence, it is incumbent on their masters to ensure that they desist from any work on the Sabbath like Jews (*O.H., ccciv.*1). But servants who did not commit themselves to the observance of even the "seven laws of Noah" may be excluded from the Sabbath rest enjoined on slaves (*Ex. xx.*10; *xxiii.*12; and *Deut. v.*14) and therefore be employed to assist the Jewish sick on the same terms as other non-Jews; see *M.B., a.l.,* 1.

92 Nachmanides, quoted in *Shittah Mekubbetzeth,* on *Baba Metzi'a* 90a; for further sources, see Kahana, *op. cit., p.*232.

93 See also *supra, p.*79; and note 43 above.

94 But *cf. supra, p.*79; and note 72 above.

95 The ointment of old (closed) wounds is merely "an enjoyment", not a cure, and therefore forbidden (*ib.*).

96 In this respect the care for sick animals is even less handicapped by religious considerations than the attention to human ailments, for similar exercises for the relief of man are forbidden (*O.H., cccxxviii.*42); see notes 36 and 43 above.

97 Preuss (*p*.349) identifies the complaint with plethora; cf. *supra*, *chpt*.IV (note 6).

98 This law, of talmudic origin (b*Shabbath* 128b), is of special interest in view of the statement by Jesus: "What man shall there be among you, that shall have one sheep, and if it fall into a pit on the Sabbath day, will he not lay hold on it, and lift it out?" (*Matth. xii*.11; cf. *Luke xiv*.5); see J. Wohlgemuth, "Das Leid der Tiere", in *Jeschurun*, *vol.xv* (1928), *p*.264 (note 1).

99 This law is first codified by Asheri (*Baba Metzi'a, ii*.29). Cf. note 75 above.

100 Because it involves an undue exertion incompatible with the Sabbath rest (Rashi, *Shabbath* 128b). But it may be permitted to render such assistance if the dam bears for the first time and her life is in danger; see *P.M.*, *'Eshel 'Avraham*, *O.H.*, *cccxxxii*.2; and *M.B.*, *Bi'ur Halakhah*, on *cccxxxii*.1.

101 On these aids, see Preuss, *p*.499; and Krauss, *vol.ii*, *p*.114. From a discussion in the Talmud (b*Shabbath* 128b) on this and the following law it is not clear whether these concessions apply only to festivals (as evidently assumed by Karo) or also to the Sabbath (as explicitly held in the *Tur, O.H.*, *cccxxxii* and *dxxiii*).

102 The explanations added in brackets are based on the source of this law in the Talmud (b*Shabbath* 128b); see Preuss, *p*.499 *f*. Krauss (*vol.ti, pp*.114 and 505 [note 783]) wrongly infers that such "compassion" was shown only to, not by, clean animals.

103 *M.A.*, *dxxxii*.2.

104 See Preuss, *p*.323; and Krauss, *vol.i*, *p*.239.

105 But this allowance does not extend to the second day of New Year, since both days of that festival enjoy the status of "one prolonged sanctity" (*ib*.).

106 *M.B.*, *a.l.*, 5.

107 Cf. note 96 above.

108 *M.A.*, *cdl*.9.

109 See Preuss, *p*.277; and Krauss, *vol.i*, *p*.258.

110 Including eggs (*O.H.*, *cdlxii*.4).

111 In this connection it is of interest to learn that Amatus Lusitanus, describing his treatment of the celebrated 16th century rabbi-physician and historian Azariah di Rossi, writes of having "advised him to avoid as much as possible unleavened bread; if, however, he cannot refrain from it at the feast of Passover, according to the rules of his religion, then he shall have it prepared with sugar and eggs, so as to make it lighter and more easily digestible" (*Centuria iv*, *cur*.42; quoted by Friedenwald, *p*.399).

112 But he may dilute it well with water (*M.A.*, *a.l.*, 12).

113 See *infra*, *p*.92.

114 Because "he who is engaged on one religious precept is exempt from another" (b*Sukkah* 25a).

115 See *Lev. xxiii*.42.

116 Provided the complaint is likely to be aggravated by this observance (*M.B.*, *a.l.*, 9). The extension of this concession to people who are only slightly indisposed is due to the law's insistence that the booth is to replace the dwelling in which one would live under the same circumstances for the rest of the year; this excludes accommodation made inadequate by any form of ill-health (b*Sukkah* 26a).

117 Unless the patient is dangerously ill (*M.B.*, *a.l.*, 11).

118 See note 2 above.

119 Eating and drinking are biblically prohibited by the commandment:

" . . . and ye shall afflict your souls" (*Lev. xxiii*.27). While the refusal to observe the other restrictions certainly constitutes no capital offence as does eating or drinking (*O.H., dcxi*.1), it is disputed whether they are of biblical or merely rabbinic status; see *M.B., a.l.*, 3.

[120] See *supra, pp*.59 *ff*. and 69 *f*. Cf. also *supra, p*.51 *ff*. That class includes, of course, lying-in women within three days of the birth (*O.H., dcxvii*.4); see *supra, p*.61. According to Achai Gaon (*She'eltoth, no*.149), such women must not fast for thirty days following the birth, but this view is disputed by all other authorities (see *Beth Yoseph, O.H., dcxvii* [end]). See Loew, *Lebensalter, p*.76.

[121] This law is first codified by Asheri (*Yoma, viii*.7) in the name of a Gaon.

[122] Except if required for grave medical reasons (*Beth Yoseph, O.H., dcxiii*).

[123] This is, in fact, forbidden on every public fast (*O.H., dlxvii*.3; and *Ba'er Hetev, O.H., iv*.6). But see *M.A., dlxvii*.6 for another view.

[124] Although four of these fasts are mentioned in a Prophetical book (*Zech. viii*.19), they only enjoy the status of an accepted "custom"; see Maimonides, *Hil. Ta'aniyoth, v*.5; and *Maggid Mishnah, a.l.* But Karo describes their observance as an obligation, adding "it is forbidden to break the fence [protecting these regulations]" (*O.H., dl*.1).

[125] Neither the Prophets nor the Talmud mention this fast; see *Maggid Mishnah, loc. cit.*

[126] These exemptions are not set out in the same detail as those of the Day of Atonement, due probably to the non-biblical status of the Ninth of Av.

[127] Such a formal release is necessary if one has undertaken to fast regularly on certain days, since such an undertaking assumes the character of a vow.

[128] See C. Capellmann, *Pastoral-Medizin*, 1878, *p*.94.

[129] Capellmann, *op. cit., p*.92 *f*.

[130] *I.e.* the "*Shema*", in conformity with the law to read it "when thou liest down" (*Deut. vi*.7; and *xi*.19). See Singer, *Prayer-Book, p*.97.

[131] In the Talmud (b*Mo'ed Katan* 15a) this view is based on an interpretation of *Lev. xiii*.45. But later authorities have contested this opinion; see *SHaKH, cccxxxiv*.12.

[132] This token of mourning is rabbinically enacted (*SHaKH, cccxl*.2) on the basis of *Lev. x*.2; see b*Mo'ed Katan* 24a.

[133] *SHaKH, a.l.*, 1.

[134] Whether the departed was related to him or not (*SHaKH, a.l.*, 2).

[135] See Preuss, *p*.405.

[136] *Cf. supra, p*.61; and note 2 above.

[137] They may place a small cushion underneath them (*SHaKH, ccclxxxvii*.1).

[138] *Cf.* the ban on fasting during the plague; see *supra*, Introduction (notes 46 and 73).

[139] See Preuss; *p*.506; and Krauss, *vol.i, p*.256 f. The mainly vegetarian origin of medicinical products is evidently also assumed by Ben Sirach in his statement "God bringeth up medicines from the earth" (*Ecclus. xxxviii*.4) and in the *Targum* on *Eccl. ii*.5.

[140] While the *Shulhan 'Arukh* devotes 175 chapters to the Sabbath (*O.H., ccxlii–cdxi*), the dietary laws occupy 138 chapters (*Y.D., i–cxxxviii*), apart from the many incidental references to food items, *e.g.* among the laws on Passover, vows, idols, etc.; of these *Y.D., i–cx* deals only with meat and the slaughtering of animals.

141 For instance, while leaven on Passover (*O.H.*, *cdxlii*.1) and meat boiled with milk falls into this category (*Y.D.*, *lxxxvii*.1), blood and other forbidden animal substances may be sold to non-Jews or put to any other advantage (except eating).

142 For example, by using forbidden food to strike a plaster, or by offering a patient a bitter drink containing an admixture of a prohibited substance, so that the palate experiences no enjoyment (Maimonides, *Hil. Yesodei Hatorah*, *v*.8). Cf. also *supra*, *chpt.*V (note 10).

143 Because the Bible, in prohibiting these articles (*Ex. xxiii*.19; and *Deut. xxii*.9), does not refer specifically to "eating" them (b*Pesahim* 24b).

144 Because "the ashes of whatever must be burned [due to its prohibited nature] are permitted" (b*Temurah* 34a); see r*RIVaSH*, *no.*265; and *SHaKH*, *clv*.19.

145 The express reason for the rabbinical ban on the consumption of cooked food and certain strong drinks prepared by Gentiles is the fear that the resultant social intimacy may lead to intermarriage; see b*Avodah Zarah* 31b; and Rashi, *'Avodah Zarah* 35b. Cf. *Y.D.*, *cxiv*.1. See also *supra*, *chpt.*V (note 38).

146 Originally the talmudic ban on all non-Jewish wines included their use for any benefit whatever (m*Avodah Zarah*, *ii*.2; see Tosaphoth, *'Avodah Zarah* 29b [top]), a position still accepted by Karo (*Y.D.*, *cxxiii*.1). The enactment against drinking was to serve as a barrier against intermarriage (*cf.* preceding note), while that against other uses was prompted by the suspicion that such wine might have been dedicated to idolatrous purposes (*TaZ* and *SHaKH*, *a.l.*, 1). But since, due to the disappearance of ritual wine-libations among non-Jews, the second consideration became inapplicable, Isserles limited the prohibition to drinking only (*ib.*, gloss). Hence he permits sick people to use it for bathing purposes, though for healthy persons such use is still forbidden within the category of drinking (*SHaKH*, *clv*.17).

147 Wine-baths as a cure, especially for children, were already known to the Talmud (t*Shabbath*, *xii*.13); see Preuss, *p.*511.

148 It is also permitted to sprinkle such wine to perfume the air (*Y.D.*, *cviii*.5, gloss), as was the practice in talmudic times; see Krauss, *vol.i*, *p.*77.

149 For a summary of some opinions on this question, see *D.T.*, *clv*.23.

150 Liqueurs dearer than wine are suspected to contain an admixture of wine; hence they must not be bought from a non-Jewish merchant unless discharged from the barrel in the buyer's presence (*ib.*, 4). But this is waived in the case of professional dealers, as it is assumed they would not wish to harm their reputation of reliability (*ib.*, 5).

151 See *supra*, *p.*57.

152 See S. W. Baron, *The Jewish Community*, 1942, *vol.ii*, *p.*109.

153 For examples of the medicinal use of human milk among primitive peoples, see Ploss and Bartels, *Woman*, *vol.iii*, *p.*233 *ff.* Galen and Pliny, too, commended it; see Zimmels, *p.*243 (note 10). But the discussion in the Talmud (b*Kethuboth* 60a) on the drinking of human milk ignores its medical use.

154 *SHaKH*, *a.l.*, 7; citing Luria, *Yam shel Shelomo*, *Hullin*, *viii*.102.

155 The weaning age among the ancient Jews was at two to three years; see Loew, *Lebensalter*, *p.*120; Preuss, *p.*471; and Krauss, *vol.ii*, *p.*9 *f.* Jerome (*Quaest. Hebr.*, *Gen. xxi*.14) speaks of Jewish children sometimes weaned as late as in the fifth year.

156 *Novellae of RaSHBA*, on *Yevamoth* 114a; so also *RaN*, on *'Avodah Zarah*, *ii* (beginning). They believe that a Jewess's milk transmits "the Jewish qualities of compassion and bashfulness—engendered by the con-

stant performance of divine precepts—and helps to rear similar natural features". See also Loew, *loc. cit.*; and Zimmels, *p.*74.

[157] Josephus, *Antiquities*, ii.9,5.

[158] *Ex. Rabbah*, i.25. The Talmud also relates the story (b*Sotah* 12b); see Preuss, *p.*474 *f.*

[159] This story, though somewhat at variance with the Palestinian Talmud's express sanction (j*'Avodah Zarah*, ii.1; *cf. RaN, loc. cit.*), derived from the Prophet's vision that "their queens [shall be] thy nursing mothers" (*Is. xlix.*23) is used by Adreth (*loc. cit.*) to prove that the opposition to the employment of non-Jewish nurses is based only on piety, not on any legal prohibition. For a discussion on these and other rabbinic sources, see *Bi'ur HaGRA, Y.D., lxxxi.*31 and 32.

[160] A word rendered by Karo into the Arabic *"shumr"* (*ib.*) and possibly connected with the *"phanag"* drug, identified by Zimmels (*p.*126) with balsam (probably *"panax"*); *cf. Ez. xxvii.*17. But Epstein (*A.H., a.l.,* 23) states: "We do not know what this [herb] is, but we can conclude... the consumption of medicines does not count as eating at all."

[161] See *Deut. xxii.*9.

[162] See *Lev. xix.*19.

[163] See *infra*, chapter IX (end).

[164] See *Deut. xviii.*3.

[165] For instance, as a cure against fever (*Levush, a.l.*), a popular custom recorded in the Talmud (b*Sanhedrin* 47b). But it is not indicated how the dust was used; see Preuss, *p.*184.

[166] Preuss (*p.*277) records a talmudic view that this was forbidden, but he omits to state that this was not accepted in the final ruling of the Talmud (b*Makkoth* 21a).

[167] *TaZ, a.l.,* 1.

[168] This law is first mentioned in the 15th century by Israel Isserlein, *responsa, no.* 160; and in *'Issur Vehetter, no.*59. In more general terms the decision already appeared in *Piskei Tosaphoth, 'Avodah Zarah, i*; see Wohlgemuth, *op. cit., p.*256. None of these sources actually specify any particular medical uses to which living animals can be put. But early in the 18th century Jacob Reischer (r*Shevuth Ya'akov*, part *iii, no.*71) used this ruling to permit a Jewish physician to test the effects of a new drug on an animal before applying it to human beings; see Zimmels, *p.*16. In the present century, several scholars have concluded that Jewish law does not object to vivisectionist experiments on animals for medical purposes, provided no unnecessary suffering is inflicted on them; see J. D. Eisenstein, in *OY, vol.ix, p.*50; Wohlgemuth, *op. cit., p.*248 *f.*; J. M. Breisch, r*Helkath Ya'akov, nos.*30 and 31 (quoting the view of J. Weinberg); and Zimmels, *p.*17. *Cf. infra, p.*102 *f.*

[169] See *supra, p.*32 *ff.*

[170] See *infra*, chapter X.

[171] See *supra, p.*55 *f.*

[172] See *infra*, chapter XV.

[173] See *supra, chpt.*III (note 65).

[174] This is presumed to occur after three days (*ib.*)—an observation based on the Talmud (b*Niddah* 67a); see Preuss, *p.*293.

[175] See *Deut. xxv.*7 *ff*; and note 86 above.

[176] *Cf.* also *supra, p.*87.

[177] See Singer, *Prayer-Book, p.*238a *f.*

[178] *Nu. vi.* 24—26. In particular, priests are disqualified from the rite if certain conspicuous blemishes affect their face or hands, since that may cause the congregation to look at them (*O.H., cxxviii.*30); this should

(CHAPTER VI)

not be done (*ib.*, 23), so as not to distract one's attention from the blessing (*M.A.*, *a.l.*, 35).

[179] For some details, see Preuss, *p*.318 *ff.*; and *OY*, *vol.viii*, *p*.35.

[180] See Preuss, *p*.337 *f.*; Krauss, *vol.i*, *p*.246; and *OY*, *vol.iv*, *p*.314. The legal disabilities of the deaf-dumb are entirely due to the mental dementia resulting from their inability to communicate audibly with their environment. But in view of the modern advancement in the treatment of such cases, it has been suggested that their religious and legal status may now be modified; see Zimmels; *pp*.21 and 165 *f*. For a full survey of the rabbinic literature on the subject, see *Sedei Hemed*, *vol.i*, *s.v.* "*Heth*", *nos*.30, 31, 103, 106—108 and 114—116.

[181] See Preuss, *p*.362; and *OY*, *vol.x*, *p*.64 *f*. Cf. also *infra*, chapter X (end).

[182] See Preuss, *p*.343 *ff*. *Cf*. Zimmels, *p*.111. See also *supra*, chpt.IV (note 33); and *p*.104.

Chapter Seven

[1] *Cf. JE*, *vol.v*, *p*.454.

[2] Series of purely ethical or social laws are interrupted at random by precepts of a distinctly ritual or religious character in the Pentateuch (*e.g.*, *Ex. xxiii*; *Lev. xix, xxiv*; and *Deut. xxii ff.*) and in the Decalogue itself (*Ex. xx*.2—17; and *Deut. v*.6—18). *Cf.* also Isaiah's denunciation of hypocritical fasts and his entreaty "to deal thy bread to the hungry..." together with his plea for the joyful observance of the Sabbath in the same chapter (*Is. lviii*).

[3] Thus the Midrash (*Mekhilta*, on *Ex. xxi*.1; so also Rashi, *a.l.*) comments on the close association between the laws on the altar (*Ex. xx*)—a ritual precept *par excellence*—and the social ordinances (*Ex. xxi*): this teaches that "as the former are from Sinai, so are the latter from Sinai" —*i.e.* whence they equally derive their validity.

[4] j*Shekalim*, *iii*.2 (end).

[5] According to Obadiah of Bartinura (on m'*Avoth*, *i*.1), the tractate *Ethics of the Fathers* (rather than the first Mishnah tractate) is introduced by the statement "Moses received the Law from Sinai and handed it down to..." in order to emphasise the Sinaitic origin particularly of laws which may be thought to have been "invented by the philosophers". Similarly, the rabbis stress the significance of the reference to Sinai (*Lev. xxvi*.1) in the preamble to an important group of social laws (see *Sifra* and Rashi, *a.l.*). Again, the duty to "love thy neighbour as thyself" (*Lev. xix*.18) is imperative only because "I am the Lord" (*ib.*)—that is, "because I have commanded it" (Abarvanel, *a.l.*). *Cf.* M. Lazarus, *Die Ethik des Judenthums*, 1904, *vol.i*, *p*.85 *ff*.

[6] Maimonides, *Mishnah Commentary*, on *Hullin*, *vii*.6.

[7] See S. W. Baron, *A Social and Religious History of the Jews*, 1937, *vol.i*, *pp*.66 and 72.

[8] *Cf. e.g.* the warnings in *Deut. xvii*.7, 13 and elsewhere, indicating the social nature of the crimes perpetrated, in the first instance, against God.

[9] Thus, the comprehensive list given by Maimonides (*Hil. Sanhedrin*, *xv*.10—13; and *xix*) of all capital crimes and the 207 offences carrying corporal punishment consists of numerous laws in either category; all are subject to the same juridical procedure.

10 David Halevi, in fact, regards the statement of this law as altogether superfluous (*TaZ, a.l.*, 21). According to another commentary (*Beth Lehem Yehudah, a.l.*), it may have been recorded to teach that in such circumstances it is lawful to borrow on interest from a Jew so as to avoid any delay, even if a non-Jewish dealer is at hand to advance the money required a little later.

11 See *supra*, p.73.

12 See *Lev. xix.*32. If a patient nevertheless rose out of respect, he should not be told "sit down!" as is normally done, because such a request may be understood as "[continue to] sit in your sickness!" (*O.H., ccclxxvi.*2; *cf. supra*, p.). But this motivation of the law is not mentioned in its talmudic source (b*Mo'ed Katan* 27b); hence, one commentator explains its meaning to the effect that people who are ill or in mourning, in contrast to others, need not await the order to sit down, being exempted from the duty to stand up in the first place (R. Hananel, in Tosaphoth, *a.l.*).

13 This is an extension of the original purpose of the law: to prevent the promiscuous mixing of the sexes through disguise; see *Targum* and Rashi, *a.l.*

14 See Preuss, *p.*426. He adds that this operation is enforced as religious law among Mohammedan women and commonly practiced among men, too.

15 Because the ban applies only to acts performed for the sake of enjoyment or beautification (Tosaphoth, *Sotah* 59a).

16 See *supra*, Introduction (note 74).

17 So as not to disturb the concentration on one's studies (*TaZ, a.l.*, 6).

18 The Talmud (m*Baba Metzi'a, ii.*10) and the codes (*H.M., loc. cit.*) require bypassers to assist the animal only if the owner himself lends a hand; but if he is old or sick, they must help the animal without his assistance.

19 See *infra*, chapter IX.

20 Unless it is the custom to render medical aid free (*ib.*). Otherwise, the favour received would offend against the vow; *cf. supra*, p.50.

21 This definition is added by Moses Ribkes (*Be'er Hagolah, a.l.*) in the name of Asheri. It is based on the statement in the Talmud (b*Shabbath* 41a) that "he who washes in hot water without drinking of it is like an oven heated from outside but not from inside". Such water was evidently drunk during the bath (see Krauss, *vol.i, pp.*210 and 230). But the reference may also be to drinking of wine and various spice mixtures to strengthen the body after the bath, as was common among the Romans (see Preuss, *p.*636; and Krauss, *vol.i, p.*231 f.).

22 See *supra*, p.83.

23 *Cf.* the lifting, for similar reasons, of the ban on administering divorces on the Sabbath (*supra*, p.80 f.).

24 See V. Kurrein, "Kartenspiel und Spielkarten im juedischen Schrifttume", in *MGWJ, vol.lxvi* (1922), *p.*205; and Baron, *op. cit., vol.ii, p.*317.

25 b*Baba Kamma* 60b. For further sources on the subject, see *TE, vol.v, p.*457.

26 Tosaphoth, *Baba Kamma* 60b. *Cf.* also b*Sanhedrin* 74a.

27 Asheri, *Baba Kamma, vi.*12; see also *SeMA, H.M., ccclix.*10.

28 See *supra*, p.53 ff.

29 Rashi, *Baba Kamma* 60b. For a talmudic argument in support of Rashi's interpretation, see J. Ettlinger, r*Binyan Tziyon, no.*167. But it is doubtful whether even Rashi would in practice dispute the unequivocal right to save one's life through theft if necessary; hence, it is assumed

that the circumstances envisaged in his interpretation were such as to provide an alternative way to escape death or that the difficulty raised by his interpretation could be otherwise resolved (see sources cited in the two following notes).

30 Nachmanides, cited in *Shittah Mekubbetzeth*, on *Kethuboth* 19a. See B. H. Auerbach, *Nahal 'Eshkol*, 1868, part *ii*, p.118 *ff*.; Moses Schick, r*MaHaRaM Shik*, Y.D., nos. 347 and 348; and *Sedei Hemed*, vol.*i*, *s.v.* "*Aleph*", no.16.

31 The same source is also cited (again as an "extraneous *Boraitha*") in the name of R. Aaron Halevi (*Kovetz al Yad*, on Maimonides, *Hil. Yesodei Hatorah*, v.5) and R. Abraham ibn Daud (see Z. H. Chajes, *Glosses of MaHaRaTZ*, on *Baba Kamma* 60b).

32 The view is attributed to the tannaitic sage, R. Me'ir. The opinion is not found in our version of the Talmud, but it has been suggested that the reference may be to a passage in the Palestinian Talmud (*j'Avodah Zarah*, *ii*.2) which teaches that one must rather give up one's life than to obey an order to attack or to kill a man (Chajes, *loc. cit.*). Only one source considers the suggestion that these views may denote an acknowledgement of a distinction in principle between religious and moral obligation (r*Beth Yehudah*, Y.D., no.47; cited in *Sedei Hemed*, *loc. cit.*). See also J. L. Unterman, *Shevet Miyehudah*, 1955, p.59 *ff*.

33 See r*MaHaRaM Shik*, *loc. cit.*

34 b*Baba Kamma* 119a.

35 See *Nahal 'Eshkol*, *loc. cit.*; and other sources cited in note 30 above. They argue that this ruling follows logically from the generally accepted law that one is in duty bound—and, in fact, compelled by the court—to save one's fellow-man from danger, even if one thereby incurs financial loss (H.M., cdxxvi), albeit that the person so saved must afterwards recompense his rescuer if he has the means to do so (*Tur*, H.M., cdxxvi). The same applies to the redemption of captives (Y.D., cclii.12, gloss). Hence, one may obviously also use another's money to escape from death.

36 Karo, *Beth Yoseph*, H.M., cdxxvi; and *Keseph Mishneh*, on *Hil. Rotze'ah*, *i*.14.

37 Karo, *loc. cit.* Cf. *supra*, p.45.

38 See *SeMA*, H.M., cdxxvi.2.

39 So *SeMA*, *loc. cit.*; and *Be'er Hagolah*, a.l., 2. For further details on the argument, see Unterman, *op. cit.*, p.19 *ff*.

40 Ibn Chabib, *Tosaphoth Yom Hakippurim*, on *Yoma* 82b; so also Menachem Recanati, cited in P.T., Y.D., clvii.15. They reason that, in the attempt to defend one's life, one must stop short only of actual murder, "because one does not destroy one life to save another" (see *supra*, p.54 f.); but this principle was never extended to include the loss of limbs or organs.

41 r*RaDBaZ*, part *iii*, no.627. He ruled that, if faced with the alternatives of being killed oneself or of cutting off a limb or organ of another person, one need not sacrifice one's life (though if done, it would be an act of extreme piety). One of his arguments is that "the laws of the *Torah* are bound to be in harmony with reason and logic, and how could it enter our mind to suggest that a person would allow his eye to be blinded, or his arm or leg to be severed, so that ⌈others⌉ shall not kill his neighbour?" For a similar view, see D.T., clvii.58.

42 In modern rabbinic literature, this problem is generally treated only in regard to the use of parts removed from dead bodies (see *supra*, chpt.I ⌈note 93⌉)—a practice which the church considers "certainly licit" (J.

McCarthy, in *Irish Ecclesiastical Record*, *vol.lxvii* [1946], *p.*197). For earlier, more remote parallels, *cf.* Zimmels, *p.*152.

43 So Noldin (*Theol. Moral.*, *ii*, n.328) and Jorio (*Theol. Moral.*, *ii*, n.200), cited by McCarthy, *op. cit.*, *p.*192 *ff.*

44 So B. J. Cunningham, *The Morality of Organic Transplantation*, 1946, *p.*71.

45 So Vermeersch (*Theol. Moral.*, *ii*, n.323), cited by McCarthy, *loc. cit.*

46 The ban on self-mutilation is based on the Talmud (m*Baba Kamma*, *viii.*6).

47 See Preuss, *p.*603 *ff.*; and *JE*, *vol.xi*, *p.*581 *f*. The prohibition includes endangering one's life, *e.g.* by fighting to death, walking on ice, etc. (*Sepher Hasidim*, no. 675) or saving one's possessions at the risk of life (*ib.*, no.677). *Cf. supra*, *p.*7.

48 Thus, Maimonides (*Hil. Mamrim*, *ii.*4) compares the temporary suspension of a religious precept by the Jewish supreme court (to safeguard the religious life of the community) to the physician's amputation of a limb for the preservation of the patient's life. On the right to "injure" a person, if necessary in the course of his medical treatment, *cf.* also the view of Nachmanides, cited *supra*, *p.*4.

49 This is an exception to the usual rule forbidding such incisions for the dead (*Lev. xix.*28; and *Y.D.*, *cixxx.*1 *ff.*), because the mourner is here considered to mark the loss, not of the deceased, but of his religious scholarship (*SHaKH*, *a.l.*, 10; based on Asheri, *Mo'ed Katan*, *iii.*93).

50 See *Ex. xxi.*6. This was, of course, only a symbolic operation. See also *supra*, *chpt.*VI (note 91).

51 r*ROSH*, no.18, §13. According to S. W. Baron (*The Jewish Community*, 1942, *vol.ii*, *p.*223), this penalty and similarly cruel methods of mutilating the bodies of criminals had been adopted by the Jews of medieval Spain and Germany from their neighbours; such acts "had been totally unknown to their talmudic predecessors".

52 By an edict of Frederick III, adulteresses and mothers who prostituted their daughters were to have their noses amputated. The municipal laws of Augsburg of 1276 decreed a similar punishment for "vagrant girls or *'Huebschlerinnen'*, if they roamed about the streets during Lent or on Saturday nights, except when distinguished foreigners were present in the town"; see Puschmann, *Medical Education*, *p.*305.

53 McCarthy, *op. cit.*, *p.*196.

54 The statement that "man has no rights over his body [to smite it]" was made by Shene'ur Zalman ("Tanya", late 18th century) in his *Shulhan 'Arukh* (*H.M.*, *Hil. Nizkei Haguph*, 4). In a similar context, Maimonides had already asserted that human life was "the possession of the Holy One, blessed be He" (*Hil. Rotze'ah*, *i.*4). For a detailed review of these and allied sources, see S. J. Zewin, *Le'or Hahalakhah*, 1946, *p.*188 *ff.*

55 See I. J. Unterman, "The Law on the Saving of Life and its Definition", in *Hatorah Vehamedinah*, 4th series (1952), *p.*24. According to *Hagga'oth Maimuni* (on *Hil. Yesodei Hatorah*, *v.*7), the principle based on "How do you know that your blood is redder than your neighbour's?" (see *supra*, *p.*55) also operates in reverse, viz., "How do you know that his blood is redder than yours?"; *i.e.* you have no right to sacrifice your life for the sake of his.

56 Unterman, *op. cit.*, *p.*29. Similarly, the *Sepher Hasidim* (quoted in *D.T.*, *clvii.*51) ruled that if heathens threatened to kill one of two persons, of whom the one is a scholar and the other a common man, the latter should offer to lay down his life.

57 See Me'iri, *Beth Habehirah*, on *Sanhedrin, viii* (*ed.* A. Schreiber, Frankfurt, *p*.270), quoted in *D.T., clvii*.55.

58 m*Terumoth, viii*.12; see also j*Terumoth, viii* (end).

59 See 2 *Sam. xx*.1 *ff.*

60 Maimonides, *Hil. Yesodei Hatorah, v.*5.

61 Evidently leaving the decision at the discretion of the group's members, as the action in surrendering the guilty person, though lawful, may not be in accord with the principles of equity; see *TaZ, a.l.,* 7. Another explanation is offered in *P.T., a.l.,* 14. For further sources on the subject, see *TE, vol.i, p.*282.

Chapter Eight

1 Pain affecting the whole body invokes the concessions applicable to proper sickness; see *supra, p.*73.

2 So explicitly Mordecai, *Shabbath, xiv.*382. See also *supra, p.*73.

3 See *supra,* chpt.VI (note 1). For numerous examples of concessions for the relief of pain, see especially *supra,* chapters VI and VII.

4 r*Havath Ya'ir, no.*164.

5 Azulay, *Birkei Yoseph, O.H., xxxviii.*6 and *cdlxxii.*10; citing Joseph Iskapa, in *Rosh Yoseph,* on *O.H., cdlxxii.* Cf. also commentaries on *O.H., cdlxxii.*

6 b*Shabbath* 118b.

7 b*Shabbath* 12b.

8 See *M.A., a.l.,* 1.

9 The ordinary formula is: "May the All-present have compassion over you among the sick in Israel" (*Y.D., cccxxxv.*6). Its plaintive character renders it unfit for the Sabbath.

10 That is, if prices dropped by two-fifths and the depression affected the livelihood of the majority of the citizens (*O.H., dlxxvi.*10); see b*Baba Bathra* 91a.

11 *TaZ, a.l.,* 5; and *M.A., a.l.,* 14. But in practise such prayers are generally recited, though the authorities can find little justification for doing so (*M.A., loc. cit.;* and *A.H., O.H., cclxxxvii.*2).

12 So Jacob Molin, *Likkutei MaHaRIL;* cited by Samuel Halevy, r*Nahalath Shiv'ah, nos.*39, where this view is fully discussed—and opposed (see also *ib., nos.*77—80); see *S.T., cclxxxviii.*3.

13 According to Abraham ibn Daud (*Sepher Ba'alei Hanephesh, Sha'ar Hakedushah*), the frequency of intercourse "is fixed for every person according to his strength and his pleasure [in it]"; so also Jacob Emden, *Siddur Ya'avetz* (Prayer-Book) "*Beth Ya'akov*", Zitomir, 1880, *p.*333. Cf. supra, p.   .

14 Cf. *supra,* chpt.VI (note 65).

15 See *supra, p.*80.

16 According to the Talmud (m'*Avodah Zarah, ii.*1), Maimonides (*Hil. 'Avodah Zarah, ix.*16) and Karo (*Y.D., cliv.*2), a Jewess should not suckle a non-Jewish child so as not to "rear an infant unto idolatry". In medieval times the ban was justified by the fear "lest the child will fall ill or die, and a blood-libel will be levelled against the Jewess" (note on *Y.D., loc. cit.*). Cf. also *infra,* chpt.XV (note 13).

17 See *He.M., a.l.,* 2.

18 Maimonides, *Hil. 'Ishuth, xxi.*11.

[19] Glosses on *RAVeD*, *a.l.*; and *Tur*, *E.H.*, *lxxx*.

[20] b*Kethuboth* 60b. That passage simply states that if only a little food was assigned to her she may yet eat more, to which R. Shesheth adds that she must, however, provide the extra food herself.

[21] See *Maggid Mishnah* and *Keseph Mishneh*, on Maimonides, *loc. cit.*; and *Beth Yoseph*, *E.H.*, *lxxx*. But Moses Lima (*He.M.*, *a.l.*, 22) asks: "If the child is in danger, and the mother is exposed to pain only, on what grounds may the child be endangered so as to avoid her suffering?", to which Samuel Uri (*B.S.*, *a.l.*, 15) replies by referring to an analogous case in the Talmud (b*Nedarim* 80b). Another commentator (*Haggahoth MaHaRIM*, on *E.H.*, *lxxx*.12) suggests that in Maimonides's ruling the reference is to a pregnant, not a nursing, woman. In that case, the consideration of the mother's pain comes before the life of her fruit, since legally the status of life does not attach to an unborn being.

[22] But Isserles (*ib.*, gloss) holds that she ought to suckle both. This ruling is contested by most authorities; hence, it should be accepted merely as a recommendation, provided the mother is able to care for both infants; see *He.M.*, *a.l.*, 23.

[23] See *infra*, chapter XV.

[24] See *Beth Yoseph*, *Y.D.*, *cclxii*, in the name of Adreth; and *TaZ*, *a.l.*, 3. *Cf. Gen. xxxiv.25.*

[25] Thus, "on account of the infant's pain", one omits to insert the words ". . . in Whose abode is joy. . ." in the Grace after Meals, as is done on other festive occasions (see Singer, *Prayer-Book*, *p*.300); see b*Kethuboth* 8a. Some authorities advance the same reason for the omission of the benediction ". . . Who hast kept us in life. . ." usually recited when fulfilling a precept for the first time (see Singer, *op. cit.*, *p*.292); see Mordecai, *Shabbath*, *xix*.422; and Zimmels, *p*.162; but *cf. Hagga'oth Maimuni*, *Hil. Milah*, *iii*.4, expressing a contrary opinion. See also *Y.D.*, *cclxv*.7 and gloss. According to Shabbatai Cohen (*SHaKH*, *cclxv*.24), one should say Psalm *xx* in the morning prayer on the day of the circumcision, since the concern for the infant's pain overrides the general rule to omit that prayer on festive days (see Singer, *op. cit.*, *p*.73). Some French rabbis are even quoted as permitting mourners to attend a circumcision banquet (against the usual debarring them from participation in such festivities; see *Y.D.*, *cccxci*.2, gloss), because the joy is impaired by the child's pain. But Yomtov Ishbili (*Novellae of RITVA*, on *Kethuboth* 8a), citing this view, rejects it himself.

[26] b*Yevamoth* 47b; see Preuss, *p*.284.

[27] *Levush*, *Y.D.*, *cclxviii*.2.

[28] See *supra*, chpt.VI (note 91).

[29] *BaH*, *a.l.*; based on Maimonides, *Hil. 'Avadim*, *ix*.8.

[30] For full details, see I. Jakobovits, "The Medical Treatment of Animals in Jewish Law", in *The Journal of Jewish Studies*, *vol.vii* (1956), *nos*.3 and 4, *p*.207 *ff*. On the Jewish attitude to the treatment of animals generally, see *JE vol.iv*, *p*.376; *OY*, *vol.ix*, *p*.49 *ff*.; *JL*, *vol.v*, *p*.945; and especially the articles by J. Wohlgemuth, "Vom Tier und seiner Wertung", in *Jeschurun*, *vol.xiv* (1927), *p*.585 *ff*.; "Das Leid der Tiere", in *Jeschurun*, *vol.xv* (1928), *pp*.245 *ff*. and 452 *ff*.; and "Einfuehlung in das Empfindungsleben der Tiere", in *Jeschurun*, *vol.xvi* (1929), *pp*.455 *ff*. and 535 *ff*. For some biblical data, see B. Heller, "Tierschaetzung im Bibelwoerterbuch", in *MGWJ*, *vol.lxxviii* (1934), *p*.41 *ff*.; and M. L. Bamberger, "Ueber Tierschutz nach den Lehren der Torah", in *Jeschurun*, *vol.ii* (1915), *p*.80 *ff*.

[31] A talmudic sage taught that it was forbidden to buy an animal or

bird unless one had first assured the necessary supply of its food (j*Kethu-both, iv.*8). Greater legal force was attached to the teaching: "It is unlawful for man to taste anything until he has provided food for his cattle" (b*Gittin* 62a; based on *Deut. xi.*15). This law is recorded in some codes; see Maimonides, *Hil. 'Avadim, ix.*8; Abraham Danzig, *Hayei 'Adam, xlv.*1; and Gumbiner, *M.A., clxvii.*18. On its extension to the feeding of birds, see Azulay, *Birkei Yoseph, O.H., clvii.*4; and *S.T., clxvii.*2.

32 See *Ex. xxiii.*5; *Deut. xxii.*4; and the talmudic treatment of these laws in b*Baba Metzi'a* 32a *ff.* Even the regulation regarding the hired servant "In the same day shalt thou give him his hire" *Deut. xxiv.*15) is homiletically applied to the beast (*Ex. Rabbah, xxxi.*7).

33 See *supra*, pp. 36, 39, 79 and 81.

34 Based on *Ex. xxiii.*5. In the Talmud (b*Baba Metzi'a* 32a *f.*) there is a dispute on whether the prohibition is biblical or rabbinic. Isserles accepts the more stringent view of Maimonides ('*Hil. Rotze'ah, xiii.*9; *cf. Keseph Mishneh, a.l.*). For a contrary view, see Joseph Babad, *Minhath Hinnukh*, commandment *no.*80.

35 Azulay, *Birkei Yoseph, Y.D., ccclxxii.*2. Maimonides (*loc. cit.*) evidently also supports this view, since he assumes that legally it is no more lawful to cause pain to a fellow-Jew than to an animal; see *SeMA, cclxxii.*13. For a similar opinion, see also Adreth, r*RaSHBA, nos.* 252 and 257.

36 r*Havath Ya'ir, no.*191. The very argument used by Bacharach (*viz.*, the animal's lack of reason) to assign to the animal special rights not enjoyed by man is used by the Church to deprive animals of any strict rights; see J. McCarthy, in *Irish Ecclesiastical Record, vol.lxxi* (1948), *p.*266 *ff.* There is also a talmudic parallel to the view that, in some respects, greater legal protection is extended to the animal than to a man. The law "Thou shalt not muzzle the ox when he treadeth out the corn" (*Deut. xxv.*4) carries the biblical penalty of flagellation only in respect of animals, but not for the imposition of similar restraints on human workers (*Sifri* and Rashi, *a.l.*; b*Baba Metzi'a* 88b; and Maimonides, *Hil. Sekhiruth, xiii.*2). This discrimiantion, too, is due to the fact that "a human worker is different, because he is gifted with intelligence" (*A.H.. H.M., cccxxxvii.*2). For a similar reasoning, see also David ibn Zimra, r*RaDBaZ*, part *i, no.*728. *Cf. supra*, chpt.VI (note 96).

37 Legally this question arises only when the fulfilment of a religious precept would involve exposure to serious pain or discomfort; for example, if a priest, by leaving his house as soon as a death has occurred in it, must suffer the severe cold outside without adequate protection until the corpse is removed or alternative shelter becomes available. The verdict would then be affected by the status of the offence to inflict pain on human beings; see sources in the preceding two notes.

38 Sigerist, *Medicine*, p.34.

39 Genicot, *Theologiae Moralis Institutiones*, Louvain, 1902, *vol.i*, p.162; quoted by O'Malley and Walsh, *Essays*, *p.*118.

40 For Simpson himself that event marked the victorious conclusion of his fight against the moral and religious opposition to painless births; see H. L. Gordon, *Sir James Young Simpson*, 1897, *p.*123 *ff.*; and J. Duns, *The Life of Sir James Young Simpson*, 1873, *p.*215 *ff.*

41 E. S. Cowles, *Religion and Medicine in the Church*, 1925, *p.*18.

42 *Viz.*, "In pain shalt thou bring forth children" (*Gen. iii.*16). This also served as the principal argument against Simpson's advocacy of chloroform. He countered it by referring to the sanction implied in 1 Timothy *iv.*4 and, above all, in *Gen. ii.*21; see sources cited in note 40

above. Among Jewish scholars, this reference never presented any difficulty, as Eve was cursed, not commanded, to suffer. *Cf.* Zimmels, *p*.7.

43 C. Capellmann, *Pastoral-Medizin*, 1878, *p*.37 f.

44 See *Daily Telegraph*, September 19, 1949, *p*.1; cited by Zimmels, *p*.6.

45 Zimmels, *p*.7.

46 So Luria (*Yam shel Shelomo, Yevamoth, vi*.44), Sirkes (*BaH, E.H., v*) and Epstein (*A.H., E.H., v*.24). For details, see *infra*, chapter XIII.

47 J. McCarthy, in *Irish Ecclesiastical Record, vol.lxi* (1943), *p*.345 f.

48 *CE, vol.v, p*.630.

49 See *infra*, chapter XI (beginning).

50 b*Sanhedrin* 43a; see Preuss, *p*.277. *Cf.* Mark *xv*.23. The Talmud derives the regulation from the verse "Give strong drink to him that he is ready to perish, and wine unto the bitter soul" (*Prov. xxxi*.6), but elsewhere (b*Sanhedrin* 45a) the Golden Rule is adduced as proof for the duty to "choose an easy death" for the capital convict.

51 Maimonides, *Hil. Sanhedrin, xiii*.2.

52 According to one version (b*Sanhedrin* 43a), the drink was given "so as not to distract his mind"; according to another (*Semahoth, ii*.8), "so that he should not be in pain". It was administered immediately after the final confession (Maimonides, *loc. cit.*).

Chapter Nine

1 The talmudic sources are discussed by Preuss (*p*.515 *ff.*), Krauss (*vol.i, p*.264) and particularly Hamburger (*RE, vol.ii, p*.653 *ff.*).

2 b*Shabbath* 127a. On the importance of this duty, *cf.* also *Matth. xxv*.36 and 43.

3 See Singer, *Prayer-Book, p*.5.

4 "'Ye shall walk after the Lord, your God' (*Deut. xiii*.5): Can a man walk after the Divine Presence?... but [the meaning is:] imitate the qualities of the Holy One, blessed be He... Just as He visited the sick— as is written 'And the Lord appeared unto him [*viz.*, Abraham, following his circumcision]' (*Gen. xviii*.1)—so shall you, too, visit the sick" (b*Sotah* 14a); see also Rashi, on verses cited; and *Tur, Y.D., cccxxxv*.

5 b*Nedarim* 40a. So also Maimonides, *Hil. 'Avel, xiv*.4.

6 According to the Talmud (b*Nedarim* 39b), each visitor reduces the illness by one sixtieth—provided he loves the patient as himself (*Lev. Rabbah, xxxiv*.2). The argument that 60 visitors should then be able to restore the patient completely is countered in the Talmud (*loc. cit.*) by the explanation that every visitor merely removes one sixtieth of the sickness left over from the previous visit. But a caller born under the same planetary influence of the zodiac as the patient not only removes, but actually transfers to himself, a sixtieth of the disease (b*Baba Metzi'a* 30b). Maimonides (*loc. cit.*), omitting the reference to coevals, simply states: "Whoever visits a sick person is as if he took away part of the disease and relieved him of it".

7 For full sources, see S. W. Baron, *The Jewish Community*, 1942, *vol.i, p*.362 f., and *vol.ii, p*.327 *ff.*, with corresponding notes in *vol.iii*. For references to such societies in the responsa, see Zimmels, *p*.270 (note 55).

8 See I. Abrahams, *Jewish Life in the Middle Ages*, 1932, *p*.354.

9 See *supra*, *p*.20.

10 *Tur, loc. cit.*; based in b*Nedarim* 40a, and Rashi, *a.l.* See Preuss, *p*.516.

11 Nachmanides, cited in *Beth Yoseph, Y.D., cccxxxv*.

12 Jacob Molin, r*MaHaRIL, no*.197; cited by Isserles, *Y.D., cccxxxv*.2, gloss.

[13] Maimonides (*Hil. 'Avel, xiv.*5) does not record this part of the regulation given in the Talmud (j*Pe'ah, iii* [end]), but Karo (*Keseph Mishneh, a.l.*) could find no reason for this omission. See also following note.

[14] See *supra, p.*39 f. The fear of ominous consequences does not apply to visits by people in regular contact with the patient.

[15] Because, as talmudic proverb has it, "when the day rises, the patient is high; when the day sinks, the patient comes low" (b*Baba Bathra* 16b); see Preuss, *p.*517. Maimonides (*loc. cit.*) discountenances visits during the first and last three hours of the day, "because [the attendants] are then engaged with looking after the needs of the sick". David ibn Zimra *RaDBaZ, a.l.*), commenting on this divergence from the talmudic motivation of the law (b*Nedarim* 40a) as accepted by Karo, suggests that Maimonides advanced his own reason "in view of his competence in medical matters."

[16] "Out of reverence for the Divine Presence—like a person sitting in fear without turning sideways" (Rashi, *Shabbath* 12b, where this law first appears).

[17] See *supra, chpt.*I (note 4).

[18] Folowing Tosaphoth, *Shabbath* 12b.

[19] See *supra, p.*100.

[20] *Cf. supra,* pp. 50 and 94 f.

[21] *TaZ, a.l.,* 19.

[22] See Preuss, *p.*517; and Krauss, *vol.i, p.*264.

[23] b*Nedarim* 41a; in the name of the physician Samuel.

[24] On the various interpretations of this condition, see *infra, chpt.*XV (note 55).

[25] The more likely motive is, however, the protection of the patient, since the Talmud mentions Samuel's dictum in support of the law not to call on patients who may be troubled by visits.

[26] r*ReMA, no.*19 (end). So also Chayim Benevisti, *Keneseth Hagedolah;* cited in *Sedei Hemed, vol.i, s.v. "Beth", no.*116.

[27] So Joseph Molko, *Shulhan Gavo'ah;* cited in *Sedei Hemed, loc. cit.;* and Samuel di Medina, r*RaSHDaM, H.M., no.*346; see J. D. Eisenstein, *Otzar Dinim Uminhagim,* 1917, *p.*49; and Zimmels, *p.*231 f. For further sources, see Grunwald, *Kol Bo, p.*17 (note 5).

[28] But Elijah Hacohen (*Midrash Talpiyoth, s.v. "'Aaron"*) advises visitors to plague-ridden patients not to sit, but to walk to and fro until they leave; for, according to a tradition received from his teachers, "the angel of death then has no licence to dominate and strike [his victim]".

[29] So *Shulhan Gavo'ah;* cited in *Sedei Hemed, loc. cit.*

[30] J. C[assuto], "Aus dem aeltesten Protokollbuch der portugiesisch-juedischen Gemeinde in Hamburg", in *JJLG, vol.x* (1912), *pp.*252 and 280 (in minutes dated 1664 and 1666).

[31] See A. O'Malley, "The Priest in Infectious Diseases", in O'Malley and Walsh, *Essays, p.*177 f.

[32] Liguori, *Theolog. Moral., liv.v, tr.*5, *no.*710; cited by O'Malley, *loc. cit.*

[33] Of Joseph Colon, r*MaHaRIK, no.*128. For numerous other rabbinic sources on the duty to support the poor sick, including the right to divert a gift or legacy for the building of a synagogue to aiding the sick, see Baron, *op. cit., vol.iii, p.*211 (note 44).

[34] See *supra, p.*53. Moreover, it is wrong to have compassion with a person doing so, for since he shows no mercy for himself, he will certainly have no consideration for others (j*Pe'ah, viii* [end]).

[35] The general provisions on the liability to taxation (by the Jewish

community) are already mentioned in the Mishnah (*Baba Bathra, i.*5); they apply, of course, only to an autonomous Jewish society. On Jewish communal taxation in talmudic and medieval times, see Baron, *op. cit., vol.i, p.*136 *ff.*; and *vol.ii, p.*246 *ff.*

[36] In the Talmud (b*Baba Bathra* 23a) the reference is to blood-letting. That passage merely deals with damage to fruit-trees caused by the attracted ravens, but Maimonides (*Hil. Shekhenim, xi.*8) extends it also to the disturbance of ailing people.

[37] Healthy people cannot raise objection to noise coming from a near-by shop, once they allowed a precedent to be created without protest (*H.M., clvi.*2); but any subsequent illness invalidates the precedent (Jacob of Lissa, *Mishpat Hakohanim, a.l.,* 7).

[38] For further references to the sick in civil law, see *H.M., lv.*1; *cxxv.*10; *clxxv.*34; *ccvii.*15; *ccciii.*2; and *cccxxxiii.*5.

[39] See *supra, p.*20 *ff.*

[40] The Talmud (b*Shabbath* 12b) explains the insistence on Hebrew when praying in the absence of the patient as due to the ignorance of the angels (through whom the prayer is transmitted) of any other language, particularly Aramic. But in the sick-room, where the Divine Presence Itself dwells, any language can be used. The same distinction applies to ordinary prayers: only when these are read in public (that is, in the company of the Divine Presence) may one resort to languages other than Hebrew (*O.H., ci.*4). But this argument has been criticised by Tosaphoth (*a.l.*) on the grounds that, if the angels know all human thoughts, they should certainly be familiar with all languages. See also Chajes, *Glosses* of *MaHaRaTZ, a.l.* in support of this view. *Cf.* also *OY, vol.vi, p.*213. Maimonides, however, omits both rulings.

[41] See *supra*, chpt.VIII (note 9).

[42] *SHaKH, a.l.,* 4; following Rashi, *Shabbath* 12b.

[43] *Cf. supra*, chpt.I (note 128).

[44] See *supra, p.*20 *f.*

[45] *Cf. supra*, chpt.VI (note 142).

[46] *Cf. supra, p.*51 *f.*

[47] Since the patient cares only for their healing properties, not their origin (*A.H., a.l.,* 22).

[48] See *supra, p.*20.

[49] See *supra, p.*16 *ff.*

[50] See *supra, p.*20 *f.*

Chapter Ten

[1] See Ploss and Bartels, *Woman, vol.ii, p.*633 *ff.*

[2] See Preuss, *p.*11 *f.*; citing Galen, *De locis affect., vi.*40; and referring to C.A. Boettinger, *Kleine Schriften archaeologischen und antiquarischen Inhalts,* ed. Sillig, 1938, *vol.iii, p.*6.

[3] See Ploss and Bartels, *op. cit., p.*637.

[4] See P. Diepgen, "Zur Frauenheilkunde im Byzantinischen Kulturkreis des Mittelalters", in *Abhandlungen der Geistes- und Sozial-wissenschaftlichen Klasse,* 1950, *p.*10.

[5] See Ploss and Bartels, *op. cit., p.*633.

[6] See Haggard, *Devils, p.*29. For later examples of this puritan attitude, see J. Fletcher, *Morals and Medicine,* 1955, *p.*30 *f.*

[7] See Haggard, *Devils, p.*40 *ff.*; and Preuss, *p.*12.

[8] See Lecky, *European Morals, vol.ii, p.*344; and Loren M. McKinney,

"Medical Ethics and Etiquette in the Early Middle Ages", in *Bulletin of the History of Medicine, vol.xxvi* (1952), *p.*4.

[9] See Garrison, *An Introduction, p.*175.

[10] See LaWall, *Pharmacy, p.*219.

[11] See *The Healing Art the Right Hand of the Church*, 1859, *p.* 266 *f.*

[12] *Ib.*

[13] See Ploss and Bartels, *op. cit., p.*651; and H. Haeser, *Lehrbuch der Geschichte der Medizin*, 1875, *vol.i, p.*562.

[14] See Puschmann, *Medical Education, p.*280 *f.; cf.* also McKenzie, *Infancy, p.*44.

[15] See Garrison, *An Introduction, p.*169.

[16] C. Capellmann, *Pastoral-Medizin*, 1878, *p.*85 *f.*

[17] *CE, vol.x, p.*143.

[18] Except when a doctor treats his own wife and she is in a state of ritual impurity (see *supra, p.*56). Lately some rabbis have ruled that in urgent cases the doctor should then feel his wife's pulse through a cloth; see *P.T., Y.D., cxcv.*16; and *D.T., a.l.*, 56. But this exception, related solely to the stringent laws of ritual uncleanliness, is obviously irrelevant to the medical relations between the sexes in general.

[19] A. H. Israels, *Testamen hist.-med. inaug. exhibens collect. gynaecol. ex Talmude Babyl.*, Groeningen, Leer, 1845; cited by Ploss and Bartels, *op. cit., p.*635.

[20] Krauss, *vol.ii, p.*429 (note 44).

[21] Preuss, *p.*12.

[22] Ploss and Bartels, *loc. cit.*

[23] b*Ta'anith* 21b.

[24] See *infra, p.*224.

[25] b*Niddah* 47a; see Preuss, *p.*12.

[26] See Friedenwald, *p.*22; and I. Simon, "Le 'Serment Médicale' d'Assaph, Médecin Juif du VIIe Siècle", in *Révue, no.*9 (1951), *p.*38.

[27] Zahalon, *Otzar Hahayim*, Venice, 1683, *Introduction*; see Friedenwald, *p.*273.

[28] *Cf. Nu. xv.*39. See Friedenwald, *p.*277; and *cf. supra, p.*17.

[29] See S. W. Baron, *The Jewish Community*, 1942, *vol.ii, p.*328.

[30] See Friedenwald, *pp.* 218 and 542.

[31] Thus, at the end of the 14th century Arnaldo de Vilanova complained that even convents were visited only by Jewish male physicians; see *JE, vol.iv, p.*35.

[32] L. Lewin, "Juedische Aerzte in Grosspolen", in *JJLG, vol.ix* (1911), *p.*415, where a number of Jewish doctoresses in Germany and Turkey during the 14—17th centuries are listed. See also Friedenwald, *pp.* 217 *ff.* and 542; and Zimmels, *p.*31 *f.*, dealing with Jewish woman-doctors in the responsa.

[33] See Zimmels, *p.*32, referring to a Turkish woman-doctor mentioned in a 16th century responsum by Yomtov Zahalon (*no.*40).

[34] See C. Roth, "The Qualification of Jewish Physicians in the Middle Ages", in *Speculum, vol.xxviii* (1953), *p.*842.

[35] *E.g.*, b*Niddah* 22b; see Preuss, *p.*12. For references to some of the numerous instances in the responsa literature, see Zimmels, *p.*191 *f.*

[36] To establish whether the effect of wine, used instead of water, on intertwining the hair would lead to an unlawful interposition during a ritual bath; see Preuss, *p.*424 *f. Cf. supra, p.*92.

[37] So *SHaKH, cxcv.*20. For further sources, see J. Ettlinger, r*Binyan Tziyon, no.*75; and *D.T., clv.*8.

[38] Eybeschuetz, *Kerethi Upelethi*, on *Y.D., cxcv.*

39 Ettlinger, *loc. cit.*

40 See Friedenwald, *p.75.*

41 This consisted of seating the woman on a wine-barrel; if the smell of wine then escaped from her mouth, it indicated that she had been deflowered. This popular diagnosis was also advocated, with slight variations, by Hippocrates, Aetius, Albertus Magnus and others; see Preuss, *p.560.*

42 b*Kethuboth* 10b; see Preuss, *p.559 f.* The Talmud (b*Yevamoth* 60b) also mentions a miraculous method to test the maturity of the women to be slain "in the matter of Peor" (see *Nu. xxxi.*17; and Rashi, *a.l.*)—evidently again an indication of the reluctance to submit women to ordinary gynecological examinations. But priests, charged with diagnosing signs of leprosy, had to view personally the entire body of female as well as male suspects; see m*Nega'im, ii,* 4.

43 Since Maimonides (*Hil. 'Ishuth, xi.*12) does not stipulate that the test prescribed in the Talmud must be used, it is assumed (*Maggid Mishnah, a.l.*) that he would regard any reliable method to ascertain virginity as valid. The commentaries, too, maintain that "we are no longer competent" to rely on the talmudic test; see *He.M., lxviii.*3; and *Ba'er Hetev, a.l.,* 1. *Cf. supra, p.xl f.*

44 *I.e.,* the cancelation of her endowment rights determined in the marriage contract; see *E.H., lxviii.*1; and *He.M., a.l.,* 1.

45 Known as "דורקטי" in the original. This is variously derived from τρωκτή, "raw" (see Jastrow, *Dictionary, p.*290), or τραχῶδης, "dry, hard wood" (see Kohut, *Aruch Completum, vol.iii, p.*162). In the Talmud (b*Kethuboth* 10b), as in the gloss to *E.H., lxviii.*5, the word is aggadically interpreted as "דור קומע", "a cut-off race; that is, a family whose members are barren and through whom the procreation of children is cut off". See Preuss, *p.*561.

46 "These are the symptoms of barenness: any woman who has no breasts, has pain during coitus, is abnormally formed at the lower abdomen [probably referring to languets and *mons veneris*], and whose voice is coarse and indistinguishable from that of men" (*E.H., clxxii.*4), or who shows any of these defects (*ib.,* gloss). For further details, see Preuss, *p.*261.

47 *I.e.,* particularly the growth of two pubic hairs (*E.H., clv.*12). See Preuss, *p.*146.

48 They cannot otherwise have conjugal relations (*ib.*). *Cf.* Preuss, *p.*141 *ff.*

49 *Cf. supra,* chpt.VI (note 86).

50 A woman comes of age either with the appearance of pubic hair (to be certified by women) or with the development of her breasts (to be ascertained by men, unless she is over twelve years old); see *B.S., a.l.,* 7.

51 For the law mentions only the evidence of the midwife, the father and the mother as acceptable to determine the first-born of twin children (*ib.*).

52 *'Avel Rabbathi, xii.*

53 Karo, *Beth Yoseph, Y.D., cccxxxv.*

54 Jaffe, *Levush, a.l.*

55 *Cf. supra,* chpt.III (note 69).

56 Isserles, *Darkei Mosheh, Y.D., cccxxxv.*4.

57 Falk, *Derishah, a.l.,* 4.

58 Sirkes, *BaH, a.l.*

59 b*Sanhedrin* 85b. See also Rashi, on *Ex. xxi.*15.

60 RaMBaN, *Torath Ha'adam;* cited by Karo, *Beth Yoseph, Y.D., ccxli.*

61 *Cf. supra, p.*4. Hence, several recent authorities permit a doctor to

give injections or similar treatments to his own patient at the latter's request; see J. Gershuni, in *Hapardes, vol.xxx, no.*3 (Dec. 1955), *p.*15 *ff.*; and I. J. Weisz, r*Minhath Yitzhak, nos.* 24—25.

⁶² Maimonides, *Hil. Mamrim, vi.*10. He bases this ruling on a story about a sage in similar circumstances related in the Talmud (b*Kiddushin* 31b).

⁶³ *RAVeD, a.l.*

⁶⁴ So Falk, *Derishah, Y.D., ccxl.*2; and *TaZ, a.l.,* 14.

⁶⁵ That is, if the mental illness struck her after her marriage; otherwise she cannot be married at all (*B.S., a.l.,* 9); see *infra, p.*156.

⁶⁶ If she is incompetent "to guard her deed of divorce", a divorce is biblically invalid (since she cannot perform any legal act), and her husband remains fully responsible for her maintenance. But if she is merely incapable of "looking after herself", she can be divorced according to biblical law, though the rabbis, to protect her, objected to this. In that case, Karo and Isserles differ on whether the husband, if he leaves her, must still provide for her subsistence and medical attention (*E.H., cxix.*6) or not (*ib.,* gloss); see *B.S., a.l.,* 10. But *cf.* also *He.M., a.l.,* 9.

⁶⁷ Even though a wife could normally be divorced against her will. But following the ban on such divorces by R. Gershom (*ib.,* gloss), no authority disputes an insane wife's claims for maintenance and other expenses against her husband (*He.M., loc. cit.*; and 12). Hence, Karo's decision (see preceding note), anyhow, is no longer valid.

⁶⁸ The enactment is of talmudic origin (b*Yevamoth* 113b); see *JE, vol.vi, p.*605.

⁶⁹ Only thus can the objection raised by Ibn Daud be overcome.

⁷⁰ For some sources, see Preuss, *p.*366.

⁷¹ m*Baba Kamma, viii.*4; see also Preuss, *p.*366. On the legal status of idiots, *cf.* also *supra, p.*92.

Chapter Eleven

¹ See *supra, p.*46 *ff.*

² m*'Avoth, iv.*22; see Singer, *Prayer-Book, p.*200.

³ m*'Avoth, iv.*21; see Singer, *loc. cit.*

⁴ Karo (*Beth Yoseph, Y.D., cccxxxv*) derives this law from a passage in *Semahoth*. But this is not found in our version of the tractate; see *Bi'ur HaGRA, a.l.* 9.

⁵ So *Tur* and *Beth Yoseph, Y.D., cccxxxv. Cf. supra, p.*51.

⁶ Samuel Strasson (*Novellae of ReSHaSH,* on *Berakhoth* 60a) actually expresses surprise that one should even contemplate a fatal outcome of the illness, considering that the Talmud urges one "not to invite misfortune by ominous words" (b*Berakhoth* 60a) and "not to despair of divine mercy even when a sharpened sword is laid upon one's throat" (b*Berakhoth* 10a).

⁷ This formula, which may be extended at will (*ib.,* gloss), goes back to a tradition first recorded by Nachmanides; see *Beth Yoseph, Y.D., cccxxxviii.*

⁸ *Cf.* also *supra, p.*87.

⁹ *SHaKH, a.l.,* 1. Any other act in anticipation of the expected demise is also frowned upon, such as the provision of funeral pipers and lamenting women, or of a coffin (*Y.D., cccxxxix.*1) or a grave (*ib.,* gloss).

¹⁰ *Midrash Rabbah,* on *Eccles. v.*6; see Preuss, *p.*32 *f.*

11 *Ib.* In this connection, Preuss (*p*.33) suggests that it may be significant that only the Hebrew language derives the term for "doctor" (רופא) from a root (רפה) denoting to "ease", "to assuage", whereas other tongues link the word for "physicians" with the meaning "to conjure", or "to know". *Cf.* Friedenwald, *p*.10.

12 Galen, *ed.* Kuehn, *vol.xvii, p*.145 *f.*

13 See Diepgen, *Die Theologie, p*.49, where reference is also made to the Jewish view.

14 *E.g.,* in the *Gratian Decretals, C.xxiii, qu*.3, *c*.11; quoted, together with other sources, by Diepgen, *loc. cit.*

15 See Diepgen, *op. cit., p*.48 *f.*

16 See Diepgen, *op. cit., p*.53 *f.* For some modern views on telling the truth to patients, see Joseph Fletcher, *Morals and Medicine*, 1955, *p*.34 *ff.*

17 See Diepgen, *op. cit., pp*.50 *f.* and 55 *f.*, where this attitude is also illustrated by many other sources. The nearest parallel to this view in Jewish writings is the suggestion by Me'iri that the violation of the Sabbath may be permitted to enable an otherwise lost person to make his confession; see *supra, p*.48.

18 Joshua Falk (Perishah, *Y.D., cccxxxix*.5) considers the maximum duration of this state (which affects certain legal issues) to be three days. This is also assumed in the ruling that one must mourn for a relative three days after he was seen in a dying state (*Y.D., cccxxxix*.2), since he is presumed dead by then (*ib.*, gloss).

19 Isserles bases this interpretation on the *Targum* rendering (גססיהן) for "side" (*i.e.* chest) in *Is. lx*.4 ("and thy daughters are borne on the *side*").

20 Apart form certain legal disabilities.

21 On the performance of these acts after death, see m*Shabbath, xxiii*.5. *Cf.* John *xix*.39.

22 Accroding to Servius, this served to revive a body which may only have been apparently dead; see Preuss, *p*.602.

23 To prevent the intrusion of air through the nose and rectum into the body (b*Shabbath* 151b); see Preuss, *p*.601; and Krauss, *vol.ii, p*.55.

24 Originally this act, performed after death on the Sabbath, served to place the corpse on the floor without touching it (which is forbidden on the Sabbath); see m*Shabbath, xxiii*.5; and Krauss, *loc. cit.* Later this act was believed to hasten death by removing feathers from the dying, as recorded by Isserles. Maimonides omits this item altogether in his list of these laws (*Hil. 'Avel, iv*.5).

25 To cool the corpse and prevent its quick decomposition (j*Shabbath, iv*.6); see Preuss, *p*.601; and Krauss, *loc. cit.*

26 To cool it and thereby prevent it from swelling up (b*Shabbath* 151b).

27 Preuss, *p*.601.

28 Caspar Questel, *De pulvinari morientibus non subtrahendo. Von Abziehung Sterbenden Hauptkuessen*, 1678.

29 Joshua Boaz Baruch of Italy, *Shiltei Gibborim*, on Alfasi, *Mo'ed Katan, iii*.1237.

30 Jaffe, *Levush, a.l.* See also *JE, vol.iv, p*.486.

31 b*Shabbath* 151b; and *Semahoth, i*.4.

32 For a discussion on the relevance of this to the two last-mentioned acts, see *BaH* and *Derishah, Y.D., cccxxxix.*

33 Even after death the body should not be moved immediately, lest it be merely in a swoon (*SHaKH, a.l.*, 5; following Maimonides, *Hil. 'Avel, iv*.5).

34 But care should be taken to prevent the patient from shifting a limb

out of his bed (*cf. Gen. xlix.*33); see Abraham Danzig, *Hokhmath 'Adam, cli.*19.

35 See Israel Lipschuetz, *Tiphereth Yisra'el, Yoma, viii* (*Bo'az,* 3). Similarly, "if the dying person claims he cannot depart unless they put him in another place, they must not remove him" (*Sepher Hasidim, no.*723).

36 See *Sepher Hasidim, no.*724.

37 b*'Avodah Zarah* 18a. Yet the sage abjured the executioner to add to the fire and to remove the tufts of wool from his heart, so that he would die more quickly (*ib.*).

38 *Sepher Hayashar;* see M. Steinschneider, *Hebraeische Bibliographie, vol.xvii* (1877), *p.*61; and A. Marx, "The Scientific Work of Some Outstanding Medieval Jewish Scholars", in *Essays and Studies in Memory of Linda R. Miller,* 1938, *p.*145.

39 On the admission of doctors that they practise euthanasia, see Fletcher, *op. cit., p.*205 f.

40 *rRaDBaZ,* part *i, no.*695. Cf. Loew, *Lebensalter, p.*60; and Zimmels, *p.*69.

41 Cf. *Tiph'ereth Yisra'el, loc. cit.*

42 *Sepher Hasidim, no.*723; see also *Shiltei Gibborim, loc. cit.* According to one rabbinic view (*rBeth Ya'akov, no.*59), even medicines must not be used to "delay the departure of the soul"; see *Gilyon MaHaRSHA,* on *Y.D., cccxxxix.*1.

43 *Sepher Hasidim, no.*234.

44 See b*Sanhedrin* 78a; and Maimonides, *Hil. Rotze'ah, ii.*7. The law distinguishes between killing persons dying "by the hand of Heaven" and such as are in a dying state "by the hand of man"; only the former act is liable to capital punishment. The acquittal (from the death penalty) of a man who kills a person dying by an act of violence is simply due to the "biblical decree" which considers a person so injured as already legally dead, since his vitality has been impaired. But if the victim had been in a sinking condition for natural causes, his murderer is fully liable, since there had been no previous *action* to diminish life, and in Jewish law it makes no difference whether the victim is a child or an aged person with only a short while to live (*cf. supra, p.*46); see *Minhath Hinnukh,* commandment *no.*34; and *TE, vol.v, p.*395 f.

45 For instance, would it be lawful to withdraw insulin injections from a diabetic who developed inoperable cancer and is in great pain? A Catholic moralist sanctions this only if the insulin itself contributes to the acute pain resulting from the cancer (J. McCarthy, in *Irish Ecclesiastical Record, vol.lviii* [1941], *p.*552 ff.). For a recent rabbinical study of this problem, and on the Jewish legal attitude to euthanasia generally, see I. Jakobovits, in *Hapardes, vol.xxxi, no.*1 (October 1956), *p.*28 ff., and *vol.xxxi, no.*3 (December 1956), *p.*16 ff.

46 In 1923 a rabbi expressed the view that one must not withdraw food from an incurable to expedite his death, even if the absence of food would relieve his agony, "for a doubtful contingency [*viz.,* the doctors' verdict that the disease will prove fatal] cannot legally disestablish a certainty [*viz.,* the patient's death if the food is withdrawn]" (D. Z. Katzburg, in *Tel Talpiyoth, vol.xxx* [1923], *p.*66). But this judgment does not necessarily determine the decision in cases where the withdrawal of a *medicament* would lead to an easier death. On the Jewish attitude to euthanasia, see also I. Rabinowitch, "Euthanasia", in *McGill Medical Journal, vol.xix* (1950), *p.*160.

47 So *RaN, Nedarim* 40a. For such prayers in the Talmud, see b*Kethu-*

both 104a; b*Baba Metzi'a* 84a; and b*Ta'anith* 23a. *Cf.* also *Tiph'ereth Yisra'el, loc. cit.*

48 Thus, an old woman seeking relief by death was advised her wish would be granted if she would not absent herself from the synagogue for three days (*Yalkut*, Proverbs, *no.*943).

49 Tosaphoth, *Gittin* 57b; and '*Avodah Zarah* 18a. *Cf.* the justification of Saul's suicide and the voluntary martyrdom of Daniel's friends in *Gen. Rabbah*, *xxxiv.*13. For a similar exception, see also *supra*, *p.*98. But Solomon Luria (*Yam shel Shelomo, Baba Kamma*, *viii.*59) endorses the view that even self-destruction to escape from an oppressor is to be condemned. On this dispute, see *Beth Yoseph, Y.D., clvii*; and more fully J. L. Unterman, *Shevet Miyehudah*, 1955, *p.*42 *ff.*

50 Several patristic writers allowed suicide to achieve martyrdom, to avoid apostacy or to retain virginity. But this sanction was later withdrawn. See Fletcher, *op. cit., p.*178.

51 The Talmud (b*Sanhedrin* 45a and 52a) uses the exact Hebrew equivalent ("מיתה יפה") to denote the "easy [quick] death" to be chosen for capital convicts; see *supra*, *p.*105.

52 Lecky, *European Morals, vol.i, xi.*233; cited in *Oxford English Dictionary, vol.iii, s.v.* "Euthanasia 3".

53 Plato, *Republic, iii.*405.

54 For other barbaric measures to rid society of "useless" individuals, see Plato, *v.*459—461.

55 L. Edelstein, "The Hippocratic Oath", in *Supplements to the Bulletin of the History of Medicine*, 1943, *p.*10 *ff.*

56 K. Deichgraeber, "Die aerztliche Standesethik des hippocratischen Eides", in *Quellen zur Geschichte der Naturwissenschaft und Medizin, vol.iii* (1932), *p.*36.

57 See Neuburger, *History, vol.i, p.*181. *Cf.* also Fletcher, *op. cit., p.*177.

58 More, *Utopia*, part *ii*, chpt.*vii*; see *ERE*, *vol.v, p.*601; and Fletcher, *op. cit., p.*179.

59 Augustine, *De civilitate Dei, i.*17 *f.* See also note 50 above.

60 Aquinas, *Summa*, II.*ii.*64, 65; see *ERE, op. cit., p.*600.

61 See *Irish Ecclesiastical Record, vol.lix* (1942), *p.*468 *f.*

62 At the 2nd Reading of the Voluntary Euthanasia Legislation Bill, 1. 12. 1936.

63 See W. G. Earengey, "Voluntary Euthanasia", in *Medico-Legal Review, vol.viii* (1940), *p.*93.

Chapter Twelve

1 According to Isserles, some authorities permit this, but it is better to adopt the more stringent view (*ib.*, gloss). *Cf.* also *infra, p.*242.

2 According to the Talmud (b*Hullin* 21a), the severence of the flesh is not essential in the case of old people to render the unclean if their neck or back is fractured; see *SHaKH, a.l.*, 1. On the legal presumption of death, *cf.* also *supra*, chpt.XI (note 44).

3 b*Yoma* 85a. See also *supra, p.*46.

4 The Talmud (b*Yoma* 85a) also records one view according to which the signs of life may also be checked at the heart (pulsation) or, following another version (j*Yoma, viii.*5), at the navel. But the respiration test is considered paramount, since its reliability is supported by the

biblical reference to "all in whose nostrils was the breath of the spirit of life" (*Gen. vii.*22). Preuss (*p.*601 *f.*) strangely states that he could find no information in the Talmud concerning the symptoms of death. For further details, see I. Simon, "La Médecine légale dans le Bible et le Talmud", in *Révue, no.*2 (1948), *p.*50 *f.*

5b'*Arakhin* 7a. See also *supra, p.xli* and *infra, p.*130 *f.*

6 b*Sanhedrin* 46a and b. In the Bible the law is stated only in the context of the disposal of bodies of persons executed for blasphemy; its extension to all corpses is based on the emphasis ". . . thou shalt *surely* bury him" (*Deut. xxi.*23). For further details, see Preuss, *p.*612; Hamburger, *RE, vol.i, p.*161; and *OY, vol.ix, p.*91.

7 Based on m*Sanhedrin, vi.*5; and *Semahoth, xi.*1.

8 See *supra, chpt.*XI (note 33).

9 For a summary of some of these controversies, see M. Dienemann, in *Die Hygiene der Juden, ed.* M. Grunwald, 1911, *p.*208 *f.*; and Zimmels, *p.*57 *f.*

10 See Friedenwald, *p.*599 (note 188).

11 See *Bikkurei Ha'ittim,* 1824, *p.*233 *ff.*; *JE, vol.iii, p.*434; *OY, vol.ix, p.*91; and literature cited in note 9 above. Mendelsohn's agreement with the civil authorities was also approvingly quoted in non-Jewish works; see, *e.g.,* J. P. Frank, *System einer vollstaendigen medizinischen Polizey, iv, vol.ii,* part *v,* § 35.

12 The argument was based mainly on two talmudic passages: According to the Mishnah (m*Niddah, x.*4), certain categories of persons (*e.g.,* those afflicted with gonorrhoea or leprosy) do not cause defilement upon their death "until the decay of the flesh has set in", because—as the Talmud (b*Niddah* 69b) explains—"they may merely have fainted and only appear to be dead"; see Preuss, p.602. The second passage indicating a distrust in the ordinary tokens of death is the reference (*Semahoth, viii.*1) to the custom of visiting the cemetery to watch the dead for three days following their burial; for "once it happened that they watched one who thereupon continued to live for 25 years and another who still had five children before dying". It was also argued that the Talmud applied the respiration test only to people buried under a pile of debris, but not to ordinary cases of death.

13 Emden, cited by Schreiber, r*Hatham Sopher, Y.D., no.*338; see *P. T., Y.D., ccclvii.* 1. These authorities reject the argument from the Mishnah (see preceding note) as irrelevant, and the proof from *Semahoth* as inconclusive, because the occurances mentioned there are "remote incidents which may happen once in a thousand years" and which are recorded only to justify the custom of visiting the graves for three days (which would otherwise be forbidden as a heathen superstition). Moreover, they argue, the context in which the Talmud refers to the establishment of death by the cessation of breathing clearly proves the applicability of that test to all deaths, since a sudden and violent death (as dealt with in the Talmud) is more likely to be "apparent" than a lingering death following illness.

14 r*Hatham Sopher, loc. cit.*; see *OY, vol.ix, p.*91.

15 See Krauss, *vol.ii, pp.*55 and 473 (note 411).

16 This belief is also encountered among other ancient peoples, *e.g.,* the Persians; see A. O'Rahilly, "Jewish Burial", in *Irish Ecclesiastical Record, vol.lviii* (1941), *p.*133 *f.*; citing G. Maspero, *Histoire ancienne, vol.iii, p.*589.

17 *Gen. Rabbah, c.*7; *Lev. Rabbah, xviii.*1; *Midrash Rabbah,* on *Eccles. xii.*6; and j*Mo'ed Katan, iii.*5.

[18] Based on m*Yevamoth, xvi.*3. This law is explicitly connected with the belief in the soul's association with the body for three days; see *Gen. Rabbah, lxv.*20; and *Eccles. Rabbah, loc. cit.*

[19] Falk, *Perishah, a.*l., 3. See note 12 above. See also Gloss on Asheri, *Mo'ed Katan, iii.*39, in the name of *'Or Zaru'a*; and Hamburger, *RE, vol.i,* p.161.

[20] For references to the views which follow, see O'Malley and Walsh, *Essays,* p.164; W. M. Drum's Appendix "The Moment of Death" to A. E. Sandford, *Pastoral Medicine,* 1904; J. McCarthy, in *Irish Ecclesiastical Record, vol.lviii* (1941), p.369 *ff.*; F. J. Connell, "How Soon May Embalming Begin?", in *American Ecclesiastical Review, vol.xxix* (1948), p.230; and G. Kelly, in *Theological Studies, vol.x* (1949), p.88 *f.*

[21] See *supra,* p.88.

[22] Moses Gruenwald, r*'Arugath Habosam, vol.ii,* Y.D., no.251.

[23] Jacob Reischer, r*Shevuth Ya'akov,* part *ii,* no.97; see *P.T.,* Y.D., *-cclxiii.*5; and Zimmels, p.58.

[24] *Sepher Hasidim,* nos. 451 and 1542; see *Ba'er Hetev,* Y.D., ccclii (end).

[25] See O'Malley and Walsh, *Essays,* p.185.

[26] See *supra, Introduction,* p.xli and notes 88–92.

[27] For a summary of the sources, see *Sedei Hemed,* part *iv, s.v. "Aveluth",* no.141; S. Schachna, *Mishmereth Shalom (Hayim Uverakhah),* 1930, part *ii,* p.61 *f.*; and Grunwald, *Kol Bo,* p.49 *f.*

[28] See, *e.g.,* Moses Teitelbaum, r*Heshiv Mosheh, O.H.,* no.13; and most of the responsa cited in the following notes.

[29] See, *e.g.,* Meir Posner, *Beth Me'ir,* on Y.D., ccclxiv.4; and Shalom Mordecai Schwadran, r*MaHaRSHaM,* part *ii,* no.159.

[30] So J. Piek, cited in *Mishmereth Shalom, loc. cit.*

[31] See, *e.g.,* Eleazar of Pielz, r*Shemen Roke'ah,* part *ii,* no.13; cited in *P.T.,* Y.D., ccclxiv.5. But others permit such a delay only if the woman actually died in labour; see, *e.g.,* Chayim Judah Leib, r*Sha'arei De'ah,* no.70; cited by Zimmels, p.69. See also *Sedei Hemed, loc. cit.*

[32] See r*Shemen Roke'ah,* and *Mishmereth Shalom, loc. cit.* Teitelbaum (*loc. cit.*) quotes a lengthy formula to be recited three times in Hebrew and in the vernacular to induce the corpse to deliver the foetus. If this fails, the woman should be asked for forgiveness and be buried without further efforts to extract the child.

[33] See sources cited in note 29 above.

[34] See, *e.g.,* Chayim Halberstam, r*Divrei Hayim,* part *ii,* Y.D., no.134; cited by Zimmels, p.69. Halberstam forbids the doctor to use instruments in the attempt to deliver the child. For further sources, see *Kol Bo, loc. cit.*

[35] Instead she is to remain clothed as she was at her death, so that any discharge from her body is buried with her; see *SHuKH, a.*l., 11.

[36] See M. Verdier, *La Jurisprudence particulière de la Chirurgie en France,* 1764, *vol.ii,* p.262 *f.*; cited by G. Wolff, "Leichenbesichtigung und Untersuchung bis zur Carolina als Vorstufe Gerichtlicher Sektion", in *Janus, vol.xlii* (1938), p.260.

[37] See *The Healing Art the Right Hand of the Church,* 1859, p.266.

[38] See Ploss and Bartels, *Woman, vol.iii,* p.82; citing *Opera, De Synodo Dioecesana, lib.xi, cap.vii,* 13, *vol.xi,* p.418.

[39] See Haggard, *Devils,* p.27.

[40] See Ploss and Bartels, *loc. cit.*

[41] See J. Needham, *A History of Embryology,* 1934, p.182 (note).

[42] F. E. Cangliamila, *Embryologia sacra*, 1763, *lib.ii, cap.xvi.* On the popularity of this work, see *supra, p.xxxv.*

[43] See Needham, *loc. cit.*; and C. Capellmann, *Pastoral-Medizin*, 1878, *p.*25.

[44] So, *e.g.*, A. M. Vering, *Handbuch der Pastoralmedizin*, 1835, *p.*257.

[45] The decision is not usually mentioned in current manuals on Catholic medical ethics.

[46] M. Macher, *Pastoralheilkunde fuer Seelsorger*, 1860, *p.*338.

[47] Capellmann, *op. cit., p.*24.

[48] In Christianity, one of the principal factors bearing on this subject is to save the child for baptism; see Wolff, *loc. cit.* On the Christian horror at the death without baptism of infants, whether born or unborn, see W. E. H. Lecky, *History of the Rise and Influence of the Spirit of Rationalism in Europe*, 1870, *vol.i, p.*360 *ff.*; and *European Morals, vol.ii, p.*23 f.; E. Westermark, *Moral Ideas, vol.i, p.*417; and *Christianity and Morals*, 1939, *p.*244; and *infra, p.*175 *f.*

[49] See Cumston, *An Introduction, p.*43. But the practice was later forbidden; see *ib., p.*46.

[50] A. Macalister, "Archaeologia Anatomica", in *Journal Anat. & Phys., vol.xxxii, p.*775; cited by Campbell, *Arabian Medicine, vol.i, p.*8 (note).

[51] See McKenzie, *Infancy, p.*18. He considers that the practice must post-date the *Ebers Papyrus* (*ca.* 1560 B.C.E.), since its close attention to external diseases strongly contrasts with the "shallow guess-work" on internal diseases, suggesting a lack of anatomical knowledge at that time.

[52] See G. Maspero, *The Dawn of Civilisation: Egypt and Chaldea*, ed. A. H. Sayce, 1910, *p.*216; Puschmann, *Medical Education, p.*23; and Castiglioni, *History, p.*59, where the view is expressed that, according to Diodorus Siculus, the stoning was merely symbolic.

[53] See Puschmann, *op. cit., p.*57. But *cf.* Osler, *Evolution, p.*69. The claim is based on Aristotle's mention of dissection for determining the cause and extent of diseases (*De part. anim., iv.*2), but is weakened by his admission that "the inward parts of man are known least of all" and that he had never seen the human kidneys or uterus (*Hist. anim., i.*16).

[54] Based on comment of Chalcidius (6th century C.E.) on the *Timaeus*; see Allbutt, *Greek Medicine, p.*98.

[55] See Singer, *Anatomy, p.*16.

[56] See Wolff, *op. cit., p.*228 *f.*

[57] See Neuburger, *History, vol.i, p.*150.

[58] Osler, *Evolution, p.*73. On the religious restraints to anatomical studies in pre-Alexandrian Greece, see Puschmann, *op. cit., p.*57; and W. H. Haggard, *The Doctor in History*, 1935, *pp.*74 and 92.

[59] On the charge that these physicians practised vivisection even on human beings—first made by Celsus (*Proem*) and repeated by Tertullian (*De anima, cap.x*) and Augustine (*De anima et eius origine, iv.*3 and 6) —see Puschmann, *op. cit., p.*78; Thorndike, *Magic, vol.i, p.*147 (note 7); and L. Edelstein, "Die Geschichte der Sektion in der Antike", in *Quellen und Studien zur Geschichte der Naturwissenschaften und der Medizin*, 1932, *p.*102. But according to Singer (*Anatomy, p.*34 *f.*), the justice of the charge is placed in doubt by Galen's silence on it.

[60] C. Singer, "Galen as a Modern", in *Proceedings of the Royal Siciety of Medicine, vol.xlii* (1949), *p.*565.

[61] Some hold that Galen may have studied anatomy very occasionally on human corpses—probably of hostile soldiers, criminals and still-born or exposed children; see Puschmann, *op. cit., p.*101 *f.*; Neuburger, *History, vol.i, p.*254; Thorndike, *Magic, vol.i, p.*147 *f.*; and H. E. Sigerist, "Die

Geburt der abendlaendischen Medizin", in *Essays, ed.* Singer and Sigerist, *p.*201.

62 E. A. Wallis Budge, *Syrian Anatomy, Pathology and Therapeutics*; or *"the Book of Medicines"*, 1913, *vol.i, p.clxii f.* Many passages prove that the author attached great value to dissection; *e.g.*, "those who dissect will call these 'soft' as you know" (*vol.ii,* p.107), and "this we can only learn from those who dissect the body..." (*vol.ii,* p.129).

63 See Budge, *op. cit., vol.i, p.xlvii.*

64 See Puschmann, *op. cit., p.*14.

65 The *Susruta* (*iii.*5) mentions that very occasionally the body would be exposed in river water for seven days, so that the friction of the soft parts would reveal the internal organs for anatomical examination; see Castiglioni, *History, p.*88; and Neuburger, *History, vol.i, p.*48.

66 See Campbell, *loc. cit.*

67 See Neuburger, *op. cit., p.*62 *f.* Castiglioni (*History, p.*102) adds that, according to the teaching of Confucius, the body is sacred, so that the study of anatomy was hindered to the present. Yet, the dissections on criminals were occasionally practised at the time of the Sung dynasty (10th–13th centuries).

68 Philo, *De special, leg., iii.*117; see translation by F. H. Colson, *Loeb Classical Series, vol.vii, p.*549 *f.*

69 By E. Carmoly, *Histoire des médecins juifs,* 1844, *p.*12.

70 By R. Landau, *Geschichte der juedischen Aerzte,* 1895, *p.*15.

71 Preuss, *p.*45. Carmoly based his allegation on a passage in the Talmud (bSanhedrin 47b) in which the use of earth from Rav's grave is justified for the cure of fever (*cf. supra, p.*91); ostensibly that indicated the people's desire to avenge Rav's (alleged) dissection of the dead by destroying his grave. In fact, the passage evidently describes some kind of saint-cult; see Preuss, *p.*184.

72 So Puschmann, *op. cit., p.*30; and A. H. Israels, *Collectanes gynaecologica ex Talmude Babylonico,* 1845; cited by Ploss and Bartels, *Woman, vol.i, p.*380 *f.*

73 See S. Muntner, *Ba'ayath Hanethiha Yehokhmath Habittur Beyisra'el,* 1955, *p.*13 *ff.*

74 H. Baas, *Outlines of the History of Medicine,* 1899, *pp.*37 and 295 (note 2). Altogether, the survey of talmudic medicine given by Baas is somewhat inaccurate.

75 t*Niddah, iv.*17. The account appears with slight variations in b*Niddah* 30b.

76 Needham, *op. cit., p.*47.

77 Pliny, *Nat. Hist., xix.*27 (*ed.* Harduin, *vol.iii, p.*588); see Preuss, *p.*44.

78 b*Bekhoroth* 45a.

79 Hebrew: (שלק). This is translated as "slit", "anatomised", or "dissected" by Levy (*Woerterbuch, vol.iv, p.*566), Kohut (*Aruch Completum, vol.viii, p.*90) and Jastrow (*Dictionary, p.*1588). But Preuss (*p.*47 *f.*), supported in a note by I. Loew (*a.l.*), maintains that the word should here—in common with its usual meaning—be rendered "cooked" or "boiled hard" and that this may be the only mention of boiling as a method of dissection in antiquity, if one disregards a concealed reference by Galen (*De ossib. ad tiron., cap.vi, xi* [*ed.* Kuehn, *vol.ii, pp.* 754 and 762]) to the dissolution of the jaw bone and the vertebra by boiling—observations probably carried out in the kitchen. Preuss assumes that the boiling of corpses for anatomical ends was only introduced by Vesalius, though it had been used to facilitate the long-distance transport of dead crusaders

(see *infra*, p.139). But Preuss overlooked the employment of this method by Mondino early in the 14th century (see *infra*, p.140).

80 I. L. Katzenelsohn, *Hatalmud Veharephu'ah*, 1928, p.237 f.

81 m'*Oholoth*, i.8.

82 The argument is also endorsed by I. M. Rabinowitch (*Post-Mortem Examinations and Jewish Law*, 1945, p.25 [note]) who avers that the talmudic figure—at 248 to 252 bones—approximates more closely to the findings of modern anatomy (assigning 270 to the new-born, 350 at the age of 14 years, and 206 after middle age) than the number given by Hippocrates (111) and Galen (over 200). But Preuss (p.69 f.) doubts the reliability of these counts, as ossification is varied and difficult to define.

83 b*Berakhoth* 4a, in a statement attributed to King David praising himself before God by contrasting his unpalatable work on putrid substances with the sumptuous parties enjoyed by other kings at the time.

84 b*Niddah* 24b.

85 With the exception of the last-mentioned statement, all the accounts deal with observations made for ritual purposes. The formation of the foetus affects the laws of uncleanliness in cases of miscarriage. The number of bones in the human body determines the defilement caused by touching a skeleton made up of at least the majority of all bones. The examination of blood and other uterine discharges is necessary to decide whether a woman is ritually pure or not.

86 Cf. *supra*, p.97.

87 This consideration also accounts for the Jewish opposition to cremation; see Rabinowitch, *op. cit.*, p.19. Cf. also Preuss, p.615 f.

88 b*Hullin* 11b. The passage sets out to find biblical support for the principle that a fact known to be true in a majority of cases is legally regarded as a certainty, even if no test to confirm it is made in individual cases. The argument runs as follows: The Bible insists on the execution of a murderer. Yet, the victim may have previously suffered from a fatal disease or injury, thus freeing the murderer from capital guilt as the killer of a virtually dead man (*cf. supra*, chpt.XI [note 44]). But since the murderer is nevertheless convicted, we must presume that such a contingency may be ignored and that the victim is legally deemed to have been healthy like most men. The Talmud then challenges the conclusiveness of this argument with the question: Let us examine the body to establish its integrity (without having to rely on the majority principle)? Answer: That would be a disgrace to the dead. Counter-question: But perhaps a body may be disgraced to save a human life (*viz.*, of the murderer, by establishing the inviability of his victim)? Answer: The autopsy might in any case prove inconclusive, as the victim's fatal injury could have been at the point of entry of the murderer's sword.

89 So Rabinowitch, *op. cit.*, p.28. See also Preuss, p.46.

90 The Talmud (b*Baba Bathra* 154a) forbids heirs to open the grave of a person to establish whether he was a minor or had reached his majority (by the appearance of pubic hair); the reasons given are that this would constitute a desecration of the dead and that, moreover, the signs to be ascertained may have changed after death. See Rabinowitch, *op. cit.*, p.27; and note 192 below.

91 See Wolff, *op. cit.*, pp. 226 and 285.

92 See *supra*, p.8 f.

93 The pioneer of modern anatomy, Andreas Vesalius (*De Fabrica Corporis Humani*, 1543, Preface), himself attributed the decline of dissection and anatomy since ancient times to the practice of entrusting

manual operations to barbers "who were too ignorant to read the writings of the teachers of anatomy"; see translation by Benjamin Farrington, in *Proceedings of the Royal Society of Medicine, vol.xxv* (1932), *p.*1357 *ff.*; cited by Stern, *Society, p.*13.

94 Augustine, *The City of God, lib.xxii, cap.xxiv* (*A Select Library of the Nicene and Post-Nicene Fathers of the Christian Church,* ed. Ph. Schaff, 1903, *vol.ii, p.*503); see Stern, *Society, p.*179 *f.*

95 See Singer, "Galen as a Modern", *op. cit., p.*570.

96 Sigerist, "Die Geburt", *op. cit., p.*196.

97 See Puschmann, *op. cit., p.*144.

98 See Puschmann, *op. cit., p.*202.

99 This belief, already found in the Talmud (b*Ta'anith* 21b), has survived to modern times, though Tyson had dismissed it as a "vulgar error" in 1683; see F. J. Cole, *A History of Comparative Anatomy,* 1944, *p.*49.

100 See D. Riesman, *Medicine in Modern Society,* 1939, *p.*94.

101 See Puschmann, *op. cit., p.*244.

102 See Mary N. Alston, "Attitude of the Church to Dissection before 1500", in *Bulletin of the History of Medicine, vol.xvi* (1944), *p.*255 *f.*

103 See Osler, *Evolution, p.*146.

104 See Singer, *Anatomy, p.*71.

105 See Singer, *Anatomy, p.*73; and Puschmann, *op. cit., p.*244 *f.*

106 See Puschmann, *op. cit., p.*247.

107 See Sigerist, "Die Geburt", *op. cit., p.*196 *f.*

108 *Ib.* To these "feasts" the civil and ecclesiastical authorities were often invited as special guests; see Castiglioni, *History, p.*375.

109 See Rashdall, *Universities, vol.i, p.*245.

110 See Puschmann, *op. cit., p.*249 *f.*

111 See Osler, *Evolution, p.*116.

112 See Osler, *Evolution, p.*148; and Rashdall, *Universities, vol.i, p.*148.

113 See Singer, *Evolution, p.*111 *ff.*

114 See Garrison, *Introduction, p.*282.

115 See Garrison, *Introduction, p.*398.

116 See Puschmann, *op. cit., pp.* 328 and 407.

117 For the text of this Bull, see J. J. Walsh, *The Popes and Science,* 1912, *p.*32 *ff.*

118 r*RaSHBA, no.*369; see Zimmels, *p.*58; and *infra, p.*144 *f.*

119 R. Virchow, "Morgagni and the Anatomical Concept", in *Bulletin of the History of Medicine, vol.vii* (1939), *p.*981. He regards the popular opposition to dissection as having been "fortified by canonical interdiction", so that "the real difficulty lay with the Church".

120 R. Park, *An Epitome of the History of Medicine,* 1903, *p.*93. He considers that the Bull "operated to discourage and prohibit anatomical dissection, since nearly 200 years later the University of Tuebingen was obliged to apply to Pope Sixtus IV for permission to authorise dissection".

121 Baas, *op. cit., p.*295; and *Grundriss der Geschichte der Medizin und des heilenden Standes,* 1876, *p.*237. His express reference to a papal prohibition of dissection in 1300 plainly contradicts the claim of the *Catholic Encyclopedia* (*vol.i, p.*458 *f.*) that Baas shared the opposite view.

122 Puschmann, *op. cit., p.*245. He believed that the Bull "robbed anatomical enquiry... of an aid the loss of which was keenly felt".

123 Alston (*op. cit., p.*221 *ff.*) claims that of recent authors only A. D. White maintained the charge of Church opposition to dissection.

124 Allbutt, *Greek Medicine, p.*476. He states that "the first attempts at dissection made by Mundini in 1406 were interrupted... by an edict of Boniface IV [sic!]".

[125] Stern, *Society*, *p.*177 *ff.* He holds the Church largely responsible for delaying the practice of dissection and adduces proofs from Boniface's Bull and other sources.

[126] Singer, *Anatomy*, *p.*85 *f.* He believes that Mondini's reluctance to clean certain human bones completely and to boil parts of the corpse was based on the Bull, which "was not directed against anatomists, but told against them".

[127] H. Haeser, *Lehrbuch der Geschichte der Medizin*, Jena, 1875, *vol.i*, *p.*736.

[128] J. L. Pagel; cited in *CE*, *loc. cit.*

[129] M. Neuburger, *Geschichte der Medizin*, 1906, *vol.ii*, *p.*432.

[130] Walsh, *op. cit.*, *p.*28 *ff.* in chapter on "The supposed papal prohibition of dissection".

[131] Garrison, *Introduction*, *p.*161; and *CE*, *loc. cit.* He follows Neuburger and Walsh in assuming that the Bull was simply a mandate to prevent the bodies of crusaders from being boiled and dismembered before returning them to their relatives. See also E. von Rudloff, *Ueber das Conservieren von Leichen im Mittelalter*, Freiburg diss., 1921.

[132] Rashdall, *Universities*, *vol.i*, *p.*244 *f.* Though he speaks of "religious prejudice" as responsible for the opposition to dissection, he regards it as erroneous to assume that Boniface legislated against the practice.

[133] Castiglioni, in his *History*, omits the reference to the Bull altogether.

[134] B. C. A. Windle, *The Church and Science*, 1920, *p.*23.

[135] Alston, *op. cit.*, *p.*224. But the author asserts (*p.*231) that the Bull did not apply to bodies used for anatomical purposes, as proved by the itemised account of dissections at the Medical Faculty in Paris (1491) which includes expenses for subsequent burial in consecrated ground and for having mass said.

[136] The work was issued by the Benedictiones of St.-Maur and continued by members of the Institute of France; see *CE*, *loc. cit.*; and Walsh, *op. cit.*, *p.*53 *f.*

[137] See *The Fasciculo di Medicina* (Venice, 1493), *ed.* C. Singer, 1925. *p.*96.

[138] Alston, *op. cit.*, *p.*225 *f.*

[139] The statement is quoted in full by E. Wickersheimer, "L'Anatomie de Guido de Vigevano", in *Sudhoff's Archiv fuer die Geschichte der Medizin*, *vol.vii* (1914), *p.*1 *ff.*

[140] Rashdall, *loc. cit.*

[141] Puschmann, *op. cit.*, *p.*327.

[142] J. P. MacMurrich, "Leonardo da Vinci and Vesalius", in *Medical Library and Historical Journal*, *vol.ix* (1906), *p.*344; cited by Stern, *Society*, *p.*177.

[143] See Cole, *op. cit.*, *p.*57.

[144] See M. Forster, *History of Physiology*, 1901, *p.*17.

[145] Sigerist, "Die Geburt", *op. cit.*, *p.*197.

[146] See P. Diepgen, "Die Bedeutung des Mittelalters fuer den Fortschritt der Medizin", in *Essays*, *ed.* Singer and Sigerist, *p.*107; Diepgen, in *Janus*, *vol.xxvi* (1922), *p.*91; and Wolff, *op. cit.*, *p.*263 *ff.* Wolff (*p.*252) also mentions that the viewing of corpses for legal purposes was already introduced in 1209 under Innocent III (*Decret. Gregor.*, *ix*, *lib.v*, *fol.*293, Basileae, 1511).

[147] See Singer, *Anatomy*, *p.*85 *f.*; Castiglioni, *History*, *p.*368; and note 120 above.

[148] See A. H. Buck, *The Growth of Medicine from the Earliest Times to about 1500*, 1917, *p.*346.

149 See G. Sarton, *Introduction to the History of Science*, 1927, *vol.ii*, pp.783 and 1081. See also Puschmann, *op. cit.*, *p.94*; cited by Stern, *loc. cit.*

150 See M. Roth, *Andrea Vesalius Bruxellensis*, 1892, *p.33*; cited by White, *Warfare*, *vol.ii*, *p.46*.

151 In the 18th century, the naturalist Albrecht von Haller could not obtain human bodies for dissection at Tuebingen, where students had to use dogs; see H. E. Sigerist, *Great Doctors*, 1933, *p.192*. In England the ban on private dissections was removed only in 1745, after which date private schools of anatomy began to flourish; see C. Wall, *The History of the Surgeon's Company*, 1937, *p.86*. For further instances of public indignation against dissection in America, Britain, Ireland and France during, and even after, the 18th century, see Stern, *Society*, *p.180 ff*. In the State of New Jersey no dissections whatever are permitted to the present day, and consequently there are no medical schools there; see LaWall, *Pharmacy*, *p.133*.

152 From the 15th century onwards, experimental anatomy was greatly stimulated by the desire of artists and sculptors to portray the human body realistically. Among the great artists who engaged in dissection were Verrocchio, Andrea Manegno, Lucio Signorelli, Pollajuolo, Donatello, Leonardo da Vinci, Albrecht Duerer, Michael Angelo and Raphael; see Stern, *Society*, *p.49*; and Singer, *Evolution*, *p.90 ff*.

153 See Alston, *op. cit.*, *p.221 ff*. For the full text of the reply, see Th. Puschmann, *Handbuch der Geschichte der Medizin*, 1902, *vol.ii*, *p.227*; and Walsh, *op. cit.*, *p.58 f*.

154 Canon 2328 of the 1917 Code of Canon Law; see S. Woywood, *A Practical Commentary on the Code of Canon Law*, 1926, *vol.i*, *p.256*.

155 See Woywood, *op. cit.*, *vol.ii*, *p.479*.

156 Rashdall, *Universities*, *vol.ii*, *p.136*.

157 P. L. Burshell, *Ancient History of Medicine*, 1878, *p.18*.

158 See Haeser, *op. cit.*, *vol.i*, *p.560*; Puschmann, *Medical Education*, *p.163*; Osler, *Evolution*, *p.102*; Garrison, *Introduction*, *p.135*; Browne, *Arabian Medicine*, *p.36 f.*; and Meyerhof, "Science and Medicine", in *Legacy of Islam*, ed. T. Arnold and A. Guillaume, 1931, *p.344*.

159 See Ploss and Bartels, *Woman*, *vol.iii*, *p.8*.

160 Alston, *op. cit.*, *p.223 f*.

161 See B. Stern, *Medizin, Aberglaube und Geschlechtsleben in der Tuerkei*, 1903, *vol.i*, *p.53*.

162 See S. Muntner, "Persian Medicine and its Relation to Jewish and Other Medical Science", in *The Hebrew Medical Journal*, *vol.xxv* (1952), *p.202*. Religious scruples regarding dissection also accounted for the delay in opening a medical school at the Hebrew University in Jerusalem; *cf. infra*, *p.150 f*.

163 See Stern, *op. cit.*, *p.54*.

164 See Castiglioni, *History*, *p.284*.

165 Friedenwald, *p.192*. He alleges that Maimonides was fettered chiefly by "the thrawldom of authority and the prohibition of anatomical study".

166 See Friedenwald, *p.251*. Astruc (1684–1766) was himself of Jewish descent.

167 The charge occurs, for instance, in *The Healing Art the Right Hand of the Church*, 1859, *p.111 f.*; and in *A General Exposition of the General State of the Medical Profession*, by "Alexipharmacus", 1829, *p.12*.

168 See Preuss, *p.45*; Rabinowitch, *op. cit.*, *p.23 f.*; and I. Simon, in *Révue*, *op. cit.*, *p.51 f*.

169 See *supra*, *p.126*.

170 Rabinowitch (*op. cit., p.*25) quotes Maimonides (*Sepher Hare-phu'oth*) for the following observation: "Those not acquainted with Anatomy think that nerves and arteries are the same, and, were it not for the study of Anatomy in which we are busily engaged, we also would not know the difference". It is hardly on the evidence of this statement that a rabbi (D. Z. Katzburg, *Tel Talpiyoth, vol.xxxi* [1924], *p.*123) expressed his conviction that Maimonides must have carried out anatomical experiments on cadavers. He supported his claim by referring to the assertion by C. J. D. Azulay (*Devash Lephi*, Livorno, 1801, *no.*20) that "Maimonides was familiar with all sciences... including anatomy". A similar statement was already made in the 15th century by Barfat (*rRIVaSH, no.*447), but this is not mentioned by Katzburg.

171 Friedenwald, *p.*334. For further references to the relations of Amatus with Judaism, see *ib., pp.* 339 (note), 342 and 381 ff.

172 Amatus, *Centuria i, cur.*52; see I. Muenz, *Die juedischen Aerzte im Mittelalter*, 1922, *p.*112 f.; and Friedenwald, *pp.* 338 and 354.

173 See Singer, "Judaism", in *The Jews, p.*1069.

174 Friedenwald, *p.*312.

175 Zahalon, *'Otzar Hahayim*, Venice, 1683; see J. Leibowitz, "On the Plague in the Ghetto at Rome in 1656", in Reprint from *Dappim Rephu'im*, 1943, *p.*3.

176 This illustration has often been reproduced; see *JE, vol.iv, p.*162; *JL, vol.iv, p.*37; and *Encyclopedia Hebraica, vol.iv, p.*406.

177 See L. Lewin, "Juedische Aerzte in Grosspolen", in *JJLG, vol.ix* (1911), *p.*419.

178 See L. Perel, "La vie de l'anatomiste Hirschfeld", in *Révue, no.*2 (1948), *p.*29 ff.

179 *Address to the Public, Drawn from Nature and Religion, against the unlimited Dissection of Human Bodies*, London, 1829, *p.*7.

180 The first objection to the manner in which Jewish bodies were used for dissection dates from 1672; see Isaac Hayim Cantarini, *Pahad Yitzhak*, Amsterdam, 1685, *p.*446 ff. Further cases occurred in 1680; see S. W. Baron, *The Jewish Community*, 1942, *vol.ii, p.*151; citing Antonio Ciscato, *Gli Ebrei in Padova*, Padua, 1901. See also *JE, vol.ix, p.*459. On the precautions taken against the theft of bodies at the Old Cemetery of the Spanish and Portuguese Congregation in London in the 18th century, see *The Jewish Chronicle*, March 25, 1925.

181 In many German cemeteries friends watched graves to prevent them from being "rolfinked" (a reference to Prof. Rolfink's avarice for corpses); see Puschmann, *op. cit., p.*400.

182 See *supra, p.*139.

183 Reference to Adreth's responsum in connection with the problem of dissection is first made by the questioner in E. Landau, *rNoda Biyehudah*, part *ii,* Y.D., *no.*210.

184 *rRaDBaZ*, part *i, no.*484; see Zimmels, *p.*58.

185 *Cf.* b*Shabbath* 152b; and *supra, p.*129. Hence also the rule to bury the dead in direct contact with the earth; see j*Kilayim, ix.*3; and Y.D., ccclxii.1.

186 Isaac Elhanan of Kovno, *rEyn Yitzhak*, Y.D., *no.*33; see Zimmels, *p.*58.

187 See *supra, p.*141. As the Jewish decision is dated Shevat 15, 5497 (corresponding to January 17, 1737), the enquiry which led to it can hardly have been stimulated by the very similar question addressed to Rome and answered in the same year.

188 Benjamin Wolf Gintzburger; he was among the first Jewish students

to graduate at a German university (1743) and to interest himself in talmudic medicine; his thesis bore the title "*Qua medicinam ex Talmudicis illustrat*"; see Friedenwald, *pp.* 99, 120 and 237; and Zimmels, *p.*30.

189 Emden, r*She'ilath Yavetz*, part *i*, *no.*41.

190 r*RaSHBA*, *no.*365. But elsewhere (*Novellae of RaSHBA*, on *Baba Kamma* 10a) Adreth expresses the view—shared by Maimonides (see *Mishneh Lemelekh*, on *Hil. 'Avel, xiv* [end])—that the benefit derived from a non-Jewish corpse is not proscribed. For a summary of the later views on this controversy, see *P.T.*, *Y.D.*, *cccxlix.*1 and 2.

191 r*Noda Biyehudah*, *loc. cit.*; see Rabinowitch, *op. cit.*, *p.*28 *f.*; and Zimmels, *p.*14.

192 Landau proves this by referring to the prohibition in the Talmud (see note 90 above), followed by the codes (*Y.D.*, *ccclxiii.*7), to open a grave for establishing the age of the deceased in support of legal claims by the heirs.

193 Rabinowitch (*loc. cit.*), discussing these arguments, concludes that they were all valid in the circumstances then prevailing, adding: "There is no doubt that had [Landau] felt that the autopsy could have served a purpose to save life that he would have permitted it. . .".

194 r*Hatham Sopher*, *Y.D.*, *no.*336.

195 For a similar attitude among the Mohammedans, see *supra*, *p.*142.

196 r*Binyan Tziyon*, *no.*170.

197 Hence, for example, the dead may be clothed in shrouds made of materials otherwise forbidden to be worn, *i.e.* if made of wool and linen (*Y.D.*, *cccli.*1).

198 See *supra*, *p.*96 *ff.*

199 r*MaHaRaM Shik*, *Y.D.*, *no.*347.

200 The Talmud (b*Sanhedrin* 46b) assumes that burial is required to prevent disgrace; hence a person's expressed wish not to be buried must not be fulfilled.

201 See *supra*, *p.*53 *ff.*

202 B. H. Auerbach (*Nahal 'Eshkol*, 1868, part *ii*, *p.*117 *ff.*); and S. Bamberger r*Zekher Simhah*, *no.*158).

203 H. Adler, *Anglo-Jewish Memories*, 1909, *p.*137.

204 A. I. Kook, r*Da'ath Kohen*, *no.*199.

205 B. Uziel, r*Mishpetei Uzi'el*, *Y.D.*, *nos.* 28 and 29.

206 Hillel Posek, in *Haposek*, *vol.xi* (1949), *no.*111 (*Av* 5709).

207 So Joseph Zweig, r*Porath Yoseph*, *no.*17; and A. A. Price, *Mishnath Avraham* on *Sepher Hasidim*, 1955, *p.*180. See also Simon Gruenfeld, in *Tel Talpiyoth*, *vol.xxxi* (1924), *pp.* 117 and 122.

208 Eliezer Duenner, *Zikhron 'Avraham Mosheh*, 1945, *p.*82 *ff.*; based on the permission to engage in sorcery for study purposes, though this is otherwise biblically forbidden (b*Sanhedrin* 68a).

209 So Bamberger, *loc. cit.*,; D. Z. Katzburg, in *Tel Talpiyoth*, *op. cit.*, *p.*130; Hillel Posek, *loc. cit.*; Uziel, *loc. cit.*; and Zweig, *loc. cit.*

210 J. L. Lewin, in *Yagdil Torah*, *vol.viii*, *no.*31; cited by J. D. Eisenstein, *'Otzar Dinim Uminhagim*, 1917, *p.*453. See also Uziel, *loc. cit.*

211 So Hillel Posek, *loc. cit.*; Duenner, *loc. cit.*; and Price, *op. cit.*, *p.*184. See also note 193 above.

212 This point was particularly stressed by Kook, *loc. cit.*

213 Y. J. Grunwald, *Kol Bo*, 1947, *vol.i*, *pp.* 40 *f.* and 44 *f.*

214 *Deut. xxi.*22–23.

215 Asher Gronis, *Pri 'Asher*, 1936, *no.*3.

216 r*Melamed Leho'il*, *Y.D.*, *no.*109.

217 See Yehudah Meir Schapira, r*'Or Hame'ir*, part *i*, *no.*74.

[218] *Ib.*; see also David Menachem Babad, r*Havatzeleth Hasharon*, Y.D., no.94; and authorities cited by Grunwald, *loc. cit.*

[219] See Eliazar Hayim Schapira, r*Minhath 'Elazar*, part *iv*, no.25; cited by Grunwald, *loc. cit.*

[220] See *Yagdil Torah*, *vol.vii*, *p.17*; and *vol.viii*; cited by Grunwald, *loc. cit.*

[221] See Moses Jonah Zweig, r'*Ohel Mosheh*, part *i*, no.4. See also Jacob Levy, "Nituhei Methim Beyisra'el", in *Hama'ayon*, *vol.iii* (1956), *p.26*.

[2] *Ib.*; and Babad, *loc. cit.*

[223] See M. J. Zweig, *loc. cit.*

[224] *Ib.*; following Malchiel Zwi Halevy of Lomza, r*Divrei Malki'el*, part *ii*, no.95.

[225] See Y. M. Schapira, *loc. cit.* See also Levy, *op. cit.*, *p.29*.

[226] See M. J. Zweig, *loc. cit.*

[227] See following pages.

[228] See Katzburg, in *Tel Talpiyoth*, *loc. cit.*; quoting Hayim Hirschson, *Malki Bakodesh*.

[229] See notes 161–164 above; and LaWall, *Pharmacy*, *p.133*.

[230] See M. D. Silberstein, "Ba'ayath Nitu'ah Hamethim Upithrona", in *Yavneh*, 1949, *p.214 ff.* (Nisan 5709); and in *Dat Yisra'el Umedinath Yisra'el*, 1951, *p.159 ff.*

[231] *Ib.*, *p.161*. The terms of the agreement are also given and fully discussed by Eliezer Judah Waldenberg (a member of the Chief Rabbinate), r*Tzitz Eli'ezer*, part *iv*, no.14.

[232] Passed on August 26, 1953, statute no.62; see official publication *Sepher Hahukim*, issue no.134, *p.162* (September 4, 1953).

[233] See Silberstein, *loc. cit.*

[234] *Ib.*

[235] Anatomy Act 1832, 2 & 3 Will. 4 c 75, sections 7, 8 and 15. That Act—which still governs the law in this matter in England—provided that any competent legal authority could order a post-mortem examination on any human body, and that any executor or other party having lawful possession of the body of any person (other than an undertaker) could permit its use for anatomical examination, provided that the person did not obect during his lifetime and that the relatives did not require its immediate burial. It also entitled a person to direct that his body be used for anatomical purposes after death, unless an objection was raised by his nearest known relative.

[236] See *Lev. xxi.*11, and Rashi, *a.l.* This point is emphasised by Levy, *op. cit.*, *p.25*.

[237] Friedenwald (*op. cit.*, *vol.i*, *p.126*) has listed the following articles: C. D. Spivak, "Post-Mortem Examination Among the Jews", in *New York Medical Journal*, June 13, 1914, *p.11*; N. Mosessohn, "Post-Mortem Examinations Among the Jews", in *Jewish Tribune*, December 18, 1914; J. Z. Lauterbach, "The Jewish Attitude Toward Autopsy", in *The Jewish Indicator*, October 30, 1925; M. Robinson, "The Advancement of Science through Autopsy", in *The Synagogue Light*, Brooklyn, February 1938; and O. Saphir, "Autopsies Among Jews", in *Medical Leaves*, 1939. To this list could be added, apart from the monographs and articles by Rabinowitch, Silberstein, Muntner and Levy already noted: H. L. Gordon, "Bedikath Methei Yisra'el al pi Dinei Yisra'el", in *Hebrew Medical Journal*, 1937, part *i*, *p.141 ff.*; M. Greiber, *Nitu'ah Hamethim Letzorkhei Limmud Vahakirah*, Jerusalem, 1943; and A. Kottler, "The Jewish Attitude on Autopsy", in *New York State Journal of Medicine*, 1957, *p.1649 ff.*

[238] Muntner, *op. cit.*, *p.3*.

(CHAPTER XII)

239 *Ib., p.*6.

240 Levy, *op. cit., p.*30. This trend was also confirmed by Professor H. Baruk of the Sorbonne (as reported in *Ha'aretz,* Elul 7, 1955); see Levy, *loc. cit.* (note 25).

241 *Ib., pp.* 21 and 30 (note 23).

242 *Ib., p.*31. In fact, Prof. Baruk offered to supply Jerusalem with all materials required for a model anatomical institute to dispense with dissection; see Levy, *loc. cit.*

243 *Ib., p.*28 *f.*

Chapter Thirteen

1 F. Galton, *Human Faculty,* 1883, *p.*44; see *Oxford English Dictionary, vol.iii, p.*319.

2 Plato, *Republic, v.*

3 On the "extremely large literature devoted to the subject", see Lecky, *European Morals, vol.ii, p.*24 *ff.*

4 See *ERE, vol.viii, p.*423 *ff., s.v.* "Marriage".

5 M. Grunwald, "Biblische und Talmudische Quellen juedischer Eugenik", in *Hygiene und Judentum,* ed. Hans Goslar, 1930, *p.*60. For bibliographical material on the subject, see *ib.;* and Friedenwald, *p.*138 *ff.* See also *Encyclopedia Hebraica,* 1949, *vol.i, p.*668 *ff.;* and Saul Munk, "Religionsgesetzliche Fragen die sich aus dem Gesetz zur Verhuetung von erbkranken Nachwuchses... ergeben", in *Nachalath Z'wi, vol.v* (1935), *p.*183 *ff.*

6 Isserles derives this from a responsum addressed to the leaders of the Tunisian Jewish community by Isaac ben Shesheth Barfat (r*RIVaSH, no.*15) which states: "... all this [*i.e.* the duty of the courts to exercise compulsion in matrimonial matters] applies according to the strict law of the Talmud; but what shall we do, not having seen [such action]in our own days nor heard of it for many generations past...".

7 The idea behind this mishnaic regulation (m*Yevamoth, vi.*6) is no doubt that a man must replace himself and his wife, or those who combined to give birth to him.

8 The Talmud (b*Yevamoth* 62b) bases this rabbinic precept on the verse: "In the morning sow thy seed, and in the evening withhold not thy hand" (*Eccl. xi.*6); "for whoever adds one soul in Israel is as if he built a world" (Maimonides, *Hil. 'Ishuth, xv.*16).

9 b*Baba Bathra* 110a. See Preuss, *p.*528; and Krauss, *vol.ii, p.*30 *ff.*

10 b*Bekhoroth* 45b.

11 Preuss (*p.*343 *f.*) accepts this law as proof for the belief in the hereditary character of leprosy and epilepsy, but he adds that the ban on marrying into such families could also be due to their being looked upon as socially inferior. I. L. Katzenelsohn (*Hatalmud Veharephu'ah,* 1928, *p.*230), however, argues that the law must be eugenically motivated, since the ban extends specifically to women in whose families the disease exists, even if they themselves are quite free from it.

12 Rashi, *Yevamoth* 64b. See Preuss, *p.*344.

13 For instance, since 1913 laws requiring pre-marital physical examinations, mainly to prevent the transmission of syphilis, existed in some States in the U.S.A.; by 1954 such legislation was enforced in 40 States; see J. K. Shafer, "Premarital Health Examination Legislation", in *Public*

Health Reports, Washington, *lxix* (May 1954), *p.*487 *ff.*; the article is reprinted, and augmented by the text of all the current laws, in *Premarital Health Legislation, Analysis and Compilation of State Laws,* U. S. Department of Health, Education, and Welfare, 1954.

14 See Krauss, *vol.ii, p.*33.

15 But lunatics can legally consummate a levirate union (*E.H., clxxii.*11 and 12), because their marriage bond is already partly established by the previous marriage contract of the levir's late brother; his death automatically binds the widow to his surviving brother(s). See *Deut. xxv.*5 *ff.*

16 *Cf. supra, chpt.*VI (note 180).

17 See b*Yevamoth* 112b; and Rashi, *a.l.*

18 I. Simon, "La gynécologie. . . dans la Bible et le Talmud", in *Révue, no.*4 (1949), *p.*54. See also Preuss, *p.*363.

19 For further limitations of this law, and their explanation, see *A. H., E.H., cliv.*27 *ff.*

20 See note 7 above.

21 See m*Yevamoth, vi.*6; and Rashi, *Yevamoth* 64a. See also Preuss, *p.*478.

22 See S. W. Baron, *The Jewish Community*, 1942, *vol.ii, p.*309; and A. A. Neuman, *The Jews in Spain*, 1948, *vol.ii, p.*53 *ff.*

23 b*Yevamoth* 64b; see Preuss, *p.*535. On the practical distinction between the two interpretations, see Joshua Falk, *Derishah, E.H., ix.*1; and *B.S., a.l.,* 1.

24 *Birkei Yoseph, a.l.,* 3; see Zimmels, *p.*91.

25 Just as the circumcision of a boy must be put off if either two brothers or two maternal cousins have previously died through the operation; see *infra, p.*198 *f.*

26 r*RaMBaM, no.*170. See H. S. Lewis, "Maimonides on Superstition", in *JQR, vol.xvii* (1905), *p.*487.

27 Maimonides, *Hil. 'Issurei Bi'ah, xxi.*31.

28 See *He.M., a.l.,* 3; and *B.S., a.l.,* 7. Both refer to Asheri (r*ROSH, no.*53, §8) as the source for this clause. Falk (*Derishah, a.l.,* 2) explains that the infection through intercourse can be transmitted only from women to men. *Cf.* note 25 above.

29 See, *e.g., Y.D., clxxxvii.*12 and 14; *ccxxxv.*1; *E.H., x.*4; and *lxxvi.*9. Hence, when some rabbis considered the advisibility of limiting the Jewish population during the Hadrian persecution in the 2nd century, they discussed the expediency of placing a temporary ban on all marriages (b*Baba Bathra* 60b), but the enforcement of continence was never even contemplated.

30 A contrary opinion, however, was expressed in the same year by the Catholic writer, Henry Davis (*Eugenics, Aims and Methods,* 1930, *p.*56).

31 According to Jacob Emden (r*She'ilath Yavetz, no.*111), the prohibition extends even to the sterilisation of fish; see *P.T., E.H., v.*8.

32 See McKenzie, *Infancy, p.*379.

33 Preuss (*p.*258), making this statement, concludes that Abucalsem—who claimed that castration was religiously proscribed—must therefore be included among the Jewish-Arabian physicians.

34 See Neuburger, *History, vol.i, p.*73.

35 See McKenzie, *Infancy, p.*378.

36 See Castiglioni, *History, p.*104.

37 For this and the preceding data, see McKenzie, *Infancy, p.*377 *ff.*; J. Fletcher, *Morals and Medicine,* 1955, *p.*143 *f.*; and Savas Nittis, "The Hippocratic Oath in Reference to Lithotomy", in *Bulletin of the History of Medicine, vol.vii* (1937), *p.*723 *ff.*

38 See W. H. S. Jones, *The Doctor's Oath,* 1924, *p.*48.

[39] M. P. Littré, *Oevres Complètes d'Hippocrate*, 1839–61, *vol.iv*, p.620.

[40] Puschmann, *Medical Education*, p.43. So also Savas Nittis, in his monographic study of the whole problem (*loc. cit.*).

[41] Jones, *loc. cit.*

[42] L. Edelstein, "The Hippocratic Oath", in *Supplements to the Bulletin of the History of Medicine*, 1943, p.25 f.

[43] *Cf. supra*, p.124 f.

[44] See Puschmann, *Medical Education*, p.44.

[45] See A. H. McNeile, *The Gospel according to St. Matthew*, 1915, p.276.

[46] See McKenzie, *Infancy*, p.380.

[47] Paul Aeginita, *On castration*, *vi.*28; quoted by Savas Nittis, "Hippocratic Ethics and Present-day Trends in Medicine", in *Bulletin of the History of Medicine*, *vol.xii* (1942), p.342.

[48] Augustine, *De Haeres.*, cap.*xxxvii.*

[49] See Savas Nittis, *op. cit.*, p.727; and A. P. Cawadias, "Male Eunuchism", in *Proceedings of the Royal Society of Medicine*, *vol.xxxix* (1946), p.502.

[50] See McKenzie, *Infancy*, p.381.

[51] See Cawadias, *loc. cit.*

[52] See Cawadias, *loc. cit.*; and Fletcher, *op. cit.*, p.144.

[53] See S. Woywood, *A Practical Commentary on the Code of Canon Law*, 1926, *vol.i*, p.533. The prohibition is classified under mutilation, not sterilisation.

[54] Holy Office reply dated February 24, 1940; see J. McCarthy, in *Irish Ecclesiastical Record*, *vol.lxx* (1948), p.1013 ff.

[55] So Pius XI, Encyclical "*Casti Connubii*", 1930; see edition and translation by V. McNabb, 1933, p.31 f. See also Davis, *op. cit.*, p.43 ff.

[56] Punitive sterilisation was originally declared unlawful in "*Casti Connubii*". But this was subsequently withdrawn in an amendment published in Fascicle 14 of the *Acta Apostolicae Sedis*, *vol.xxii* (1930), p.604. On the theological debate thus reopened, see McCarthy, *loc. cit.*

[57] The first European legislation on eugenic sterilisation was enacted in the Swiss Canton of Vaud in 1921. Apart from the far-reaching sterilisation programme carried out in Germany under the Nazis (affecting over 250,000 people during the first few years after 1933), extensive legislation was also introduced in the Scandinavian countries; see Sigerist, *Civilisation*, p.105 f.; and *Lancet*, 1942, part *ii*, p.106 f. In the United States the first such enactment dates back to 1907 (in Indiana). By now 32 States have passed sterilisation laws (26 of them providing for compulsory sterilisation, though the programme is effectively carried out only in a few of them) and 53,000 operations have been performed under these laws; see Fletcher, *op. cit.*, p.166; and B. Shartel, "Symposium on Sterilisation", in *American Practitioner*, *vol.i* (1947), no.9, p.485. On present-day legislation, see *British Encyclopedia of Medical Practice*, 1952, *vol.xi*, p.572 ff.

[58] See *British Encyclopedia of Medical Practice*, *op. cit.*, p.573.

[59] b*Shabbath* 110b. See also t*Makkoth*, *v.*6; and t*Bekhoroth*, *iii.*24.

[60] According to the Talmud (b*Shabbath* 111a), "That which hath its stones... torn, or cut..." (*Lev. xvii.*24) refers to two successive operations which are both prohibited. Rashi (*a.l.*) explains the first action as completely cutting the seminal ducts inside the scrotum, and the second as emptying it; whereas Tosaphoth (*a.l.*) applies the first to cutting them partly, and the second to severing them completely. In any case, it clearly is an offence to impair the genitals even of a castrate. Hence, Moses Schreiber (r*Hatham Sopher*, *E.H.*, no.20) concludes that the ban on

castration must be regarded as a "scriptural decree" which cannot be wholly explained as a measure to prevent the destruction of man's reproductive powers. *Cf. infra, p.*167.

61 This clause is first recorded by Maimonides (*Hil. 'Issurei Bi'ah, xvi.*12) who evidently derived it by analogy from b*Sanhedrin* 76b (note on *Maggid Mishnah, a.l.*).

62 See *infra, p.*164.

63 Hebrew   "כוס עקרין".   Loew (*Lebensalter, p.*380 [note 159]) rejects Buxdorf's translation *"poculum sterilitatis, contra sterilitatem"* as mistaken. L. Wiesner ("Kindersegen und Kinderlosigkeit im altrabbinischem Schrifttume", in *MGWJ, vol.lxvi* [1922], *p.*37 [note 2]) attributes the same error to Ploss and Bartels (*Woman, vol.ii, p.*299), the drink serving, in fact, not to cure, but to produce, sterility. Actually, as pointed out by W. Ebstein (*Die Medizin im Neuen Testament und im Talmud,* 1903, *p.*208 ff.), one type of this potion was designed to prevent sterility (*e.g.,* b*Shabbath* 10a and b), another to produce it (*e.g.,* b*Yevamoth* 65b). Krauss (*vol.ii, p.*435 [note 94]) insists on rendering "cup of roots", not "of barrenness".

64 For details of the composition, see Preuss, *p.*439; and Wiesner, *op. cit., p.*37.

65 So, *e.g.,* in the *Ebers Papyrus* (*sec.xciii; ed.* B. Ebbell, 1937, *p.*108) and Pliny (*Nat. Hist., xx.*44, 2; *xxiv.*47, 4; *xxv.*33; and *xxvii.*17.55, 3); see Ploss and Bartels, *op. cit., p.*289 ff. Justinian law (*Corpus juris civilis, ed.* Krueger, 1928, *vol.i, pp.* 852 and 676), too, assumed that conception could be prevented, as well as promoted, by medicinal drinks.

66 For examples, see Thorndike, *Magic, vol.i, p.*656; *vol.ii, pp.*470, 736, 744 and 763.

67 Thus, Solomon Ganzfried's very popular *Kitzur Shulhan 'Arukh,* first published in 1864 and often republished, still refers to the potion (*cxci.*5).

68 Jakob Horovitz, r*Mattei Levy,* part *ii, no.*31. J. L. Unterman (*Shevet Miyehudah,* 1955, *p.*285) believes that the drink produced not organic, but merely functional changes in the nervous system.

69 N. E. Himes, *Medical History of Contraception,* 1934, *p.*3. But in very recent experiments carried out in Puerto Rico, American scientists have succeeded in discovering a compound (with progestational activity) which, like the potion mentioned in the Talmud, can be taken by mouth to produce either sterility or fertility; see Robert Sheenan, "A Pill to Cur Overpopulation?", in *Life International,* July 7, 1958, *p.*35 ff.

70 Maimonides, *Hil. 'Issurei Bi'ah, xvi.*12; based on b*Shabbath* 110a and b.

71 "Because the genitals were not touched" (Moses Ribkes, *Be'er Hagolah, a.l.*).

72 See *'Otzar Haposkim,* 1947, E.H., *vol.i, p.*248 (*no.*68).

73 Maimonides (*loc. cit.*) evidently regards such sterilisation as biblically forbidden, but Me'iri (*Beth Habehirah,* on *Shabbath* 110b) states explicitly that it is only a rabbinic offence; see *'Otzar Haposkim, op. cit., p.*249 (*no.*70).

74 *She'iltoth d'rabbi 'Achai,* Emor, *no.*105.

75 Tosaphoth, *Shabbath* 110b.

76 Asheri, *Shabbath, xiv.*9.

77 *Tur, E.H., v.*

78 Because it is only in regard to work on the Sabbath that one is not culpable for an act which, while it unavoidably results in violating a law, is intended to serve legitimate ends; see *B.S., a.l.,* 13.

79 So first in *Novellae of RITVA,* on *Yevamoth* 63b. See also *Birkei*

Yoseph, E.H., v.12; A.H., a.l., 22; and *'Otzar Haposkim, op. cit.* (*no.*69). Some authorities even sanction the therapeutic sterilisation of males in the absence of danger to life, provided it is carried out by a non-Jewish surgeon; see *'Otzar Haposkim, op. cit., p.*252 (*no.*77); and, with full sources, B. M. Birg, in *No'am, ed.* M. M. Kasher, *vol.i,* 1958, *p.*257 *ff.* The problem often arises in operations on the prostrate gland. These usually impair the seminal ducts and cause sterility (thus raising doubts whether the patient may maintain his marriage; see *infra, p.*166). Wherever possible, therefore, the obstruction should be eliminated by trans-urethral prostatomy, or better still overcome by the insertion of a flexible tube (katherisation), whereby the generative functions remain intact. Where these procedures would not suffice, the surgeon should be asked to limit the operation to the gland proper, leaving the very bottom of it unexcised, so as to protect the ducts from injury. See Israel Baruch Nass, in *Hapardes, vol.xxx, no.*7 (April 1956), *p.*10 *ff.* On this and similar problems, see also Nisan Telushkin, in *Hapardes, vol.xxix, no.*8 (May 1955), *p.*26 *ff.*; Moses Feinstein, in *Hapardes, vol.xxx, no.*8 (May 1956), *p.*26 *ff.*; and especially Birg, *op. cit., p.*245 *ff.*

[80] Joseph Saul Nathansohn, r*Sho'el Umeshiv,* 2nd *ed.,* part *iii, no.*44; see Zimmels, *p.*25.

[81] Elijah Chazan, r*Ta'alumoth Lev,* Livorno, 1839, *no.*4 (*p.*13b); see *'Otzar Haposkim, op. cit., p.*249 (*no.*69).

[82] *RITVA, loc. cit.* He adds that he knew of great men who had treated themselves thus.

[83] *Birkei Yoseph, op. cit.,* 13. For further sources, see *'Otzar Haposkim,*

[84] In fact, in such circumstances, even the administration of a sterilising potion may be unlawful; see *'Otzar Haposkim, loc. cit.*

[85] *Sepher Hasidim, ed.* Mekitzei Nirdamim, 1924, *no.*18.

[86] See Preuss, *p.*254.

[87] t*Bekhoroth, v.*2.

[88] t*Sanhedrin, vii.*5; and b*Sanhedrin* 36b. This is also codified by Maimonides (*Hil. Sanhedrin, ii.*3) who adds that the ban on castrates, as indeed on any childless man, is due to the fear that they may be too cruel and possess insufficient compassion (which only parents usually have).

[89] The dispute on this goes back to the Talmud (*Sopherim, xiv.*17); see Preuss, *p.*260.

[90] So *Maggid Mishnah,* on *Hil. 'Issurei Bi'ah, xiv.*11; *cf.* Tosaphoth, *Shabbath* 111a.

[91] So Aaron Halevy, *Sepher Hahinnukh,* commandment *no.*291. But Joseph Babad (*Minhath Hinnukh, a.l.*) remarks that this would not in itself explain why women are not included in this law (seeing that animals, too—though free from the precept of procreation—must yet not be sterilised by drink). Halevy's statement, therefore, merely implies that, if the duty of propagation were incumbent on women, they then would not be allowed to take the drink for that reason. See *'Otzar Haposkim, op. cit., p.*250 (*no.*71).

[92] Since his ruling is given quite categorically (*E.H., v.*12).

[93] *TaZ, a.l.,* 7.

[94] *B.S., a.l.,* 14.

[95] Luria, *Yom shel Shelomo, Yevamoth, vi.*44.

[96] *BaH, E.H., v.*

[97] So, *e.g., A.H., a.l.,* 24.

[98] For a summary of the views on this modern responsa, see *'Otzar Haposkim, op. cit., p.*250 *f.* (*no.*72).

[99] r*Hatham Sopher, E.H., no.*20; cited in *P.T., E.H., v.*11.

[100] *Yam shel Shelomo, loc. cit.*; see Simon, in *Révue, loc. cit.*

[101] *Gen. Rabbah, xliv.*10; adverting to *Gen. xv.*2 and Psalms *cxxxix.*23.

[102] b*Berachoth* 10a. So also *Yalkut,* 2 *Sam., no.*242.

[103] *Lev. Rabbah, xx.*7; and *Tanhuma, 'Aharei,* 13.

[104] b*Yevamoth* 75b; see Preuss, *p.*255 f.

[105] b*Yevamoth* 75a and j*Yevamoth, viii*; as cited by Tosaphoth, *Yevamoth* 75b; see Preuss, *p.*256.

[106] Tosaphoth, *loc. cit.*

[107] Mordecai, *Yevamoth, viii.*70. So also Luria, *Yam shel Shelomo, Yevamoth, viii.*8.

[108] Schreiber (r*Hatham Sopher, E.H., no.*19) reasons that the condition necessitating the operation did not here affect the testicles themselves but some abdominal complaint.

[109] See Preuss, *p.*256.

[110] Azulay (*Birkey Yoseph, E.H., v.*15) cites one view according to which surgically sterilised women, too, are debarred from marriage with Jews. But this isolated opinion is refuted by many authorities as completely without foundation; see *'Otzar Haposkim, op. cit., p.*208 f. (*no.*1); and Munk, in *Nachalath Z'wi, op. cit., p.*190.

[111] Maimonides, *Hil. 'Issurei Bi'ah, xvi.*9. The Talmud (b*Yevamoth* 75b) deduces the distinction by analogy with the marriage ban on bastards (*Deut. xxiii.*3) whose disqualification is also caused by human action. A similar difference is made between congenital and artificial eunuchs due—according to one view (m*Yevamoth, viii.*4)—to the fact that the former condition can be healed, whereas the latter is incurable. But the inference drawn from the juxtaposition of our law and that of the bastard makes it quite clear that the legal distinction between "man-made" and "Heaven-made" castrates is not based on medical considerations. *Cf.* note 60 above.

[112] Rashi, *Yevamoth* 75b. But see *B.S., a.l.,* 12; and *'Otzar Haposkim, op. cit., p.*244 (*no.*58).

[113] Asheri, *Yevamoth, viii.*2.

[114] See *P.T., a.l.,* 7; and Birg, *op. cit., p.*252.

[115] So r*Hatham Sopher, E.H., nos.* 17 and 19; and many authorities cited in *'Otzar Haposkim, op. cit., p.*241 ff. (*no.*56); and especially Birg, *op. cit., p.*253 ff. See also Unterman, *op. cit., p.*284 ff.; and note 79 above.

[116] So expressly Hayim Halberstam of Zanz, r*Divrei Hayim,* part *ii, E.H., no.*31. This is also assumed by most other late authorities; see Birg, *op. cit., p.*247 f.; and *cf.* notes 60 and 111 above. But Aaron Halevy (*Sepher Hamitzvoth,* commandment *no.*559) and Jacob Emden (r'*Iggereth Bikkoreth, p.*5) appear to regard the prohibition of sterilisation and the marriage ban on castrates as based on identical considerations; see Birg, *op. cit., p.*246.

[117] *Cf. supra, p.*156. Sterility produced by a drink, too, does not disqualify a man from "entering the congregation of the Lord" (*Birkei Yoseph, a.l.,* 7; *cf.* Tosaphoth, *Sotah* 26a; and r*Hatham Sopher, E.H., no.*17). But for qualifications of this view, see *P.T., a.l.,* 9; and Birg, *op. cit., p.*250.

[118] For a historical and comparative study of the whole subject, see I. Jakobovits, "Artificial Insemination, Birth-Control and Abortion", in *The Hebrew Medical Journal, vol.xxvi* (1953), part *ii, p.*171 ff.

[119] Augustine, *De conjug. adult., lib.ii, n.*12; see S. D'Irsay, "Patristic Medicine", in *Annals of the History of Medicine, vol.ix* (1928), *p.*371.

[120] See Pius XI, Encyclical *"Casti Connubii",* 1930; and J. McCarthy, in *Irish Ecclesiastical Record, vol.lxi* (1943), *p.*267 f.

121 See F. J. Connell, "Birth-Control: The Case for the Catholic", in *Atlantic Monthly*, October 1939, *p*.471.

122 According to the findings of Professors Ogino (Japan, 1924) and Knaus (Austria, 1929), conception can only occur only between the 12th and 19th day before the next menstruation date. The Talmud (b*Niddah* 31b; *cf.* 25b), too, states that women can conceive only immediately prior to the menstrual period (according to one view), or soon after the purification following it 12 days later (according to another); see Preuss, *p*.435. This is also recorded by Gumbiner (*M.A.*, *dlxxiv*.5), although Tosaphoth (*Sotah* 27a) already recognised that such "safety" was enjoyed only by most but not all women. Himes (*op. cit.*, *p*.8) declares that the knowledge of the "safe period dates at least from Soranus". H. Sutherland (*Control of Life*, 1944, *p*.235) believes it to be assumed in the purity legislation in Leviticus.

123 Already in the last century, the "safe-period" device was recommended to the Catholic faithful by A. Ballerini (*Opus Theologicum Morale*, *vol.iv*, *p*.251) and others, "particularly when incontinence may lead to the danger of *abusus matrimonii*"; see C. Capellmann, *Pastoral-Medizin*, 1878, *p*.135. This device was also specifically excluded from Pius XI's condemnation of contraceptives (see note 55 above); see H. Sutherland, *Control of Life*, 1936, *p*.222 *f*. But according to A. Bonnar (*The Catholic Doctor*, 1948, *p*.73), a decision of the Sacred Plenitentiary dated June 16, 1888 implied that, while the restriction of intercourse to the infertile days was not sinful, it was far from ideal. For an exhaustive survey of the whole problem, see P. Ahearne, "The Confessor and the Ogino-Knaus Theory", in *Irish Ecclesiastical Record*, *vol.lxi* (1943), *p*.1 *ff*.

124 See Reports of *Lambeth Conference* of 1908, 1920, 1930 (resolution 15) and 1958.

125 See Himes, *op. cit.*, *p*.8 *f*.

126 See Himes, *op. cit.*, *p*.9.

127 Soranus, *Gynecology*, *pars.* 60 and 61; quoted by N. E. Himes, "Soranus on Birth-Control", *p*.2 *f*., reprinted from the *New England Journal of Medicine*, *vol.ccv* (1931), *no*.10, *p*.490 *ff*.

128 b*Yevamoth* 12b; and parallel passages in b*Kethuboth* 39a and b*Niddah* 45a.

129 So Rashi, *Yevamoth* 12b.

130 So R. Tam, in Tosaphoth, *Yevamoth* 12b. On the other hand, while Rashi allows the precaution to be taken even before intercourse, R. Tam holds that the tampon may only be used afterwards to remove the semen.

13.1 On the danger of conception to minor women, see Preuss, *p*.441.

132 A second conception following the original pregnancy (superfoetation), it is feared, might turn the foetus into a "sandal" (*foetus compressus*). Whether such a double pregnancy (resulting from two impregnations some days or even weeks apart) is possible has been much discussed to the present day. The possibility was assumed by Aristotle (*Hist. Anim.*, *vii*.4; and *De gener.*, *iv*.87 and 88) and Pliny (*Nat. Hist.*, *vii*.11) as well as by Hippocrates. Avicenna, too, shared the talmudic view that a superfoetation may prove dangerous; see Ploss and Bartels, *Woman*, *vol.ii*, *p*.344 *ff*. In the Talmud itself opinions are divided: while the Palestinians affirmed the possibility (j*Yevamoth*, *iv*.2), at least if the second conception occurred within forty days of the first, the Babylonians denied it (b*Niddah* 27a); see Loew, *Lebensalter*, *p*.61 *f*.; Preuss, *p*.447 *f*.; and I. Simon, "La Médecine Légale dans la Bible et le Talmud", in *Révue*, *no*.3 (1949), *p*.52 *f*. In fact, cases of superfoetation are reported in the 15th century by Simon Duran (r*TaSHBeTZ*, part *iv*, *no*.49; see

Zimmels, *p.64 f.*), in the 18th century by Tidy (see O'Malley and Walsh, *Essays, p.82*) and quite recently by H. Runge (in *Archiv fuer Gynaekologie, vol.clxxiii* [1942], *p.159 ff.*) and others (see *American Journal of Surgery, vol.lx* [1943], *p.450 ff.*). By contrast, the feasibility of super-fecundation—that is, a double pregnancy produced by two men within a few days of each other (*i.e.*, before the first sperma has fructified the female ovum)—is generally conceded in medical sources (see Ploss and Bartels, *Woman, vol.ii, p.347*) as well as in the Palestinian Talmud (*loc. cit.*).

[133] The loss of the mother's milk resulting from a conception during lactation might lead to the suckling's starvation; see Preuss, *p.471*. This fear explains the rabbinic ban on marrying a divorced or widowed woman who is pregnant or lactating until the child is twenty-four months old (*E.H., xiii.*11).

[134] This, too, is a dispute between Rashi and R. Tam (see notes 129 and 130 above).

[135] This verse is usually applied to justify some relaxation of the law (see *supra*, Introduction [note 78]), not a more rigorous interpretation of it. Consequently, it is likely that the verse is used here, too, to support a more lenient ruling (*i.e.*, of not insisting on, while yet sanctioning, the precaution).

[136] So, e.g., Solomon Zalman of Posen, r*Hemdath Shelomo, E.H., no.*46; Simchah Bunam Schreiber, r*Shevet Sopher, E.H., no.*2; J. Horovitz, r*Mattei Levy*, part *ii, no.*31; and Hayim Ozer Grodzinsky, r*Achi*ezer, E.H., no.*23.

[137] So, e.g., Epstein, *A.H., E.H., xxiii.*6.

[138] So, *e.g.*, Joseph Modena, r*Rosh Mashbir*, Salonica, 1840, part *ii, no.*69 (*p.*93b); see *Sedei Hemed, s.v. "Ishuth", no.i.*32. Cf. also '*Asiphath Zekeinim*, on *Kethuboth* 39a, in the name of Nachmanides and Aaron Halevy.

[139] Such surprise is expressed by Meir Posner, *Beth Me'ir*, on *E.H., xxiii*.

[140] The only mention of the subject is the reference, among the laws of vows, to a woman "turning herself [by violent motions] after inter-course so as to avoid a conception" (*Y.D., ccxxxv.*4), a practice common only among prostitutes (*E.H., xiii.*6).

[141] Luria, *Yam Shel Shelomo, Yevamoth, i.*8.

[142] So, *e.g.*, in addition to the authorities cited in note 136 above, S. M. Schwadron, r*MaHaRSHaM*, part *i, no.*58; and D. Hoffmann, r*Melamed Leho'il, E.H., no.*18.

[143] Originally Eger (*responsa, no.*71) held that the wife must not render the husband's act ineffective under any circumstances, since she, too, is commanded not to destroy his seed, a view also confirmed by Jacob Ett-linger (r*Binyan Tziyon, no.*137) in 1864. But in a subsequent responsum (*no.*72), Eger decided to permit the absorption of the semen after inter-course.

[144] r*Hatham Sopher, Y.D., no.*172. Most Hungarian rabbis agreed with this more stringent ruling; for a full list of the relevant responsa, see H. Klein, "Geburtenregelung: Eine halachische Betrachtung", in *Nachalath Z'wi, vol.i* (1931), *p.*258.

[145] So Klein, *op. cit., p.*260; and J. J. H. Horowitz, in *Rosenheim Fest-schrift*, 1932, end. For similar reasons some rabbis favour chemical sperm-icides in preference to tampons or pessaries; see Meir Arik, r'*Imrei Yosher*, part *i, no.*131; Menachem Mannes, r*Havatzeleth Hasharon*, note following *E.H.* part; and Klein, *op. cit., p.*259.

[146] See r*MaHaRSHaM*, part *iii*, *no.*268; r*Shevet Sopher*, *loc. cit.*; and Klein, *loc. cit.*

[147] Justifying the practice in some places to extend the period of impurity following childbirth from 7 days after male births and 14 days after female births (*Lev. xii.*2 and 5) to 40 and 80 days respectively (*Y.D.*, *cxciv.*1, gloss), Jacob Reischer (r*Shevuth Ya'akov*, part *iii*, *no.*77; cited in *D.T.*, *a.l.*, 7) comments: "...they saw that the generations progressively lose their strength, and it might be feared that, if women would be quick to purify themselves after their confinement, they would [soon] become pregnant again and, having no strength yet for a further childbirth, their renewed pregnancy might lead to their death...". Cf. also Meir Katzenellenbogen's significant observation on the enactment against polygamy pronounced by R. Gershom of Mayence at the turn of the first millenium: "...anxiety was felt... for the daughters of Israel because, in view of our exile, a man who marries many women and has many children may be unable to provide for them" (r*MaHaRaM Padua*, *no.*16; cited in *'Otzar Haposkim*, *op. cit.*, *p.*15 [*no.*61]).

Chapter Fourteen

[1] Ploss and Bartels, *Woman*; cited by McKenzie, *Infancy*, *p.*305 *f.*

[2] For details, see *ib.*

[3] *Report of Inter-Departmental Committee on Abortion*, London, July 1939; see *British Encyclopedia of Medical Practice*, Supplement 1950, *p.*294.

[4] See R. Haehnel, "Der kuenstliche Abortus im Altertum", in *Sudhoff's Archiv fuer die Geschichte der Medizin*, *vol.xxix* (1936), *p.*225.

[5] *Sacred Laws of the Aryas*, in *Sacred Books of the East*, 1897, *vol.ii*, *pp.* 74 and 281; cited in *ERE*, *vol.vi*, *p.*55.

[6] See Haehnel, *op. cit.*, *p.*224 *f.*

[7] *Vendidad*, *xv.*9-14. See Haehnel, *op. cit.*, *p.*227 *f.*; Puschmann, *Medical Education*, *p.*32; Neuburger, *History*, *vol.i*, *p.*37; and Ploss and Bartels, *Woman*, *vol.ii*, *p.*520. But it is claimed that the Avesta religion fought unsuccessfully against this evil, as "people were satisfied with having prohibited abortion" (*ib.*, *p.*635).

[8] *Assyrian Code*, §53; see Driver and Miles, *The Assyrian Laws*, *pp.* 115-117; cited by D. Mace, *Hebrew Marriage*, 1953, *p.*206 *f.* Cf. E. Neufeld, *Ancient Hebrew Marriage Laws*, 1944, *pp.* 250 and 267.

[9] See Castiglioni, *History*, *p.*58. But Haehnel (*op. cit.*, *p.*227) doubts if abortion was legally punishable in Egypt, since infanticide was quite freely tolerated.

[10] *Ebers Papyrus*, *sec.xciv*; *ed.* B. Ebbell, 1937, *p.*109.

[11] *Code of Hammurabi*, §§209-210; see V. Aptowitzer, "The Status of the Embryo in the Jewish Law of Punishment", in *Sinai*, *vol.vi* (1942), *p.*13. See also Neufeld, *loc. cit.*

[12] Neufeld, *op. cit.*, *p.*252.

[13] See B. Ritter, *Philo und die Halacha*, 1879, *p.*37. Cf. Michaelis, in *Magazin der Wissenschaft*, 4th year; cited by L. Wiesner, "Kindersegen und Kinderlosigkeit im altrabbinischem Schrifttume", in *MGWJ*, *vol.lxvi* (1922), *p.*36 *f.* See also M. W. Rapaport, in *JL*, *vol.i*, *p.*59; and *infra*, *p.*181 *f.*

[14] Ovid, *De nuce*, 22-23; *cf.* note 31 below.

15 Seneca, *Ad Helv.*, *xvi.*

16 Favorinus, *Aulus Gellius, Noct. A.H.*, *xii.*1.

17 Plutarch, *De Sanitate Tuenda.*

18 Juvenal, *Sat.*, *vi.*592 *f.* See also Ploss and Bartels, *Woman, vol.ii,* p.504.

19 Lecky, *European Morals, vol.ii,* p.21 *f.*

20 Aristotle, *Politic, vii.*16, 1335; cited by Neufeld, *op. cit.,* p.252 (note 3).

21 See *ERE, vol.vi,* p.54 *ff.*

22 See L. Edelstein, "The Hippocratic Oath", in *Supplements to the Bulletin of the History of Medicine,* 1943, p.16. *Cf. infra,* p.174 *f.*

23 See Edelstein, *loc. cit.*

24 Edelstein, *op. cit., pp.* 12 and 55 *ff.* See also Puschmann, *Medical Education,* p.42.

25 C. Singer; cited by J. Needham, *A History of Embryology,* 1934, p.57.

26 W. H. S. Jones, *The Doctor's Oath,* 1924; cited by Needham, *loc. cit.*

27 Garrison, *Introduction,* p.96.

28 This discrepancy may resolve the apparent conflict between the Oath and the advice given by a Hippocratic writer to a harp-player to procure abortion by leaping (*Oevres Complètes d'Hippocrate,* ed. M. P. Littré, 1838-61, *vol.vii,* p.490). See also Neuburger, *History, vol.i,* p.159. Siebold and Littré, however, simply attribute the contradictory passages to different authors; see Haehnel, *loc. cit.*; and *cf.* K. Deichgraeber, "Die aerztliche Standesethik des hippocratischen Eides", in *Quellen und Studien zur Geschichte der Naturwissenschaften und der Medizin,* 1932, p.36.

29 See Haehnel, *op. cit.,* p.240. See also V. Aptowitzer, "Observations on the Criminal Law of the Jews", in *JQR, vol.xv* (1924), p.90 (note 126).

30 See Ploss and Bartels, *Woman, vol.i,* p.482 *ff.*

31 Ovid, *Amores, ii.*14; *transl.* G. Showerman, *Loeb Classical Library,* 1914, p.425 *f.*

32 See Ploss and Bartels, *loc. cit.*

33 See Castiglioni, *History,* p.227.

34 See Ploss and Bartels, *Woman, vol.ii,* p.521.

35 See Ploss and Bartels, *Woman, vol.iii,* p.78.

36 *Ib.,* p.79.

37 See Preuss, p.490.

38 Soranus Ephesius, *ed.* Dietz, p.113. *Cf. supra,* chpt.XIII (note 127).

39 See Haehnel, *op. cit.,* p.238.

40 See Soranus, *ed.* J. Ilberg, *C.M.G., vol.iv* (1927), p.45 *ff.*

41 See Castiglioni, *History,* p.202; and Neuburger, *loc. cit.*

42 Ploss and Bartels, *Woman, vol.i,* p.482 *ff.*

43 "And if men strive together, and hurt a woman with child, so that her fruit [*lit.* children] depart, and yet no harm [Hebrew: "אסון"]; follow, he shall be surely fined, according as the woman's husband shall lay upon him; and he shall pay as the judges determine. But if any harm follow, then thou shalt give life for life" (*Ex. xxi.*22-23). The *Septuagint* renders: "And if two men strive and smite a women with child, and her child be born imperfectly formed, he shall be forced to pay a penalty... But if it be perfectly formed «'Εὰν δε ἐξεικοσμέον ἦ» he shall give life for life". This translation, also followed in the Samaritan and Karaite versions, is evidently based on reading "צורה" or the Samaritan "סורה" (meaning "form") for "אסון" see *Kaufmann Gedenkschrift,* 1900, p.186; and note 99 below.

44 Preuss (p.450) particularly refers to the comprehensive summaries by Plutarch (*De placitis philos., lib.v, cap.*15) and Hansen (*De termino*

animationis foetus hum. Wann das Kind im Mutterleibe die Seele emp-faengt, Halle, 1724).

45 Needham, *op. cit.*, p.9.

46 Aristotle, *De anim. hist., vii.*3; *cf.* Pliny, *Nat. Hist., vii.*6. See *CE, vol.i*, p.46 *ff.*

47 This distinction, possibly by a pure coincidence, corresponds exactly with the respective periods of impurity following childbirth laid down in the Bible (*Lev. xii.*2-5); that may have contributed to the acceptance of Aristotle's assumption by the Church. See H. Vorwahl, "Die Beseelung des Menschen", in *Sudhoff's Archiv fuer die Geschichte der Medizin, vol.xiii* (1921), p.126.

48 See *ERE, vol.vi*, p.56.

49 See Spangenberg, "Verbrechen der Abtreibung der Leibesfrucht", in *Neues Archiv des Criminalrechts, vol.ii*, p.22 *f.*; cited by Westermark, *Moral Ideas*, p.415.

50 See *ERE, loc. cit.*

51 Philo (*Vit. Mos., i.*11) attributes this view to «οἱ πολλοί» ; see R. E. Goodenough, *The Jurisprudence of the Jewish Courts in Egypt,* 1929, p.116.

52 See note 23 above. The Buddhists also believed in the entry of the soul at conception; hence they counted their age from that moment. See Vorwahl, *loc. cit.*

53 See Needham, *op. cit.*, p.57; and *CE, loc. cit.*

54 Tertulian, *De anim., cap.*23 *f.*; cited by Harnack, *Medizinisches,* p.51 *f.*

55 Tertullian, *Apol., cap.*9; cited in *ERE, loc. cit.*

56 See *CE, loc. cit.*

57 Augustine, *Quaest. in Exod.*, 80; cited by Westermark, *op. cit.*, p.416. See also E. Westermark, *Christianity and Morals*, 1939, p.243.

58 But a glossarist of the code adopted the Roman formula fixing the 40th day for both sexes. See Westermark, *loc. cit.*; and Ploss and Bartels, *Woman, vol.i*, p.483 *f.*

59 For a reproduction and detailed description of the picture, see C. Singer, *From Magic to Science*, 1928, p.226 *f.*

60 See Ploss and Bartels, *loc. cit.*; and *CE, vol.ii*, p.266 *f.*

61 Fulgentius, *De Fide*, 27; see *ERE, loc. cit.* On the emphasis in Christianity on saving the child for baptism, see Westermark, *Moral Ideas*, p.417, and *Christianity and Morals*, p.244; and G. Wolff, "Leichenbesichtigung und Untersuchung bis zur Carolina als Vorstufe gerichtlicher Sektion", in *Janus, vol.xlii* (1938), p.260.

62 See W. E. H. Lecky, *History of the Rise and Influence of the Spirit of Rationalism in Europe*, 1870, *vol.i*, p.360 (note 2); and Westermark, *loc. cit.*

63 See Lecky, *op. cit.*, p.360 *ff.*; and *European Morals, vol.ii*, p.23 *f.*

64 See *supra*, p.131.

65 See Needham, *op. cit.*, p.182 *f.* The instrument, first recommended in 1733 by Doctors of Divinity at the Sorbonne, is mentioned by Gury, *Compendium theologiae moralis, tom.ii*, p.156; cited by Capellmann, *Pastoral-Medizin*, 1878, p.104 *f.* See also S. Woywood, *A Practical Commentary on the Code of Canon Law*, 1926, *vol.i*, p.533 (note).

66 Canon 747; see J. McCarthy, in *Irish Ecclesiastical Record, vol.lv* (1940), p.341 (note).

67 See Westermark, *Moral Ideas, vol.i*, p.411.

68 For the sources on the data mentioned in this paragraph, see A.

Bonnar, *The Catholic Doctor*, 1948, *p*.78 *f*.; and Ploss and Bartels, *Woman*, *vol.i*, *p*.484.

[69] See Allbutt, *Greek Medicine*, *p*.391.

[70] See Haehnel, *op. cit.*, *p*.249 *f*.

[71] Tertullian, *De anim.*, *cap*.25; see Neuburger, *History*, *vol.i*, *p*.315; and Preuss, *p*.490. For the complete quotation of the passage, see S. D'Irsay, "Patristic Medicine", in *Annals of the History of Medicine*, *vol.ix* (1928), *p*.367 *f*.

[72] See *CE*, *vol.i*, *p*.47. For the texts of the Holy Office decrees on abortion, see O'Malley and Walsh, *Essays*, *p*.49 *ff*.

[73] See Bonnar, *op. cit.*, *p*.82. All current works on medical ethics re-affirm this position; see, *e.g.*, G. Kelly, *Medico-Moral Problems*, 1950, part *i*, *p*.10 *ff*.

[74] O'Malley (*Essays*, *p*.20 *ff*.) describes the decree as "by no means clear". For its text in full, see also J. McCarthy, *op. cit.*, *p*.59 *ff*.

[75] So Fr. Sabetti, cited by O'Malley, *Essays*, *p*.26.

[76] See T. L. Bouscaren, *Ethics of Ectopic Operations*, 1944, *p*.57; and Bonnar, *op. cit.*, *p*.89.

[77] So Capellmann, *op. cit.*, *p*.15.

[78] A. Klarman, *The Crux of Pastoral Medicine*, 1912, *p*.135. For a summary of the conflicting views, see also P. A. Finney, *Moral Problems in Hospital Practice*, 1935.

[79] O'Malley, *Essays*, *p*.54.

[80] Bonnar, *op. cit.*, *p*.84. Capellmann (*op. cit.*, *p*.19) likewise states: "There is absolutely nothing left to [the physician] but to await the death of the child or even of the mother, if he is not in a position to avert it by permitted means...".

[81] See, *e.g.*, *Ethical and Religious Directives for Catholic Hospitals*, issued by the Catholic Hospital Association of the U.S. and Canada, 1949, *p*.4.

[82] This slogan was coined by P. Tiberghien, "Principes et conscience morale", in *Cahiers Laennec*, October 1946, *p*.13 *ff*.; see G. Kelly, "Current Theology", in *Theological Studies*, *vol.x*, *no*.1 (March 1949), *p*.82.

[83] See Cumston, *An Introduction*, *p*.24.

[84] See LaWall, *Pharmacy*, *p*.219. The formula may suggest that thera-peutic abortions were occasionally sanctioned, although this oath, like the previous one, opened with a promise "to live and die as a Christian".

[85] Tacitus, *Germania*, *xix*.

[86] *Visigothic Code. iv.*4.

[87] For references to the preceding data, see Ploss and Bartels, *Woman*, *vol.i*, *p*.481 *f*., and *vol.ii*, *p*.522.

[88] See Ploss and Bartels, *Woman*, *vol.i*, *p*.485 *f*. On animation, see *supra*, *p*.174 *f*.

[89] See Ploss and Bartels, *Woman*, *vol.ii*, *p*.523.

[90] *Fleta*, *lib.i*, *cap*.23; see Ploss and Bartels, *Woman*, *vol.ii*, *p*.522.

[91] The Act (43 Geo III *c*.58) provided for the death penalty if the woman was "quick with child", and for transportation and imprisonment if she was not. The supreme penalty for abortion was abolished by a further Act only in 1837. See L. A. Parry, in *British Medical Journal*, 1938, *p*.541.

[92] See Ploss and Bartels, *loc. cit.*

[93] See Ploss and Bartels, *Woman*, *vol.i*, *p*.486; and *Report... on Abortion*, *op. cit.*, *p*.26 *f*.

[94] See Ploss and Bartels, *loc. cit.*

[95] See Westermark, *Moral Ideas*, *vol.i*, *p*.413.

96 For a comprehensive summary of the abortion laws among civilised peoples at present, see Theodor v. Miltner, "Die Gesetzgebung der Kulturvoelker zum Problem der Fruchtabtreibung", in *Archiv fuer Gynaekologie*, *vol.cxlii* (1930), *p.133 ff.*

97 In England the distinction was abolished by the Act of 1837; see Parry, *loc. cit.*

98 In England, for instance, the Infant Life Preservation Act of 1929 legalises abortion to save the mother's life or health if the seventh month of pregnancy has been reached; see D. W. Roy, in *British Encyclopedia of Medical Practice*, *vol.i*, *p.61 f.*; *ib.*, *Suppl.*, 1950, *p.2*; and Justice Humphreys, "Abortion—Should the Law be Reformed?", in *Medico-Legal Review*, *vol.vi* (1938), *p.177.*

99 See note 43 above. On the Samaritan attitude, see also A. Geiger, *Urschrift*, 1857, *p.439*; and *Hebraeische Aufsaetze*, ed. S. A. Poznanski, *vol.i*, *p.119*. The Karaite condemnation of abortion as murder is found in *'Eshkol Hakopher*, Alphabet 270 (*p.103b*) and 275 (*p.104b*); *Mibhar* and *Kether Torah*, on *Ex. xxi.22-23*; and *Gan Eden*, *p.177b*. See Loew, *Lebensalter*, pp. 44 and 70; and Aptowitzer, in *JQR*, *op. cit.*, *p.85* (note 113), and in *Sinai*, *op. cit.*, *p.10.*

100 Philo, *De spec. legibus*, *iii.*108-110.

101 *Ib.*, 117-118; so also in *De virtut.*, 138.

102 Philo, *Hypothetica*; see S. Belkin, *Philo and the Oral Law*, 1940, *p.137.*

103 Goodenough, *op. cit.*, *p.117.*

104 I. Heinemann, *Die Werke Philos*, 1910, *vol.ii*, *p.217*. So also in editorial note on Wiesner's "Kindersegen...", in *MGWJ*, *op. cit.*, *p.36 f.*

105 Josephus, *Antiquities*, *iv.*8, 33.

106 Josephus, *Contra Apionem*, *ii.*202.

107 Weyl, *Die juedischen Strafgesetze bei Fl. Josephus*, pp. 50-52 and 57 *f.*; cited by Aptowitzer, in *Sinai*, *op. cit.*, *p.11* (note 7).

108 Loew, *loci cit.*

109 Ploss and Bartels, *Woman*, *vol.ii*, *p.521.*

110 Zipser, *Josephus Flavius' Schrift gegen Apion*, *p.164 f.*; cited by Aptowitzer, *loc. cit.*

111 Heinemann, in *MGWJ*, *loc. cit.*

112 Aptowitzer, *loc. cit.*

113 In contrast to the *Septuagint*, the rabbis—like the *Vulgata* and the *Peshita* (see Aptowitzer, in *JQR*, *op. cit.*, *p.86* [note 116])—apply the reference to "harm" in *Ex. xxi.22-23* to a fatal injury sustained by the mother (*Mekhilta*, *a.l.* [*Mishpatim*, §8]). For further sources, see Aptowitzer, in *Sinai*, *op. cit.*, *p.11*. *Cf.* note 160 below.

114 This is based on the more general principle that, if one committed two actionable offences simultaneously, one suffers the severer penalty only; see, *e.g.*, b*Gittin* 52b *f.*

115 b*Sanhedrin* 57b. So also *Gen. Rabbah*, *xxxiv.*19, in the name of R. Hanina. For a summary of the principal views on this subject, see *TE*, *vol.iii*, *p.351.*

116 Instead of the usual translation: "Whoso sheddeth the blood of man, *by man* [i.e. through a human court] shall his blood be shed".

117 See *supra*, *p.135.*

118 Loew, *Lebensalter*, *p.70.*

119 Aptowitzer, in *JQR*, *op. cit.*, *p.114* (note 187); and in *Sinai*, *op. cit.*, *p.28* (note 59).

120 I. H. Weiss, *Dor Dor Vedarshav*, 1924, *vol.ii*, *p.23.*

121 Maimonides, *Hil. Melachim*, *ix.*4.

[122] Tosaphoth, *Sanhedrin* 59a, and *Hullin* 33a.

[123] See *infra*, p.186 f. Tosaphoth, too, argue in another passage (*Niddah* 43b) that no formal ban on the killing of embryos by Jews may, in fact, exist.

[124] See note 13 above.

[125] Weiss, *loc. cit.*

[126] "Do not administer to an adulterous wife an abortifacient"; see Friedenwald, p.22; and I. Simon, "Le Serment Médical d'Assaph", in *Révue*, no.9 (1951), p.38.

[127] "No woman has ever brought about an abortion with my aid"; see Friedenwald, p.369.

[128] "[Let me not be enticed] to perform an abortion on a pregnant woman"; see I. Simon, "La Prière des Médecins de Jacob Zahalon", in *Révue*, no.25 (1955), p.44 f. Friedenwald (*p.277*) wrongly renders the Hebrew passage: "... to administer a... drug to injure... some pregnant woman".

[129] See note 13 above.

[130] J. J. Walsh, *Religion and Health*, 1920, p.316.

[131] See S. W. Baron, *The Jewish Community*, 1942, *vol.ii*, p.315.

[132] See Neuburger, *History*, *vol.i*, pp. 379 and 387.

[133] *Cf. supra*, Introduction (note 92).

[134] b*Sanhedrin* 91b.

[135] *Gen. Rabbah*, xxxiv.10. On this argument, see Preuss, p.450; and especially W. Hirsch, *Rabbinic Psychology*, 1947, p.143 ff.

[136] b*Sanhedrin* 110b; and j*Shevi'ith*, iv. end. *Cf. Midrash Shoher Tov* and *Yalkut*, on *Ps. xxii*.31, where the souls of embryos are excluded from immortal life.

[137] *RaN*, on *Sanhedrin* 110b.

[138] The contention by Preuss (*p.450*) that the question of the soul's entry has no practical significance in the Talmud is disputed by Aptowitzer (in *JQR, op. cit.*, p.115 ff.; and in *Sinai, op. cit.*, p.32), He seeks to prove that only those teachers who held that the soul was united with the seed at conception regarded the embryo as a separate being—an assumption for which the Talmud itself lacks all evidence. Again, regarding the argument on the title to immortality, one commentator (Samuel Jaffe) even expresses surprise at its inclusion in the Talmud, asking: "What practical difference results from these views; do we then deal with messianic regulations?", to which another scholar (Israel Eisenstein) replies that the discussion may affect the question whether an infant should be circumcised posthumously; see '*Amudei Yerushalayim*, on j*Shevi'ith*, iv. end. The dispute, therefore, was definitely not thought to affect the issue of abortion in any way.

[139] See b*Berakhoth* 50a; t*Sotah*, vi.4; and Mekhilta, on *Ex. xv*.1.

[140] The Midrash (*Shoher Tov*, on *Ps. viii*.3) relates that at the time of the giving of the Law at Sinai even the embryos were pledged to submit to it. Similarly, the Talmud (b*Niddah* 30b) holds that all children are abjured before they are born to be righteous in life.

[141] Thus, even unborn children are said to curse flatterers (b*Sotah* 41b) and persons who withhold a teaching from their disciples (b*Sanhedrin* 91b f.).

[142] *Gen. Rabbah*, lxiii.6; see Rashi, on *Gen. xxv*.22.

[143] See b*Berakhoth* 10a.

[144] See *supra*, p.168.

[145] See *supra*, chpt.XIII (note 133).

[146] See *supra*, p.61. *Cf.* also the permission to wear the "preserving

stone" on the Sabbath to guard against miscarriages; see *supra, p*.35.

147 See *supra, chpt*.IV (note 38).

148 So Tosaphoth, *Niddah* 44b. But Jacob Emden (*glosses, a.l.*) observes: "Who would permit killing an embryo without reason, even if there is no death penalty for doing so?"

149 See *supra, p*.46 and *chpt*.XI (note 44).

150 See, *e.g.*, b*Hullin* 58a. For further sources on the embryo's human status, see *TE, vol.i, p*.75. The codes generally accept the view that the embryo is a part of the mother and does not enjoy legal rights. Hence, the proselytisation of gravid women effects the conversion to Judaism of their fruit (*Y.D., cclxviii*.6) and the sale of pregnant slaves or animals includes their unborn offspring (*H.M., ccxx*.10); the father's marriage of his unborn daughter is (at best) of doubtful validity (*E.H., xl*.8; see Loew, *loc. cit.*); and a foetus has no right of acquisition (*H.M., ccx*.1) except to inherit its father (*H.M., cclxxvi*.5; see Loew, *op. cit., p*.68 *f.*). For the same reason, still-born cirldren need not to be shown the usual respects due to the dead (*Y.D., cccxliv*.8) nor may the second day of a festival be violated for their burial (*O.H., dxxvi*.10, gloss; and *Y.D., cclxiii*.5, gloss).

151 So Aptowitzer, in *JQR, op. cit., p*.111 *f.*; and in *Sinai, op. cit., p*.26 *f.* Two conditions must be fulfilled before a murderer can be sentenced to death in Jewish law: The victim must have been an independent human being, and he must also have been fully viable (see *infra, p*.188). Hence, reasons Aptowitzer, the killer of an embryo cannot be executed; for even if the Palestinian teaching may satisfy the first condition, the second cannot be fulfilled until after the child's birth.

152 Aptowitzer (in *JQR, op. cit., p*.114 *ff.*; and in *Sinai, op. cit., p*.28 *f.*) believes that the distinction was introduced by the *Septuagint* and Philo as a compromise between the Greek school of Academy (Plato), which held that the embryo was a separate being, and the school of the Stoa, which taught that it was part of the mother. The rabbis of the Talmud, therefore, followed the argument of the earlier Greek philosophers. *Cf.* also note 172 below.

153 m'*Oholoth, vii*.6. See Preuss, *p*.488 *f.*

154 So j*Shabbath, xiv*.4; and j'*Avodah Zarah, ii*.2. Elsewhere (j*Sanhedrin, viii*. end) the head and the greater part of the body are mentioned. In the codes, too, the legal definition of the precise moment of birth varies. The rights of the first-born take effect with the appearance of the forehead only (*H.M., cclxxvii*.3; *cf. Y.D., cccv*.22). A mother's impurity following childbirth, too, commences with the emergence of the forehead, or the greater part of it, even if not completely free but only outside the lower end of the uterus (*Y.D., cxciv*.10). The moment when the head appears outside the birth canal (or when the natal cries are heard) determines the date of the child's circumcision eight days later (*Y.D., cclxii*.4). But to qualify as a levir for marriage to the deceased brother's widow (the law requires the brothers to have lived simultaneously) his head or the greater part of his body must have been delivered at the time of the brother's death (*E.H., clvii*.1). In animals, too, birth is reckoned from the moment the head (*Y.D., xiv*.1) or the greater part of the body is delivered (*ib.*, 3).

155 b*Sanhedrin* 72b.

156 The law of pursuit–based on *Lev. xix*.16 (*cf.* Rashi, *a.l.*; and see b*Sanhedrin* 73a) and *Deut. xxv*.11 and 12 (see b*Sanhedrin* 74a)–provides that it is the right and duty of any person who witnesses another pursuing,

with intent to kill, his fellowman to disable the aggressor, if necessary by a fatal blow (*H.M., cdxxv.*1).

[157] Rashi, *Sanhedrin* 72b.

[158] Maimonides, *Hil. Rotze'ah, i.*9. He presumably derives this by inference from the talmudic discussion; see Aptowitzer, in *Sinai, op. cit., p.*17 (note 23).

[159] Bacharach, *rHavath Ya'ir, no.*31.

[160] See *Mekhilta* and Rashi, *a.l.* Cf. also note 151 above, and *infra, p.*188.

[161] Landau, *rNoda Biyehudah,* part *ii, H.M., no.*59; see Aptowitzer, *loc. cit.*

[162] See *supra,* chpt.XI (note 44). For further attempts to resolve the difficulty, see J. L. Unterman, *Shevet Miyehudah,* 1955, *p.*26 ff.

[163] m*'Arachin, i.*4.

[164] The reason for the immediate execution of a pregnant mother is to avoid the agonising suspense (branded an "oppression of justice") of any delay following the verdict (Tosaphoth, *'Arachin* 7a; and Maimonides, *Hil. Sanhedrin,* xii.4); see Aptowitzer, in *Sinai, op. cit., p.*17 ff.

[165] b*'Arachin* 7a. See Preuss, *p.*490 ff.; and Loew, *op. cit., p.*60.

[166] See note 164 above. This law operates only if the woman's pregnancy was not recognised until after the death sentence was pronounced; but if it became known before or during the trial, the execution had to be postponed until the child was born, as the "oppression of justice" applies only to the suspense between the completion of the trial and the execution (b*Sanhedrin* 35a, and Rashi, *a.l.*); see Tosaphoth, *loc. cit.*; and *Mishneh Lemelekh,* on *Hil. Sotah, ii.*7.

[167] See I. Jakobovits, in *Hapardes, vol.xxx, no.*7 (April 1956), *p.*20 ff. Unterman (*op. cit., p.*50), who mentions a similar argument to explain the ruling of Maimonides in the name of another scholar (*Sepher 'Ahi'ezer,* part *iii, no.*72), himself rejects it as he regards the status of the embryo to be conditioned by its potential development into a man, not by its present function as a part of the mother. But cf. Israel Lipschuetz, *Tiph'ereth Yisra'el, 'Oholoth, vii.*6 (*no.*10).

[168] See Aptowitzer, in *JQR, op. cit., p.*94 (note 139). This important conclusion is clearly indicated by the wording in the Mishnah itself: "For we do not set aside one life for [the sake of] another" (but possibly for two lives we would!).

[169] Trani, *rMaHaRIT,* part *i, no.*99; quoted by Lampronti, *Pahad Yitzhak, s.v.* "*Nephalim*" (*ed.* Mekitzei Nirdamim, Lyck, 1864, letter "N", *p.*79b).

[170] Lampronti, *loc. cit.*

[171] This view is almost the complete reverse of the attitude of the Catholic Church which never tolerates the operation if directed at the child as the cause of the danger ("direct abortion"), though the treatment of a pregnant mother leading to her fruit's abortion may be sanctioned if the condition to be treated resulted from an illness ("indirect abortion"); see *supra, p.*176 *f.*

[172] In Jewish law, the legal distinction between viable and inviable embryos is altogether unknown (*cf.* note 152 above). Hence, any religious concession granted to preserve the life of a viable embryo (see *supra, p.*183) applies even to a foetal growth of under 40 days; see *Korban Nethan'el,* on Asheri, *Yoma, viii.*13.

[173] See Mordecai L. Winkler, *rLevushei Mordekhai,* 2nd *ed., Y.D., no.*87; H. Klein, in *Nachalath Z'wi, vol.i* (1931), *p.*254; and Zimmels, *p.*68. According to Israel Meir Mizrachi (*rPri Ha'aretz, Y.D., no.*2), a

pregnancy may also be interrupted if it is feared that the mother will otherwise suffer an attack of hysteria; see Klein, *loc. cit.* But Isaac Schorr (r*Ko'ah Shor*, *no*.20) sanctions the operation only with some hesitation, unless the mother is directly endangered by the child she carries; see Zimmels, *p*.212 (note 79).

[174] See *supra*, *p*.180.

[175] Tosaphoth, *Sanhedrin* 59a. See also *TE*, *vol.iii*, *p*.351.

[176] r*MaHaRIT*, part *i*, nos. 97 and 99; cited by Lampronti, *loc. cit.*

[177] This is analogous to the condition under which the Talmud (b'*Avodah Zarah* 26a) permits Jews to render medical aid to heathens; for no enmity is likely to be created by declining to offer professional aid free of charge (Rashi, *a.l.*); *cf. infra*, *chpt.XV* (note 13).

[178] Beneviste, *Keneseth Hagedolah*, on *Tur*, *H.M.*, *cdxxv*, *no*.6; cited in *D.T.*, *Y.D.*, *cliv*.7.

[179] Based on the talmudic interpretation of *Lev. xix.*14 (b*Pesahim* 22b).

[180] Joseph Babad, *Minhath Hinnukh*, commandment *no*.296; *cf. no*.34 (*ed.* Vilna, 1912, part *ii*, *p*.215 and part *i*, *p*.107). See also J. Z. Jalisch, *Melo Haro'im*, on *Sanhedrin* 57b.

[181] See note 168 above.

[182] Lipschuetz, *Tiph'ereth Yisra'el*, *'Oholoth*, *vii*.6 (*no*.10).

[183] Hayim Sopher, r*Mahanei Hayim*, part *ii*, *H.M.*, *no*.50.

[184] Meir of Eisenstadt, r*Panim Me'iroth*, part *ii*, *no*.8; see also Akivah Eger, on *'Oholoth*, *viii*.6.

[185] *Cf.* Rashi, *Niddah* 28a.

[186] Schick, r*MaHaRaM Shik*, *Y.D.*, *no*.155.

[187] Hoffmann, r*Melamed Leho'il*, *Y.D.*, *no*.69.

[188] See *supra*, *p*.98.

[189] This principle is already maintained in the Talmud (b*Yevamoth* 36b); see Aptowitzer, in *Sinai*, *op. cit.*, *p*.26 f. Hence, an infant under 31 days old lacks normal human status in respect of the redemption of the first-born (*Y.D.*, *ccv*.11 and 12), the exemption of a widowed mother (according to rabbinic law) from the duty to contract or dissolve the levirate bond (*E.H.*, *clvi*.4), and the laws relating to rending a garment (*Y.D.*, *cccxi*.30) and to mourning (*Y.D.*, *ccclxxiv*.8) following its death within that period, unless it had definitely been carried for a full term (*ib.*).

[190] See preceding note.

[191] Accordingly, while the Church draws the line between a viable and an inviable child during the *pre-natal* state (to permit its abortion *after* that line is passed so that it may survive its premature expulsion), Jewish law advances the line to the *post-natal* stage (to warrant the child's sacrifice *before* that line is reached as an alternative to the loss of two lives).

[192] *Zohar*, on *Ex.* (beginning); *ed.* Amsterdam, 1800, *vol.ii*, *p*.3b.

[193] See *supra*, *p*.179 f.

[194] *Sepher Hasidim*, *ed. Mekitzei Nirdamim*, *no*.1518. This work is also the first to mention the problem of monster-births which it did not wish to be destroyed (*no*.186). Early in the 19th century, Eleazar Fleckeles (r*Teshuvah Me'ahavah*, part *i*, *no*.53) ruled, against another rabbinical view, that the killing of a child born with certain animal features constituted murder; see *P.T.*, *Y.D.*, *cxciv*.5; and Zimmels, *p*.72. Luther, on the other hand, refused to baptise deformed children, believing they ought to be drowned as they had no soul; see McKenzie, *Infancy*, *p*.313.

[195] For references to the passage here mentioned, see *supra*, *chpt.XI* (note 38).

196 See references as in preceding note.

197 Bacharach, *loc. cit.* A papal decretal of 1679, too, condemned abortions to save unmarried mothers from punishment or infamy; see Bonnar, *op. cit., p.82.*

198 Emden, r*She'ilath Yavetz*, no.43. *Cf.* also note 148 above.

199 That is, any product of an adulterous or incestuous union (*E.H., iv.*13).

200 See *supra, p.*185.

201 Isaac Halevy, r*Lehem Hapanim, Kunteres 'Aharon*, no.19.

Chapter Fifteen

1 For the talmudic period, see Preuss, *p.*39; and Krauss, *vol.ii, p.*12. In the Middle Ages the position remained almost the same; see Zimmels, *p.*157.

2 Josephus, *Antiquities, xx.*2, 4. Rashi, in his Talmud commentary (*Sanhedrin* 17b; *cf. Pesahim* 7b and *Menahoth* 42a), identifies "physician" with circumciser", but his reference is probably to a surgeon performing circumcisions only; see Kohut, *Aruch Completum, vol.vii, p.*291; and Jastrow, *Dictionary, p.*1462.

3 By M. Neuburger, *Die Medizin im Fl. Josephus*, 1919, *p.*60.

4 I. Heinemann, in *MGWJ, vol.lxiv* (1920), *p.*232.

5 See *Hame'asseph*, 1898, no.65; cited in *Sedei Hemed*, chpt.ii, no.21 (*p.*115).

6 See C. E. Schapira, *Sepher 'Oth Shalom*, 1921, *p.*265.

7 For this and other German, French, Austrian and Russian regulations to ensure the medical certification of circumcisers, see Bamberger, in *Hygiene der Juden*, ed. M. Grunwald, 1911, *p.*109 *f.*; and E. Junes, "Étude sur la circoncision rituelle en Israel", in *Révue*, no.22 (1954), *p.*153 *f.* Rabbinical leaders also insisted that operators be duly authorised by an ecclesiastical court; see J.Glassberg, *Zikhron Berith Larishonim*, 1892, *p.*222 *ff.*

8 Yet if a non-Jew did perform the operation, the act is valid according to Karo (*ib.*)—because it requires no religious intention (*TaZ, a.l.,* 3)—and invalid according to Isserles (*ib.,* gloss). This difference of opinion is already reflected in the Talmud (j*Shabbath, xix.*2; *cf.* b*Menahoth* 42a); see Preuss, *p.*40.

9 Because the obligation to have their sons circumcised rests on fathers, and is not incumbent on women (*ib.,* and *cclxi.*1, gloss); see *'Oth Shalom, op. cit., p.*262.

10 Despite certain fears of accidents (see Isaac Lampronti, *Pahad Yitzhak, s.v.* "*Mohel*"), the office of circumciser is often combined with that of ritual slaughterer; see *OY, vol.vi, p.*171; and *'Oth Shalom, op. cit., p.*269 *ff. Cf.* also Zimmels, *p.*158; and *infra, p.*241. On fees charged by circumcisers, see *infra, p.*228.

11 But if a Jew performed the operation in similar circumstances, the act is valid (*Be'er Hagolah, a.l.*), since any premature circumcision carried out by a Jew is in order, provided it was not done at night (*Y.D., cclxii.*1, gloss).

12 So implied by Mordecai Jaffe, *Levush, a.l.,* and explicitly stated in *TaZ, a.l.,* 3. But *cf.* SHaKH, *a.l.,* 8.

13 That is, when necessary for the prevention of ill-feeling (*Y.D., clviii.*1;

and gloss). But in practice Jewish physicians in the Middle Ages commonly placed their services at the disposal of Jews and Gentiles alike; for
examples, see Friedenwald, *pp.* 47, 560, 564 *ff.*, 570, 591 and 622. *Cf.*
also the spirited defence of David de Pomis, *De Medico Hebraeo Enarratio
Apologica*, Venice, 1589; see Friedenwald, *p.*46 *f.* Yet the Geonim (see
Beth Yoseph, Y.D., *cclxvi* [end]) and Maimonides (*rPe'er Hador, no.*60)
were altogether opposed to the circumcision of Gentiles by Jews. Only in
subsequent centuries did the attitude become more lenient; see *'Oth Shalom*, *op. cit.*, *p.*254 *ff.*; and Zimmels, *p.* 159.

14 Fatalities are very rarely mentioned in Jewish sources, though
statistics for any but the most recent times are obviously not available.
The records of the New York City Health Department list only one death
from circumcision out of over half a million cases (including surgical
operations) for the period 1939-52; see H. Speert, "Circumcision of the
New-Born", in *Obstetrics and Gynecology, vol.ii, no.*2 (1953), *p.*171.

15 Only the act of removing the foreskin—the chief object of the operation—is of early biblical origin (see *Gen. xvii.*10-14). The additional two
acts (*viz.*, slitting the mucosa to expose the corona and sucking the wound)
are first mentioned in the Mishnah (*Shabbath, xix.*2). The first of them
was already commanded to Abraham, according to the Palestinian Talmud (*jYevamoth, viii.*1), but other teachers deny this, attributing its institution to Joshua instead (*bYevamoth* 71b). Later sources (*Yalkut,
Beha'alothkha*; Tosaphoth, *Yevamoth* 71b) regard Moses as its originator;
see *OY, loc. cit.* Modern scholars generally believe that it was introduced
at the time of the Maccabees (so Preuss, *p.*281) or after the Bar Kochba
wars (Krauss, *vol.ii, p.*438 [note 117]; and *JE, vol.iv, p.*93); see also
Glassberg, *op. cit.*, *p.*184 *f.*

16 See preceding note. The relevant statements in the Talmud serve—as
Preuss (p.281) has pointed out—not as instructions on the mode of the
operation (evidently presumed to be common knowledge), but as directives in the event of a clash between the Sabbath and circumcision laws.
As a parallel, Preuss refers to the *Koran* which does not mention circumcision, though it belongs to Islam's most important precepts.

17 See *JE, vol.iv, p.*99.

18 See I. L. Katzenelsohn, *Hatalmud Veharephu'ah*, 1928, *p.*206.

19 m*Shabbath, xix.*6.

20 Jastrow (*Dictionary, pp.* 1227 and 1235) gives both renderings: "uncovering the corona" and "splitting the membrane". So also Levy (*Woerterbuch, vol.iv, p.*128): "Die Eichel des maennlichen Gliedes entbloessen,
d.h. die sie bedeckende duenne Haut... aufreissen". Kohut (*Aruch Completum, vol.vi, p.*439) refers only to "uncovering".

21 Maimonides, *Mishnah Commentary*, on *Shabbath, xix.*2.

22 So R. Chananel, on *Shabbath* 137b; and Isaac b. Moses, r'*Or Zaru'a,
no.*97.

23 So Maimonides, *Hil. Milah, ii.*2; Abraham of Narbonne, *Sepher
Ha'eshkol*, ed. Auerbach, 1867, part *ii, p.*122; and Jacob Hagozer, *Zikhron
Berith Larishonim*, ed. Glassberg, 1892, part *i, p.*19 (*cf.* also *p.*116).
The first reference to the use of nails for this act is in Midrash *Shoher
Tov*, on *Ps. xxxv.*10; and *Yalkut*, Psalms, *no.*723.

24 So Katzenelsohn, *op. cit.*, *p.*205.

25 See *'Otzar Hage'onim*, ed. B. Lewin, 1930, *vol.ii* (*Shabbath*), *p.*134.
J. D. Eisenstein (*OY, loc. cit.*) claims that Jacob Hagozer knew of a
similar custom in Salonica.

26 See *'Otzar Hage'onim, loc. cit.*; and quotation by Z. H. Chajes,
r*MaHaRaTZ, no.*60.

[27] r*MaHaRaTZ*, loc. cit.

[28] The *Consistoire* in France, for instance, enacted a law forbidding circumcisers to use their nails; see Glassberg, *op. cit.*, p.185 f.; and Zimmels, p.163 f.

[29] Ettlinger, r*Binyan Tziyon*, no.88.

[30] See Judah Meir Schapira, r'*Or Hame'ir*, part i, no.58; D. Hoffmann, r*Melamed Leho'il*, Y.D., no.81; Glassberg, loc. cit.; and Zimmels, p.267 (note 162). For a summary of the views and arguments opposing the innovation, see '*Oth Shalom*, op. cit., pp. 275-288.

[31] See, e.g., Herman I. Kantor, "History of Circumcision: Introduction of a New Instrument", in *Texas State Journal of Medicine*, February 1953, p.77. The Orthodox Rabbinats in America, for instance, formally ruled that circumcision prepared by means of the "Gompo Clamp" were religiously invalid; see S. Gerstenfeld, in *Hapardes*, vol.xxix, no.7 (April 1955), p.14 f.

[32] b*Shabbath* 133b; see Preuss, p.282. See also note 16 above.

[33] Maimonides, loc. cit.

[34] Puschmann, *Medical Education*, p.166.

[35] Ed. Glassberg, op. cit., p.116.

[36] See *JE*, vol.iv, p.100; A. Tertis, *Sepher Dam Berith*, 1900, p.3 f.; and series of articles in *Mamelitz*, vols. iii-v (1898-1900). See also Speert, op. cit., p.169.

[37] For a German ban in 1888, see J. Horovitz, in r*Mattei Levy*, part ii, no.60. The practice was also attacked in many Jewish circles (see sources cited in preceding note), particularly at the German Reform Rabbinical Conferences of 1844, 1845 and 1846; see Bamberger, op. cit., p.110; and Zimmels, p.164.

[38] A still popular appliance is a glass-cylinder with a compressed mouth piece, first designed by a rabbi in Fulda; see *JE*, loc. cit.; Bamberger, op. cit., p.108; and S. Krauss, *Geschichte der juedischen Aerzte*, 1930, p.158. In London Tertis (op. cit., pp. 4 and 31) produced a rubber contrivance which eliminated the application of the mouth altogether; see *OY*, loc. cit.

[39] See Zimmels, p.164. This method is evidently also sanctioned by the leading 20th century scholar, Israel Meir Kagan (*M.B.*, *Bi'ur Halakhan*, on *O.H.*, cccxxxi.1) who declares this act permissible even on the Sabbath.

[40] This was justified on the grounds that the Midrash (*Tanhuma*, *Lekh Lekha* [ed. Buber, p.82]; and *Pesikta*, on *Deut.* xiv.22 [ed. Buber, p. 98a]) listed only the first two acts of the ritual; see r*MaHaRaTZ*, loc. cit.

[41] In particular, the reformers referred to a responsum attributed to Moses Schreiber (which is not among his published works of responsa); see r*MaHaRaTZ*, loc. cit.; and Kohut, *Aruch Completum*, vol.i, p.120. But others maintained that Schreiber's opinion disputing the need for carrying out the sucking by mouth was given only under duress to a certain rabbi who was faced with a complete ban on ritual circumcisers unless they suspended the oral sucking practice; see *Sedei Hemed*, "*Kunteres Hametzitzah*", part xii, chpt.i, no.11 (ed. Warsaw, 1902, vol.v, p.75); cf. chpt.ii, no.18 (p.101).

[42] Ettlinger, r*Binyan Tziyon*, no.23.

[43] See, e.g., r*Mattei Levy*, loc. cit.; Moses Schick, r*MaHaRaM Shik*, Y.D., no.244; and many sources cited by Zimmels, p.267 (note 162). The *Sedei Hemed* (loc. cit.) devotes 64 pages to the arguments in defence of the time-honoured practice, including a protest-declaration against any innovation signed by over 250 Austria-Hungarian rabbis in 1900 (chpt.iii, no.8 [p.134 ff.]).

44 Lipschuetz, *Tiph'ereth Yisra'el*, on *Shabbath, xix.*1 (*"Bo'az", no.*1). Samson Raphael Hirsch, too, ruled that a circumcision without the oral sucking act was inadmissible; see responsum published in *Nachalath Z'wi, vol.ii* (1932), *p.*192.

45 But *cf. supra, p.*59 *f.* for the general rule in the event of such conflicts.

46 See *Sedei Hemed, op. cit., chpt.iii, no.*6 (*p.*126 *ff.*). See also A. H. Merzbach, "La circoncision", in *Révue, no.*20 (1954), *p.*20 *ff.*

47 See *Sedei Hemed, op. cit., chpt.ii, no.*21 (*p.*115); and Zimmels, *p.*164. *Cf.* also note 14 above.

48 According to most talmudists, the prepuce in such cases is not really missing altogether but merely "pressed" to the corona; see Preuss, *p.*285 *f.*; and *'Oth Shalom, op. cit., p.*245 *ff.*

49 This rite performed by a needle's prick is already mentioned in the Talmud (*tShabbath, xvii.*8; *bShabbath* 135a; and *Gen. Rabbah, xlvi.*12).

50 On the consideration for the infant's pain, see *supra, p.*102.

51 But normal circumcisions and the work immediately necessary for their performance may be carried out on the Sabbath without hindrance (*Y.D., cclxvi.*2 *ff.*; and *O.H., cccxxxi.*1 *ff.*); see also *supra, chpt.*IV (note 30).

52 *Cf. supra, p.*50.

53 On the talmudic origin of these precautions, see Preuss, *p.*284 *f.*

54 The reason for this delay is perhaps not unconnected with the explanation given by the Midrash (*Deut. Rabbah, vi.*1) and Maimonides (*Guide of the Perplexed, iii.*49) for the seven-day period which must elapse after the day of birth prior to the circumcision "in order to wait until the child gains some strength".

55 See Preuss, *p.*182. In the Talmud (*bShabbath* 137a) the phrase used is "חלצתו חמה", lit: "if the heat has left him" (see Rashi, *a.l.*; and Jastrow, *Dictionary, p.*472). But in the codes the expression evidently denotes a feverish condition, as it is followed by "... or a similar illness affecting the whole body". Another explanation is offered by Nissim (*RaN, Nedarim* 41a). For a full discussion of these interpretations, see r*Mattei Levy*, part *ii, no.*52 (end).

56 See SHaKH, *a.l.*, 3. For further rabbinic sources, see Zimmels, *p.*263 (note 100).

57 Preuss (*p.*284) thinks of blennorrhoea, as assumed by Shabbatai Hacohen (*SHaKH, a.l.*, 4) who identified the condition with that described in *O.H., cccxxviii.*9; see *supra, p.*60.

58 *E.g.*, Judah Assad, r*MaHaRYA, Y.D., no.*254; and r*Mattei Levy, op. cit., no.*52. But, whereas the former responsum sanctions an additional delay of seven days after the child has gained its normal strength, the latter permits the operation as soon as the doctor declares it fit.

59 See D. Feldmann, note on *Kitzur Shulhan 'Arukh*, 1933, *clxiii.*3 (*p.*104)

60 The Hebrew word used ("ירוק") means literally "herb-like" and can denote either colour; see Jastrow, *Dictionary, p.*595.

61 This law is taken almost literally from the Talmud (*bShabbath* 134a). Rashi (*a.l.*) explains that the pale colour indicates that "the blood has not yet entered into the child [properly]; this causes it to be so weak... that it can easily faint and die".

62 The Talmud (*loc. cit.*) attributes the redness to the fact that "the blood is not absorbed in it", *viz.*, "in its flesh, so that all the blood is found between the skin and the flesh; hence, if one circumcises the child, it will lose all its blood" (Rashi, *a.l.*). The codes follow this interpretation, though (unlike Rashi) they do not explain why a fatal outcome is to be feared in the first case.

⁶³ The sources do not state whether a further seven days' delay is required after the disappearance of the symptoms here described. Chajes (rMaHaRaTZ, no.39) assumes this is not necessary, since the postponement in these cases is not due to any specific illness but to the presence of too little or too much blood, so that a circumcision may be accompanied by no loss of blood at all (invalidating the rite for religious reasons) or by excessive bleeding (leading to danger).

⁶⁴ Katzenelsohn (op. cit., p.231 f.) believes both symptoms refer to haemophilics whose condition is discussed in the Talmud in the same context.

⁶⁵ Preuss, pp. 189 and 285.

⁶⁶ Krauss, vol.i, p.255.

⁶⁷ W. Ebstein, Die Medizin im Neuen Testament und im Talmud, 1901, p.266 f. See also Junes, op. cit., in Révue, no.24 (1954), p.255.

⁶⁸ For a detailed summary of the relevant responsa, see 'Oth Shalom, op. cit., p.244 ff.

⁶⁹ For the sources, see 'Oth Shalom, loc. cit. Some authorities cited there insist on deferring the operation for seven days after the attack has subsided, because they do not regard jaundice as identical with the "green" sickness described in the Talmud. The latter's symptoms (they argue) were merely an indication of under-development and were now no longer found, whereas jaundice might be dangerous and should, therefore, be classified among the diseases requiring a seven-days' delay.

⁷⁰ bYevamoth 64b.

⁷¹ So Preuss, p.285; and Katzenelsohn, op. cit., p.266 ff. But Zimmels (p.90) points out that the sources do not necessarily attribute these deaths to excessive bleeding and that, in the responsa dealing with such cases, the cause of death was, in fact, quite often some other illness resulting from the circumcision of brothers. See also note 78 below.

⁷² By Fordyce in America; see Katzenelsohn, op. cit., p.267.

⁷³ TaZ, a.l., 1; and Bi'ur HaGRA, a.l., 4. Cf. supra, p.158.

⁷⁴ It is first reported by Karo (Beth Yoseph, Y.D., cclxiii) in the name of R. Mano'ah.

⁷⁵ Maimonides, Hil. Milah, i.18.

⁷⁶ rMaHaRaTZ, no.39.

⁷⁷ Landau, rNoda Biyehudah, Y.D., part ii, no.165; see also Preuss, p.285.

⁷⁸ Katzenelsohn, op. cit., p.233; so also Junes, op. cit., p.256. It is difficult to assume with Zimmels (p.90) that the mere postponement of the circumcision to adult age proves the brothers' deaths were due to weakness only and not to haemophilia (cf. note 71 above). This is certainly contradicted by Karo (Keseph Mishneh, on Maimonides, loc. cit.) who states expressly that the law operates "even if there was no sickness at all on account of the weakness in the blood; for if there had been any sickness, even the first son should not have been circumcised".

⁷⁹ See 'Otzar Hage'onim, op. cit., p.137 f.; and Sepher Ha'eshkol, op. cit., p.111.

⁸⁰ Asheri, Mo'ed Katan, iii.88.

⁸¹ Gen. Rabbah, xlviii.8; see L. Ginzberg, The Legends of the Jews, 1939, vol.vi, p.341 (note 118); and JE, vol.iv, p.94.

⁸² Cf. supra, p.182 f.

⁸³ Cf. Midrash Tanchuma, Lekh Lekha, xx; and Tazri'a, v.

⁸⁴ So Haggahoth Maimuni, Hil. Milah, i.10; Jacob Hagozer and his son Gershom, Zikhron Berith Larishonim, op. cit., pp. 91 ff. and 126 ff.; see also Beth Yoseph, loc. cit.; and M.A., dxxvi.20.

85 So *Sepher Ha'eshkol*, *loc. cit.*; and *Kol Bo*, cited in *Beth Yoseph*, *loc. cit.*

86 See Chajes, r*MaHaRaTZ*, *no.*27; and r*Noda Biyehudah*, part *i*, O.H., *no.*16.

87 According to Ezekiel Ellenbogen (r*Keneseth Yehezkel*, *no.*44), such an exhumation should be carried out even after a long time had elapsed since the burial; but Landau (r*Noda Biyehudah*, part *ii*, Y.D., *no.*164) permitted the opening of a grave for this purpose only immediately after the interment. See also Chajes, *loc. cit.*; *Novellae of Akivah Eger*, on Y.D., *cclxiii.*5; and *Gilyon MaHaRSHA*, on Y.D., *cccliii.*6.

88 Thus, Jacob Reischer (r*Shevuth Ya'akov*, part *ii*, *no.*82) ruled that an infant, who was sentenced to death by burning together with its mother because she had conceived it by a Christian, should be circumcised before the execution; see S. W. Baron, *The Jewish Community*, 1942, *vol.ii*, *p.*312. Cf. also Moses Schick's ruling (r*MaHaRaM Shik*, Y.D., *no.*243) that an inviable child must be circumcised.

Chapter Sixteen

1 Allbutt, *Greek Medicine*, *p.*391 (with reference to the "noble eulogy" of physicians by Basil of Caesarea in the 4th century).

2 Quoted by Friedenwald, *p.*78 *f.*

3 For the entire passage, and S. Schechter's comments on it, see Friedenwald, *p.*6 *ff.* The verse quoted here is also found frequently (with slight variations) in rabbinic literature; see j*Ta'anith*, *iii.*6; *Ex. Rabbah*, *xxi.*7; *Tanhuma, Miketz*, 10 (ed. Buber, *p.*199); *Pesikta Rabbathi*, '*Asser Te'asser*, 25 (ed. Friedmann, *p.*127a); and *Yalkut*, Job, 920. See also Hamburger, *RE, Suppl. i*, *p.*85.

4 m*Kiddushin*, *iv.*14.

5 See G. J. Litkowski, *Le Mal qu'on a dit des Médecins*, Paris, 1884. Stern, *Society*, *p.*24 *ff.*; and Charles L. Dana, "The Evil Spoken of Physicians", in *The Charaka Club*, *vol.i*, *p.*77; cited by Friedenwald, *p.*69 (note 2).

6 Galen, ed. Kuehn, *vol.xiv*, *p.*622; cited by Puschmann, *Medical Education*, *p.*124.

7 See *The Healing Art the Right Hand of the Church*, 1859, *p.*21.

8 See E. J. Withington, *Medical History from the Earliest Times*, 1894, *p.*238; quoted by Friedenwald, *p.*13 (note 25).

9 Quoted by Stern, *loc. cit.*

10 Preuss (*p.*28) mentions a special book on these interpretations by Chr. Reineke (1724).

11 Rashi, *Kiddushin* 82a.

12 So the Tosaphist Isaac Senior (on *Kiddushin* 82a). Nachmanides (*Torath Ha'adam, Sha'ar Hasakkanah*), too, regards the expression as applying only to negligent and reckless doctors. For references to further rabbinic comments, see Zimmels, *p.*170.

13 See Friedenwald, *p.*74.

14 Ibn Verga, *Shevet Yehudah*, Lemberg, 1846, *chpt.xli*; see Friedenwald, *p.*13 (note 25).

15 Duran, r*TaSHBeTZ*, part *iii*, *no.*82.

16 Edels, *MaHaRSHA*, on *Kiddushin* 82a. See Preuss, *p.*27; and Friedenwald, *p.*12.

[17] Eybeschuetz, *Kerethi Upelethi*, *Y.D.*, *clxxxviii*; cited by Kahana, in *Sinai*, *vol.xiv* (1950), *p.65* (note 21).

[18] See *supra*, *p.5*.

[19] Lampronti, *Pahad Yitzhak*, *s.v.* "*Tov*"; see Friedenwald, *p.12*.

[20] Except by some non-Jewish scholars, *e.g.* the lexicographers Buxdorf (*Lex. chaldaic.*, *s.v.* "*Rophe*") and Schenkel (*Bibellexikon*, *vol.i*, *p.252*); see Preuss, *p.28*.

[21] *'Avoth d'Rabbi Nathan*, *xxxvi.5*; see Preuss, *p.25*.

[22] Thus, Azulay, in his commentary on the passage (*Kiseh Rahamim*, *a.l.*) applies the condemnation only to physicians "who are not careful in their work".

[23] By L. Ginzberg, in a communication quoted by Friedenwald, *p.12*.

[24] The confusion is already found in the *Septuagint* which translates "רפאים" ("the shades") by "physicians" ("רופאים") and "ungodly" in the same chapter (Is. xxvi. 14 and 19 resp.). A similar error occurs in its rendering of "רפאים" in *Ps. lxxxviii.*11; see Kohut, *Aruch Completum*, *vol.vii*, *p.291*. The Samaritans made the same mistake in their translation of "רפאים" in *Deut. ii.*20; see Preuss, *p.14*.

[25] Friedenwald, *pp.* 69-83; *cf.* also *pp.* 84-98.

[26] *Ib.*, *p.83*.

[27] Abarvanel, on *Gen. xli* (beginning) in the name of earlier savants.

[28] See note 5 above.

[29] See, *e.g.*, Singer, *Prayer-Book*, *p.47*.

[30] See Friedenwald, *p.687*; and *JQR*, *vol.xiv* (1924), *p.375*.

[31] See S. Asaph, *Mekoroth Letoldoth Hahinnukh Beyisra'el*, 1930, *vol.ii*, *p.100 f.* For biographical details on Jacob Provencal, see *JE*, *vol.vii*, *p.30*.

[32] See Garrison, *Introduction*, *p.381*. *Cf. infra*, *p.212*.

[33] See C. Roth, *History of the Jews in England*, 1941, *p.132*.

[34] See L. Lewin, "Juedische Aerzte in Grosspolen", in *JJLG*, *vol.ix* (1911), *p.370* (note 3). "Doctor", like the Hebrew "rabbi", literally means "teacher". Hence the title originally belonged to university lecturers only; see Castiglioni, *History*, *p.401*. Its use to connote "medical practitioner" was, according to Puschmann (*Medical Education*, *p.262 f.*), introduced in the 13th century, and already employed in that sense by Chaucer (*Prol.* 411) in 1386; see *Oxford English Dictionary*, 1933, *vol.iii*, *s.v.* "doctor", *no.6*. But H. Haeser, (*Lehrbuch der Geschichte der Medizin*, 1875, *vol.i*, *p.828*) claims that it was first used for the medical men at Salerno.

[35] See Lewin, *op. cit.*, *p.393*.

[36] The combination of the theological and medical professions was also common in medieval Christianity (see Haeser, *op. cit.*, *p.831 ff.*), but partly for the reverse reason. Whilst the rabbis were attracted to medicine because it provided them with the income they lacked in their ecclesiastical office, medicine was drawn to the monasteries largely because of the facilities they alone offered: "To say that to the monks we owe the conservation of learning is not so true as to say that learned men betook themselves to the religious houses in order to find relief from turmoil, to secure the subsistence of life without its cares, to get access to books... When these advantages were to be had in the world, learning deserted the monasteries" (T. C. Allbutt, *Science and Medieval Thought*, 1901, *p.79* [note]).

[37] See C. Roth, *The Jewish Contribution to Civilisation*, 1943, *p.192*. See also A. A. Neuman, *The Jews in Spain*, 1948, *vol.ii*, *p.108*.

[38] See I. Muenz, *Die juedischen Aerzte im Mittelalter*, 1922, *p.117*.

[39] So McKenzie, *Infancy*, *p.43*.

CHAPTER XIV

[40] Quoted by Friedenwald, *p.*49.

[41] See Neuburger, *History, vol.i, p.*284; and Castiglioni, *History, p.*232.

[42] *Cf.* G. Sarton, *The History of Science and the New Humanism,* 1937, *p.*99 *f.* See also *supra, p.*9 *f.*

[43] D. Riesman, *Medicin in Modern Society,* 1939, *p.*4.

[44] See S. Adler, "Die Entwicklung des Schulwesens der Juden zu Frankfurt a/M bis zur Emanzipation", in *JJLG, vol.xix* (1928), *p.*250.

[45] See S. W. Baron, *The Jewish Community,* 1942, *vol.iii, p.*167 (note 18); and Zimmels, *p.*14 *f.*

[46] On the difficulties faced by Jewish students in gaining admission to European universities, even in Italy during the 16th century, see L. Lewin, "Die juedischen Studenten an der Universitaet Frankfurt a/O", in *JJLG, vol.xiv* (1921), *p.*217 *ff.*; Friedenwald, *p.*224 *ff.*; and C. Roth, "The Qualification of Jewish Physicians in the Middle Ages", in *Speculum, vol.xxviii* (1953), *p.*835.

[47] See Riesman, *op. cit., p.*5.

[48] "One has the impression that eager students, who attached themselves to distinguished scholars for the purpose of instruction on rabbinic lore, also learned what they had to teach in medical science and accompanied them on their professional visits. Thus they would attain a certain medical competence, and... could become medical practitioners themselves in due course. This was probably the means whereby most of the Jewish physicians of northern Europe, especially, obtained their training in the 12th and 13th centuries..." (Roth, in *Speculum, op. cit., p.*836).

[49] While under Moslem rule, however, Jews took up medicine through their intellectual absorption in their environment rather than through their exclusion from it; *cf.* Neuman, *loc. cit.* On the talmudic outlook as an important factor in promoting the Jewish devotion to medicine in the Middle Ages, see *supra,* chpt.I (note 145).

[50] According to Puschmann (*Medical Education, pp.* 31 and 158), medicine was probably taught at the high-schools of Tiberias, Sura and Pumpaditha. D. Hoffmann ("Mar Samuel", in *Jeschurun, vol.ix* [1922], *p.*26) did not doubt that it was included among the studies at Nehardea. Preuss (*p.*17), though he thought it unlikely that medicine was taught as a separate subject in these schools, assumed that medical matters were certainly discussed there. The Talmud itself mentions "the house of Benjamin, the Physician" (b*Sanhedrin* 99b) and "the disciples of Miniami, the Physician" at Machoza (b*Shabbath* 133b). S. Muntner believes this refers to "a special medical school"; he also speaks of "the medical schools of the Babylonian Amoraeans [which] flourished in Persian Babylon [and] entertained lively relations with Nitzovin, the capital of Roman Mesopotamia"; see his "The Antiquity of Asaph the Physician", in *Bulletin of the History of Medicine, vol.xxv* (1951), *p.*119.

[51] See I. Abrahams, *Jewish Life in the Middle Ages,* 1932, *p.*3389 *f.*

[52] Aknin, *Marpeh Lenephesh,* chpt.*vii.* See M. Guedemann, *Das juedische Unterrichtswesen,* 1873, *p.*42 *ff.*; M. Steinschneider, *Die Hebraeischen Uebersetzungen des Mittelalters,* 1893, *p.*33; and *JE, vol.vii, p.*267 *f.*

[53] Abbas, *Ya'ir Nethiv,* chpt.*xv.* See Guedemann, *op. cit., p.*147 *f.*; Steinschneider, *op. cit., p.*35; Asaph, *op. cit., p.*31; Friedenwald, *p.*222; and *JE, vol.i, p.*37 *f.*

[54] Ashkenazi, *Tzophnath Pane'ah,* MS written in 1364; see Asaph, *op. cit., vol.iii, p.*5.

[55] Hai, *Musar Haskel.* See Guedemann, *op. cit., p.*24; Asaph, *op. cit., vol.ii, p.*8; and Friedenwald, *loc. cit.*

[56] Ibn Tibbon, *Ethical Will.* See I. Abrahams, *Hebrew Ethical Wills,*

1926, *vol.i*, *p*.61; Asaph, *op. cit., vol.ii*, *p*.26; and Friedenwald, *p*.26.

[57] *Sepher Hasidim*, *no*.1469. The passage deals with a man's refusal to study medical books, as recommended by his father, on the grounds that he would then commit a sin if he did not treat the poor gratis and guilty if he caused a patient's death. He was told: "... since you were in a position to study and practise medicine but did not do so, you are regarded as if you killed [your potential patients thus dying]".

[58] Aldabi, *Shevilei 'Emunah*, Amsterdam, 1708, *chpt.iv*, *p*.45a. He declared: "All scholars must dilligently pursue the study of medicine, because we may desecrate the Sabbath as a result of a diagnosis; if somebody does not follow its advice, his blood is upon his head and he has forfeited his life. I have regarded it as right to seek and to search in the books of medicine..."; see Zimmels, *p*.1.

[59] Ibn Yachyah, *Shalsheleth Hakabbalah*, Warsaw, 1877, *p*.146. See Zimmels, *p*.2.

[60] See Asaph, *op. cit., vol.iii*, *p*.56; and Friedenwald, *p*.169.

[61] Already at about 1000 a Rabbi Abun is said to have maintained a college at Narbonne at which rabbinics and medicine were taught; see *JL, vol.iv*, *p*.31. In the 14th century medicine was a subject at a "Jewish School" in Paris which "rivalled the University of Paris"; see Friedenwald, *p*.222; and Castiglioni, "The Contribution", in *The Jews*, *p*.1026. More historically substantiated are the following two exploits. "In 1466", states C. Roth (*The Jewish Contribution, op. cit., p. 36 f.*), "the handful of Jews living in Sicily, numbering at the most no more than 100,000, received formal licence from the king to open their own properly constituted University, with faculties of Medicine, Law, and presumably the Humanities". In 1564 David Provencal published a prospectus outlining a plan for establishing in Mantua a "Jewish University" which was to include a medical school, so that Jews would not need to attend Christian colleges involving a "sinful negligence of *Torah* studies"; see M. Guedemann, "Ein Projekt zur Gruendung einer juedischen Univirsitaet aus dem 16. Jahrhundert", in *Berliner Festschrift*, 1903, *p*.171; Castiglioni, *op. cit.*, *p*.1026 f.; Baron, *op. cit., vol.ii*, *p*.191; Friedenwald, *p*.221; and Roth, in *Speculum, op. cit., p*.837 f.

[62] Adreth, *rRaSHBA*, *no*.417. See Asaph, *op. cit., vol.ii*, *p*.55; Friedenwald, *p*.680; Neuman, *op. cit., vol.ii*, *p*.131; Zimmels, *p*.20; and *JE, vol.i*.

[63] *rRaSHBA*, part *iv*, *no*.74 (*ed.* Jerusalem, 1901, *p*.28); see Zimmels, *p*.15. So also Menachem Mendel Auerbach, *'Atereth Zekeinim*, on *O.H., cccvii*.17.

[64] See Lewin, "Juedische Aerzte in Grosspolen", *op. cit., p*.395.

[65] Emden, *rShe'ilath Yavetz*, *no*.41. See Adler, *op. cit., p*.259; and Zimp.213.

[66] So Nachmanides; see R. Margulies, *Viku'ah HaRaMBaN*, *p*.9; cited mels, *p*.20. by Zimmels, *p*.1. For that reason Elijah of Vilna, though interested in all sciences, did not study medicine; see J. L. Maimon, *Sepher HaGRA*, 1954, *vol.i*, *p*.181.

[67] *Cf.* Simon Duran, *rTaSHBeTZ*, part *ii*, *no*.254; see Zimmels, *p*.15.

[68] So *Sepher Hasidim*, *no*.1470.

[69] Among the classic authors who refer to the Oath are Erotian (*c.* 50 *C.E.*) and Scribonius Largus (43 *C.E.*); see Garrison, *Introduction*, *p*.96 (note). Even in the early Middle Ages the Oath was probably known only at second hand, since the text is not found in any medical MSS of the period; see Loren M. McKiney, "Medical Ethics and Etiquette in the

Early Middle Ages", in *Bulletin of the History of Medicine, vol.xxvi* (1952), *p.*19 (note 29).

70 *Cf.* Sidney Smith, "The History and Development of Forensic Medicine", in *BMJ*, March 24, 1951, *p.*600.

71 See W. H. S. Jones, *The Doctor's Oath*, 1924, *p.*29. G. Sarton (in *Isis, vol.xx* [1932], *p.*262; and *vol.xxxviii* [1947], *p.*94 *f.*) assumes there were even earlier texts of it. The Arab version is also found in Indian literature; see E. Haas, "Hippocrates und die indische Medizin des Mittelalters", in *ZDMG, vol.xxxi* (1877), *p.*662; and R. Roth, "Indische Medizin", in *ZDMG, vol.xxvi* (1872), *p.*448.

72 So I. S. Reid, cited by Jones, *op. cit., p.*53 (note).

73 See Rashdall, *Universities, vol.i, p.*380.

74 For details on the importance of the Hebrew language in medieval medicine, see Friedenwald, *p.*146 *ff.* Already in the middle of the 9th century the influence of Jewish physicians among the Arabs was so great that Caliph Mutawakkil permitted Jewish doctors to be instructed in Hebrew or Syrian; see *JL, vol.iv, p.*26. Similar conditions evidently still existed in 1497 when King Manuel of Portugal allowed Jewish physicians and surgeons who had been, or were to be, converted and did not understand Latin to study Hebrew books; see Zimmels, *p.*176 (note); and Roth, in *Speculum, op. cit., p.*835.

75 We may here ignore the oaths of Asaf Judaeus and Amatus Lusitanus (see *supra, p.*181) which were never in practical use by Jewish students.

76 b*Nedarim* 20a and 22a. On the ethical significance of this attitude, see M. Lazarus, *Die Ethik des Judentums*, 1911, *vol.ii, p.*327 *f.*

77 Vows are praiseworthy only if they serve to strengthen the deponent's resolution to overcome a personal vice, and even then they should not become habitual (*ib.,* 7).

78 See Moses Schreiber, r*Hatham Sopher, H.M., no.*90.

79 *Cf.* Roth, in *Speculum, op. cit., p.*839.

80 *Cf.* the delay of the first Jewish member of the British Parliament taking his seat from 1847, when he was elected, to 1858, when the parliamentary oath was amended to enable a Jew to take it; see *JE, vol.x, p.*502.

81 See Friedenwald, *p.*227. A precedent for Jewish physicians swearing by the Pentateuch already existed some three centuries earlier; see Roth, in *Speculum, op. cit., p.*840.

82 So M. Meyerhof, in *Rotary Bulletin*, Cairo, February 1933; cited in *Isis, vol.xxii* (1934), *p.*222.

83 *Viz.,* rabbis (*Y.D., ccxliii.*3), judges (*H.M., viii*), ritual slaughterers (*Y.D., i*), synagogue readers (*O.H., liii.*4 *ff.*; and *dlxxxi.*1, gloss) and circumcisers (*Y.D., cclxiv.*1, gloss; see *supra, p.*192).

84 See *JE, vol.ix, p.*366 *f.*

85 Asaf Judaeus, too, abjured his pupils: "Divulge not any secret entrusted to thee", but this clause probably reflects the influence of the Hippocratic Oath rather than of Jewish sources; see Friedenwald, *p.*22; and I. Simon, "Le 'Serment Médical' d'Assaph", in *Révue, no.*9 (1951), *p.*38.

86 See *OY, vol.vi, p.*66 *f.*

87 In fact, Jewish law mentions professional secrecy only in regard to rabbinical judges: they are not permitted to divulge their dissent from a verdict reached by the majority, as such indiscretion would amount to "tale-bearing" (*H.M., xix.*1).

88 Thus, Israel Meir Kagan (*Haphetz Hayim*, ed. Hermon, Frankfurt, 1925, *p.*222 *f.*) affirms the right to disclose one's knowledge of an illness

in a person whom another intends to marry. This view is also accepted by "the better theological opinion" of the Catholic Church; see F. J. Connell, *Morals in Politics and Professions*, 1946, p.126; cited by J. Fletcher, *Morals and Medicine*, 1955, p.57 (note 31).

89 See *supra*, p.7; *cf.* also note 57 above.

90 Azulay, *Birkei Yoseph, a.l.*, 5.

91 *Tur, Y.D., cccxxxvi.*

92 But as rabbis are so restrained only if they are under 40 years of age (*ib.*, 31, gloss), it may be inferred that the restriction on physicians is similarly limited to practitioners of little experience as well as of inferior competence.

93 See *infra*, pp. 220 and 225 f.

94 *rRaMBaM, no.*27 (*ed.* Freimann, Jerusalem, 1934, p.24). Doctors living far from the synagogue were also exempted from the communal ban on holding religious services in private homes (*rRIVaSH, no.*331); see Neuman, *op. cit., vol.ii*, p.110.

95 *rRaSHBA*, cited in *Beth Yoseph, O.H., xliii. Cf. supra*, chpt.II (note 129).

96 This question was first raised in the 17th century by the French court physician Montalto, who justified his riding in a coach on the Sabbath to visit his royal patients in Paris in a lengthy dissertation; see Cecil Roth, "Elie Montalto et sa Consultation sur le Sabbat", in *REJ, vol.xciv* (1933), p.113 *ff.*; Friedenwald, p.474; and Kahana, in *Sinai, op. cit.*, p.225 *ff.* A similar decision was reached by the rabbinate in Posen in 1793; see S. Krauss, *Geschichte der juedischen Aerzte*, 1930, p.115; and Zimmels, p.182 (note 119). The problem was also discussed by Gershon Ashkenazi (*r'Avodath Hagershuni*, part *i*, no.123) in the 17th century and by Moses Schreiber (*rHatham Sopher, H.M.*, no.194) early in the 19th century; see Kahana, *loc. cit.*

97 See Hillel Posek, in *Haposek*, July 1950; and Elijah Klatzkin, *rMilu'ei 'Even, no.* 19; cited by Kahana, *op. cit.*, p.230 *f. Cf. supra*, chpt.VI (note 25).

98 This is permitted, even if another doctor is available, because "one is not destined to be healed by any [random] person" (J. Reischer, *rShevuth Ya'akov*, part *i, no.*86), and because healing the sick is like attending to "a business which cannot be put off without irretrievable loss" (*Hamudei Dani'el*, cited in *P.T., Y.D., ccclxxx.*1); see *Sedei Hemed, s.v.* " 'Aveluth", no.44. But for services rendered whilst in mourning a doctor should charge only what he needs; see Zimmels, p.182 (note 113).

99 Colon, *rMaHaRIK, no.*88; see Zimmels, p.18.

100 Hagiz, *'Eleh Hamitzvoth*, commandment *no.*262. For further details, see Kahana, *op. cit.*, p.236.

101 *Cf. supra*, p.205.

102 On the immunity from taxation granted to scholars in ancient Persia and medieval Islam, as well as to European rabbis up to the 18th century, see Baron, *op. cit., vol.ii*, p.80. Royal patrons in Spain sometimes freed their favoured physicians from taxes and granted them other privileges; see Neuman, *loc. cit.*

103 b*Baba Bathra* 21a. See Preuss, p.26 *f.*; and *JE, vol.viii*, p.409 *f.*

104 A slight variant in the reading of the *Tur* (*H.M., clvi*) may be construed as excluding from the privilege (along with secular teachers) not doctors, but teachers of medicine; see Epstein, *A.H., a.l.*, 4. But *cf.* also *TaZ, a.l.*, 1.

105 b*Sanhedrin* 17b. In the Palestinian Talmud (j*Kiddushin, iv.* end)

this prohibition is extended to all (not merely to scholars); see Preuss, p.26.

[106] Maimonides, *Hil. De'oth*, iv.23; cf. *Hil. Sanhedrin*, i.10.

[107] See Lewin, *op. cit.*, p.371 *ff*. He draws examples from numerous Polish-Jewish communities during the 16th-18th centuries.

Chapter Seventeen

[1] See Sigerist, *Civilisation*, p.102. On the whole subject, see H. E. Sigerist, "The History of Medical Licensure", in *Journal of the American Medical Association*, vol.civ (1935), p.1057 *ff*.

[2] See Puschmann, *Medical Education*, p.14.

[3] See Puschmann, *op. cit.*, pp. 97 and 121.

[4] Pliny, *Hist. Nat.*, xxix.8. See Puschmann, *loc. cit.*; and Preuss, p.32.

[5] See Sigerist, *Civilisation*, p.101.

[6] See T. Meyer-Steineg, *Geschichte des roemischen Aerztenstandes*, 1907.

[7] See Browne, *Arabian Medicine*, p.40; and Sigerist, *Medicine*, p.126.

[8] See Neuburger, *History*, vol.i, p.381 *f*. (note).

[9] See Sigerist, *Civilisation*, p.102; and *Medicine*, p.127.

[10] For the text of Frederick's law, see Robert Ritter von Toeply, *Studien zur Geschichte der Anatomie im Mittelalter*, 1898; transl. J. J. Walsh, *The Popes and Science*, 1912, p.419 *ff*.

[11] Bulaeus, *Hist. Universitat.*, Paris, 1673, tom.vi, p.11; quoted by Puschmann, *op. cit.*, p.336 *f*.

[12] See Puschmann, *loc. cit.*

[13] Henry Barnes, "On Some Extracts from the Diaries of Bishop Nicolson", in *New York Medical Journal*, vol.lxxxii (1905), p.1211.

[14] Statute 3 Henry VIII c.11 (1511). This law was virtually repealed only by Statute 18 Geo II c.15 (1745).

[15] See D. Guthrie, *A History of Medicine*, 1945, p.151.

[16] See Castiglioni, *History*, p.376; and C. Roth, "The Qualification of Jewish Physicians in the Middle Ages", in *Speculum*, vol.xxviii (1953), p.838 *f*.

[17] See Friedenwald, p.559; and Roth, *loc. cit.*

[18] By C. Wall, *The History of the Surgeon's Company*, 1937, p.22.

[19] On the history of these degrees, see R. R. James, "Licences to Practise Medicine and Surgery issued by the Archbishops of Canterbury 1588-1775", in *Janus*, vol.xli (1937), p.97 *ff*.; and *Medico-Legal Review*, vol.xi (1942), p.226 *f*.

[20] By Wall, *op. cit.*, p.23. The last Archbishop's licence was actually granted only in 1880; see James, *loc. cit.*; and *Lancet*, 1942, part ii, p.379. There are also several entries in the Diary of Bishop Nicolson (1655-1727) showing applications for licences made to him; see Barnes, *op. cit.*, p.1211.

[21] 21 & 22 *Vict.* c.90. The Act required the Archbishop to furnish the General Medical Council with information on the courses of study laid down for the candidates.

[22] See sources cited in notes 19 and 20 above.

[23] t*Baba Kamma*, ix.3.

[24] Through the rabbis the community would "control prices, supervise markets, check weights and measures, restrict speculation, assign streets to various crafts, regulate wages, hours of work and other employer-employee relations, prohibit interest, protect *bona fide* creditors, and gen-

erally... safeguard the interests of weaker members of society against the encroachments of a powerful minority" (S. W. Baron, *The Jewish Community*, 1942, *vol.i*, *p.*130; *cf. pp.* 126 *ff.*, 170 and 202 *ff.*; and *vol.ii*, *p.*208 *ff.*, *et pass.*).

25 By Abraham Ashkenazi, r*Ma'asei 'Avraham*, Y,D., no.55; see Zimmels, *p.*18 *f.*

26 Azulay, *Shiyurei Berakhah*, O.H., *cccxxviii.*9.

27 Samuel Florentin, r*'Olath Shemu'el*, Salonica, 1776, no.108. For later quotations of this statement, see Kahana, in *Sinai*, *vol.xiv* (1950), *p.*222.

28 See Castiglioni, *History*, *p.*44.

29 *Hammurabi Code*, §215-223; see Preuss, *p.*32.

30 See *The Vendidad*, ed. J. Darmsteter, in *The Sacred Books of the East*, ed. F. M. Mueller, 1880, *vol.iv*, *p.*83 *f.*; cited by Sigerist, *Civilisation*, *p.*101. See also Browne, *Arabian Medicine*, *p.*22.

31 See E. A. W. Budge. *Syrian Anatomy, Pathology and Therapeutics*, 1913, *vol.i*, *p.clxxiv.*

32 See LaWall, *Pharmacy*, *p.*120.

33 See Garrison, *Introduction*, *p.*170 *f.*

34 See Garrison, *op. cit.*, *p.*169.

35 See Preuss, *p.*32.

36 Cited by Preuss, *p.*32.

37 See note 4 above.

38 See Guthrie, *op. cit.*, *p.*111.

39 See Allbutt, *Greek Medicine*, *p.*476.

40 See *JE*, *vol.vii*, *p.*12.

41 See LaWall, *loc. cit.*

42 Castiglioni, *loc. cit.*

43 t*Baba Kamma*, ix.3.

44 t*Gittin*, iii.13.

45 *Minhath Bikkurim*, a.l.

46 t*Gittin*, iii.13.

47 See Friedenwald, *p.*20.

48 *Cf. supra*, chpt.VI (note† 91).

49 See Maimonides, *Hil. Rotze'ah*, v.6. This law, though based on the Talmud (b*Makkoth* 8a), is not codified in the *Shulhan 'Arukh*. The distinction has been thus explained: A physician whose treatment failed did not, during the fatal operation, perform a religious precept, whereas the reasonable chastisement of a child invariably constitutes a religious duty (*Yad 'Avraham*, on Y.D., *cccxxxvi.*1); see also Azulay, *Birkei Yoseph*, Y.D., *cccxxxvi.*7.

50 The reference to the penalty of "exile"—long after the withdrawal of capital jurisdiction from Jewish courts (*cf. H.M.*, *cdxxv.*1, gloss)— is rather anomalous. It can only be explained as meant to indicate the measure of guilt for which the offending physician must seek atonement by corresponding expiatory acts.

51 t*Makkoth*, ii.4.

52 See *Mechilta* and Rashi, on *Ex. xxi.*14. Cf. Azulay, *Birkei Yoseph*, Y.D., *cccxxxvi.*6 (end). But Jacob Ettlinger (r*Binyan Tziyon*, no.111) doubts whether the physician is altogether liable in these circumstances, since the accident did not involve any actionable intent or negligence.

53 Nachmanides, cited in *Beth Yoseph*, Y.D., *cccxxxvi.*

54 See *H.M.*, xxv. Cf. Baron, *op. cit.*, *vol.i*, *pp.* 128 and 142.

55 Joshua Falk, *Perishah*, Y.D., *cccxxxvi.*7.

56 Luria, r*MaHaRSHaL*, quoted in *BaH*, Y.D., *cccxxxvi.*

57 *Cf. supra*, *p.*92.

(CHAPTER XVII)

⁵⁸ According to Adreth (rRaSHBA, cited in *Beth Yoseph, O.H., cxxviii*), the exception is due to the religious character of the circumcision rite and to the possibility that the child may have been prematurely born and thus proved in any case inviable; cf. *Haggahoth Maimuni, Hil. Nesi'ath Kapayim, xv*.1. The second consideration, at any rate, does not apply to a doctor who accidentally killed his patient.

⁵⁹ See I. Jakobovits, in *Hama'or, vol.vi, no*.5 (June 1956), *p*.10 *ff*. In present-day Canon Law, a cleric who, in the absence of medical assistance, intervenes the save a human life does not incur "irregularity", even if his action resulted in the patient's death; see S. Woywood, *A Practical Commentary on the Code of Canon Law*, 1926, *vol.i, p*.534.

⁶⁰ The omission may also be connected with the exclusion from the liabilities listed in this chapter of physicians "who heal the sick with medicines, laxatives, drugs, baths and resting". According to Simon Duran (rTaSHBeTZ, part *iii, no*.82; see Friedenwald, *p*.20 *f*. [note 7]; and Zimmels, *p*.181 *f*. [note 110]), such healers cannot be sued for damages as they do not "wound" their patients, the laws of compensation applying only to surgeons "who cure wounds with the work of their hands... [or] metallic instruments".

Chapter Eighteen

¹ *Hammurabi Code*, §§215, 216, 221-223 and 227; see Preuss, *p*.34.
² See Puschmann, *Medical Education, p*.16.
³ See Puschmann, *op. cit., p*.25; Castiglioni, *History, p*.60; Preuss, *p*.15; and E. A. W. Budge, *Syrian Anatomy, Pathology and Therapeutics*, 1913, *vol.i, p.clxxiv f*.
⁴ See Castiglioni, *History, p*.66 *f*.; Sigerist, *Medicine, p*.112; and Preuss, *p*.15.
⁵ See Sigerist, *Medicine, p*.114 *f*.; and Stern, *Society, p*.7.
⁶ See Stern, *Society, p*.6.
⁷ Hippocrates, *Praecept.*, ed. Littré, *vol.ix, p*.255; cited by Preuss, *p*.35.
⁸ See Preuss, *p*.35.
⁹ Pliny, *Nat. Hist., xxix*.8.
¹⁰ See Budge, *op. cit., p.clxxv f*.; and Preuss, *p*.35.
¹¹ See Sigerist, *Medicine, p*.115.
¹² *Justinian Code, x*.53.9; see Allbutt, *Greek Medicine, p*.454.
¹³ See Diepgen, *Die Theologie, p*.23.
¹⁴ See Sigerist, *Medicine, p*.117. Cf. *supra*, chpt.XVI (note 36).
¹⁵ See Castiglioni, *History, p*.390 *f*.
¹⁶ See Garrison, *Introduction, p*.236.
¹⁷ See Garrison, *Introduction, p*.304.
¹⁸ See Sigerist, *Medicine, p*.122.
¹⁹ Josephus, *Antiquities, iv*.8.33.
²⁰ See Preuss, *p*.34.
²¹ m*Baba Kamma, viii*.1.
²² b*Baba Kamma* 85a. See Preuss, *p*.34.
²³ See Castiglioni, *History, p*.397.
²⁴ Isaac Israeli, "Doctor's Guide", *no*.40; see D. Kaufmann, "Isak Israelis Propaedeutik fuer Aerzte", in his *Gesammelte Schriften*, 1915, *vol.iii, p*.272; and Friedenwald, *p*.26.
²⁵ b*Ta'anith* 21b. See Preuss, *p*.38 *f*.

26 See Friedenwald, *p.22.*

27 *"Medicina Pauperum"*, see Ludwig Venetianer, *Asaph Judaeus*, 1917, *p.168 ff.; HE, vol.v, p.41;* and C. Roth, *The Jewish Contribution to Civilisation,* 1943, *p.193* (note). A similar book was composed by the favourite disciple of Isaac Israeli; see Ibn al Tezar, *The Book of Food for the Journey (The Poor Man's Medicine),* translated into Hebrew by Uri Barzel, in *Koroth, vol.i* (1955), *p.186 ff.*

28 Israeli, *op. cit., no.*30; see Kaufmann, *op. cit., p.*270; and Friedenwald, *p.25.*

29 See Friedenwald, *p.368.*

30 Zahalon, *'Otzar Hahayim,* Venice, 1683, Introduction; see Friedenwald, *p.273.*

31 See J. C[assuto], "Aus dem aeltesten Protokollbuch der portugiesisch-juedischen Gemeinde in Hamburg", in *JJLG, vol.xi* (1913), *p.16 f.*

32 See L. Lewin, "Juedische Aerzte in Grosspolen", in *JJLG, vol.ix* (1911), *p.406 ff. Cf.* also *supra, chpt.*XVI (note 102).

33 Nachmanides, *Torath Ha'adam, Sha'ar Hasakkanah,* ed. Warsaw, 1840, *p.*6d; see Zimmels, *p.16.*

34 *Tur, Y.D., cccxxxvi.*

35 See *supra, p.4.*

36 The Talmud (b*Berakhoth* 29a; b*Nedarim* 37a; and j*Nedarim, iv.*3) applied this principle of *imitatio Dei* originally to the gratuitous teaching and administration of the divine law, deriving the rule from the verse: "Behold, I have taught you statutes and ordinances..." (*Deut. iv.*5). The rule was then transferred to the performance of any religious precept. See Maimonides, *Hil. Talmud Torah, i.*7; and *JE, vol.v, p.*43. *Cf. supra, p.*106.

37 *Sepher Hasidim, no.*810.

38 See, *e.g.,* the early 14th century work *Kaphtor Vapherach,* by Eshtori Haparchi, *chpt.xliv* (*ed.* H. Edelmann, Berlin, 1852, *p.*100).

39 In fact, as already laid down in the Mishnah (m*Bekhoroth, iv.*6), any remuneration paid to judges invalidates their judgment.

40 See S. W. Baron, *The Jewish Community,* 1942, *vol.ii, p.*78 *ff., et pass.* According to I. Elbogen (*JL, vol.iv, p.*1205), the rabbinate was everywhere a fixed, paid office after 1350.

41 For some of the numerous arguments to vindicate the payment of regular salaries to rabbis and teachers, see Tosaphoth, *Bekhoroth* 29a; Simon Duran, r*TaSHBeTZ,* part *i, nos.* 145 and 147; Mordecai Jaffe, *Levush, Y.D., ccxlvi.*5; and Joel Sirkes, r*BaH, nos.* 51 and 52.

42 It is, of course, significant that Maimonides, who strongly denounced the professionalisation of the rabbinate (*Mishnah Commentary,* on *'Avoth, iv.*5), himself made his livelihood from the professional pursuit of medicine.

43 See Preuss, *p.15 f.*

44 See A. A. Neuman, *The Jews in Spain,* 1948, *vol.ii, p.*110 *f.*

45 See Baron, *op. cit., vol.ii, pp.* 115 and 329. *Cf. supra, pp.* 108 and 213.

46 Abraham ben Solomon ibn Tazrath (a pupil of Adreth), *Hukkath Hadayanim, no.*156; quoted by S. Asaph, *Mekoroth Letoldoth Hahinnukh Beyisra'el,* 1948, *vol.iv, p.*15.

47 Nachmanides, cited in *Beth Yoseph, Y.D., cccxxxvi.* See also *infra, p.*230.

48 See also *supra, p.*117 *f.*

49 Eleazar Fleckeles, r*Teshuvah Me'ahavah,* part *iii, Y.D., cccxxxvi.* Subsequently his verdict was used as a precedent for similar decisions by other rabbis; see Schalom Schachna, *Mishmereth Shalom,* 1930, part *ii,*

*p.*99; and David Katz (Bisteritz), *Beth David*, part *ii*, Y.D., *cccxxxvi* (ed. Vacz, 1911, *p.*306).

⁵⁰ r*RaSHBa*, no.472. Zimmels (*p.*158) found the case before Adreth as the only one of its kind.

⁵¹ Often circumcisers were so keen to perform the act that they were prepared to pay for the privilege; see Zimmels, *p.*158.

⁵² Emden, cited by J. Glassberg, *Zikhron Berith Larishonim*, 1892, *p.*193.

⁵³ Rashi, *Kiddushin* 82a; see Schachna, *loc. cit.*; and *supra, p.*203.

⁵⁴ b*Baba Metzi'a* 58a.

⁵⁵ Hence, synagogue readers should not be engaged and paid for services rendered on the Sabbath only (*O.H.*, *cccvi*.5), unless the salaried appointment is by the week or month (*ib.*, gloss); see also *O.H.*, *dlxxxv*.5; and *TaZ, a.l.,* 7.

⁵⁶ Weil's opinion is quoted by Bruna; see following note.

⁵⁷ Bruna, *responsa*, Salonica, 1798, no.114; see Kahana, in *Sinai, vol.xiv* (1950), *p.*233. On Bruna, see *JE, vol.vi, p.*667.

⁵⁸ A summary of these views is given by Kahana, *op. cit., p.*233 *ff.*

⁵⁹ So the 19th century rabbi of Smyrna, Hayim Modai; see Kahana, *op. cit., p.*234.

⁶⁰ So *Joseph Te'umim, P.M.*, on *O.H., TaZ, cccvi*.4.

⁶¹ So S. Schiffer, r*Sithri Umagini*, 1932, part *i*, no.15 (2).

⁶² Zahalon, *loc. cit.*; see Zimmels, *p.*182 (note 114).

⁶³ Schreiber, r*Hatham Sopher, H.M.*, no.194; see Kahana, *op. cit., p.*235.

⁶⁴ Moses Schick, r*MaHaRaM Shik, Y.D.*, no.343; see Grunwald, *Kol Bo, p.*58.

⁶⁵ b*Ta'anith* 20b. See Preuss, *p.*398; and *cf. supra, p.*224.

⁶⁶ b*Baba Kamma* 116b; and b*Yevamoth* 106a. See Tosaphoth, *a.l.*; and *Be'er Hagolah, Y.D., cccxxxvi*.8 and 9.

⁶⁷ Ibn Tuvvah, in r*TaSHBeTZ*, part *iv* (*Hut Hameshulash*), no.20; see Zimmels, *p.*17. On Ibn Tuvvah, see *JE, vol.xii, p.*68 *f.*

⁶⁸ Ibn Zimra, r*RaDBaZ*, part *iii*, no.986 (556). For other responsa on the subject, see Zimmels, *p.*177 (note 44).

⁶⁹ Zahalon, *loc. cit.*

⁷⁰ See LaWall, *Pharmacy, p.*352 *ff.* On the resultant wrangle between the apothecaries and the physicians and the subsequent victory of the former, see also Garrison, *Introduction, p.*294.

⁷·¹ See LaWall, *Pharmacy, p.*492.

⁷² See LaWall, *Pharmacy, p.*499.

⁷³ See LaWall, *Pharmacy, p.*524 *ff.*

Chapter Nineteen

¹ Maimonides, *Hil. Sanhedrin, ii.*1. This is not, however, directly mentioned in the Talmud among the necessary qualifications (b*Sanhedrin* 17a; and b*Menahoth* 65a).

² David ibn Zimra, *RaDBaZ, a.l.*

³ See *supra, p.*33 *f.*

⁴ For collection of the most important sources, see Kahana, in *Sinai, vol.xiv* (1950), *p.*63 *ff.*; *Sedei Hemed, Ma'arekheth Yom Hakippurim,* no.3; *'Otzar Haposkim, E.H., vol.i* (1947), *pp.* 42 and 61; Israel Lipschuetz, *Tiph'ereth Yisra'el*, on *Shabbath, xix.*2; and Zimmels, *pp.* 24 *f.*, 180 *f.* (notes 96-107) and 193 (notes 172-173).

5 A. H. Merzbach, "The Religious Physician and His Mission in the Jewish State", in *Dath Yisra'el Umedinath Yisra'el*, 1951, p.151.

6 b*Baba Bathra* 159a.

7 Maimonides, *Hil. Yesodei Hatorah, vii.*7.

8 See *JE, vol.i,* p.169 *f.*, and *vol.v,* p.277 *ff.*

9 See b*Rosh Hashanah* 21b.

10 So expressly *Maggid Mishnah,* on *Hil. Hovel Umazzik, v.*4; but *cf.* Maimonides, *Hil. Rotze'ah, iv.*8 and 9.

.11 The evidence of non-Jews is generally inadmissible (*H.M., xxxiv.*19) "even if they are presumed not to lie" (*SeMA, a.l.,* 48; based on *glosses* on Asheri, *Gittin, i.*10). This view regards non-Jews as being categorically excluded by the scriptural insistence on "his brother" (*Deut.xix.*19), *i.e.* his fellow-Jew, in connection with the laws on evidence. But others hold that the original restriction applied only to heathens whose truthfulness was always suspect; hence, their evidence would be valid in certain circumstances when their honesty would not be in question. So R. Yakar, in glosses on Asheri, *loc. cit.*; and Simon Duran, r*TaSHBeTZ*, part *i, no.*75. See also *Beth Yoseph* and *BaH, H.M., xxxiv. Cf. OY, vol.iii,* p.258; and *TE, vol.v,* p.337 *ff.*

12 See *supra, pp.* 60 and 66, and *chpt.*IV (note 45).

13 See *supra,* p.127 *f.*

14 See *supra,* p.196.

15 See Kahana, in *Sinai, op. cit.,* p.63 (note 7).

16 The fact that Maimonides, as already noted (note 1 above), required the members of the *Sanhedrin* to have some knowledge of medicine has been taken to imply that he, too, doubted the absolute validity of the physicians' evidence before rabbinical courts; see Judah Assad, r*MaHaRYA,* Y.D., *no.*193. Cf. also note 19 below.

17 See b*Baba Kamma* 91a. Cf. *supra,* p.227.

18 See m*Makkoth, iii.*11; and Maimonides, *Hil. Sanhedrin, xvii.*2 and 3.

19 See b*Sanhedrin* 78a and b. But according to Rashi (*a.l.*) and Obadiah of Bartinura (m*Makkoth, iii.*11), these estimates were made by the judges themselves (*cf.* notes 1 and 16 above). Yet Maimonides (*Hil. Rotze'ah, ii.*8) states expressly that the fatal character of certain injuries was to be determined by "the physicians". *Cf.* also *OY, vol.vii,* p.226.

20 See b*Kiddushin* 74a. But a midwife's evidence, to be valid, must be given immediately following the birth (*H.M., cclxxvii.*12). For further conditions, see *P.T., a.l.,* 5. Cf. also note 47 below.

21 See j*Shabbath, vi.*2. On the legal value of such competence, see *supra,* p.36.

22 I.e., if a gravely ill husband desired it to take effect only if he subsequently died from the illness afflicting him at the time, so that it must be ascertained whether that illness did, in fact, afterwards cause his death (and thus validate the divorce).

23 b*Gittin* 72b. So also Maimonides, *Hil. Gerushin, ix.*18.

24 r*RaSHBA*, cited in *Beth Yoseph, E.H., cxlv.*

25 See *supra,* p.xli *f.*

26 See *supra, chpt.*X (note 36).

27 See m*Bekhoroth, iv.*4 and 5. See Preuss, p.43.

28 See Preuss, p.20.

29 See m*Bekhoroth, iv.*4; and b*Sanhedrin* 33a.

30 See b*Nazi*r 52a.

3,1 b*Niddah* 22b. See Preuss, p.483.

32 The physicians concluded that the woman suffered from some internal wound or mole from which they had lost the suspicious objects (which

looked like red peals and red hairs respectively). The account then continues: "Let [the discharge] be placed in [tepid] water [for twenty-four hours]; if it dissolves, [the woman] is unclean [because the discharge proved to be congealed blood]".

33 Karo, *Beth Yoseph*, *Y.D.*, *cxci.*

34 So Asheri, *Tosaphei HaROSH*, on *Niddah* 22b; Joseph Colon, r*MaHaRIK*, *no.*159; and Meir Rothenburg, r*MaHaRaM*, *ed. Mekitzei Nirdamim*, 1891, *no.*53.

35 But the proviso is not made if the claim is corroborated by the woman's own observation (*ib.*).

36 Isserles, *Darkei Mosheh*, *Y.D.*, *cxci.*

37 So Meir of Lublin, r*MaHaRaM Lublin*, *no.*111; and Meir Eisenstadt, r*Panim Me'iroth*, part *i*, *no.*12.

38 See Kahana, in *Sinai*, *op. cit.*, *p.*63 f.

39 Schreiber, r*Hatham Sopher*, *Y.D.*, *no.*158; see also *E.H.*, part *ii*, *no.*82. For further discussions on this attitude, see Moses Schick, r*MaHaRaM Shik*, *Y.D.*, *nos.* 155 and 243; S. M. Schwadron, r*MaHaRSHaM*, part *i*, *nos.* 13, 24, 25 and 114, and part *ii*, *no.*72; Chayim Halberstam, r*Divrei Hayim*, part *ii*, *no.*77; *Sedei Hemed*, *loc. cit.*; and Kahana, in *Sinai*, *op. cit.*, *p.*65.

40 A. Gruenhut, r*Mosheh Ha'ish*, *no.*28.

41 Mordecai Banet, r*Parashath Mordekhai*, *Y.D.*, *no.*10.

42 See *supra*, *p.xli* f. Cf. r*Divrei Hayim*, part *i*, *no.*31.

43 See *D.T.*, *Y.D.*, *clxxvii.*98. Zimmels (*p.*181 [note 107]), too, quotes several authorities in support of this view.

44 So Jacob Reischer, r*Shevuth Ya'akov*, part *i*, *no.*65.

45 So r*MaHaRSHaM*, part *i*, *no.*13.

46 See *Sedei Hemed*, *loc. cit.* On the trustworthiness of non-observant Jews, see *D.T.*, *Y.D.*, *clxxvii.*97 and 98; and r*MaHaRSHaM*, part *i*, *nos.* 13 and 24. On the reliability of non-Jewish doctors, see Kahana, in *Sinai*, *op. cit.*, *p.*221 f.; and *TE*, *vol.v*, *p.*343. Cf. also note 11 above.

47 So r*MaHaRSHaM*, part *ii*, *no.*164; cited in *D.T.*, *Y.D.*, *cxci.*35. On the evidence of midwives, see also Gumbiner, *M.A.*, *dxviii.*8; and sources cited by Zimmels, *p.*193 (note 172). Cf. note 20 above.

48 For a number of sources, see Zimmels, *p.*178 (note 59).

49 Lampronti, *Pahad Yitzhak*, *s.v.* "*Holeh Beshabbath*".

50 Yomtov Ishbili, *Novellae of RITVA*, on *Shabbath* 75a; and *Maggid Mishnah*, on *Hil. 'Issurei Bi'ah*, *v.*3.

5,1 r*Hatham Sopher*, *Y.D.*, *no.*101; cited in *P.T.*, *Y.D.*, *cxcvi.*3. See also the view of David ibn Zimra, quoted *supra*, *chpt.*IX (note 15).

52 Thus, Maimonides (*Hil. De'oth*, *iv.*19), followed by Karo, warns in the name of "the medical sages" that 999 persons out of a thousand die from excessive sexual indulgence and that "man should therefore be on his guard" (*O.H.*, *ccxl.*14). Again, discussing the medical benefits of refraining from certain mixed foods, Bachya ben Asher (*Commentary on Ex. xxiii.*19 [ed. Amsterdam, 1726, *p.*112b]) observes: "It is also the view of the physicians that the mixture of boiled fish and cheese disposes to evil qualities and leprosy". A similar statement appears in several halachic works; see Daniel Tirni, '*Ikrei Dinim*, *Y.D.*, *no.*14 (§5), citing r*Hinnukh Beth Yehudah*, *no.*61, in the name of MaHaRaM of Cracow. For a like reason Jacob Reischer (r*Shevuth Ya'akov*, part *i*, *no.*65) warns against the consumption of a hen in the body of which water was found or whose legs were swollen, although that involved no religious prohibition; see Tirni, *op. cit.*, (§9). The sources cited in notes 50 and 51 also bear testimony to the influence of medical considerations on the

formation of Jewish law. L. Lewin ("Juedische Aerzte in Grosspolen", in *JJLG, vol.ix* [1911], *p.*410 *ff.*) has named (with references) twenty-seven Jewish writers in Germany and Poland during the 16th-18th centuries, mostly rabbis, who gave dietetic, medical or prophylactic rules in their works.

[53] By Zimmels, *pp.* 19 and 23 (and corresponding notes).

[54] See Zimmels, *p.*177 *f.* (note 59); citing responsa from thirteen rabbis (from the 16th to the 19th century) who "approached doctors to hear their views on medical problems or to convince themselves that their own opinions were right".

[55] See Zimmels, *p.*192 (note 167).

[56] To resolve an argument with Zvi Ashkenazi (see *rHakham Tzevi, no.*74) on the ritual fitness of a hen in which no heart could be found, Jonathan Eybeschuetz (*Kerethi Upelethi*, on *Y.D.*, *xl*) asked the medical faculty at the University of Halle in 1709 whether any creature could live without a heart or whether some extra organ could replace its function. The reply is translated in full by Zimmels, *p.*40 *f.* At about the same time, Eybeschuetz (*Benei 'Ahuvah*, Prague, 1819, part *iii*, *p.*15b *ff.*) submitted a further enquiry to the medical faculty at the University of Prague to ascertain whether the milk of a nursing mother, who had successively lost three children, might have been poisonous. The information was required to solve a religious matrimonial problem; see Zimmels, *p.*75 *f.* Zimmels (*p.*92) also refers to a question submitted by R. Akivah Eger (*responsa*, part *i*, *no.*61) to a professor in Frankfort whether there existed a particular vein leading the blood from the haemorrhoids to the uterus or not.

Chapter Twenty

[1] See *supra*, *p.*24 *f.*

[2] See especially *supra*, *pp.* xxxi and 204 *ff.*

[3] Dante, *Divina Commedia*, Canto XII, V, 135-136; see D. Riesman, "A Physician in the Papal Chair," in *Annals of Medical History*, *vol.v* (1923), *p.*296. *Cf. supra*, *chpt.*I (note 119).

[4] W. H. R. Rivers, *Medicine, Magic and Religion*, 1924, *p.*144.

[5] Rivers, *op. cit.*, *p.*116. On more recent developments in this relationship, see W. Oursler, *The Healing Power of Faith*, 1958.

[6] Preuss (*p.*18 *f.*), making this statement, rightly observes that the priest merely declared what was pure or impure (*Lev. xiii ff.*), without offering any medical advice.

[7] See especially supra, p.   .

[8] *Cf. supra*, *chpt.*XVI (note 36).

[9] The ban was pronounced by the Councils of Clermont (1130), Rheims (1131), Montpellier (1162), Tours (1163), Paris (1212), the Lateran Synods of 1139 and 1215, and in the papal decretals of Alexander III (1180) and Honorius III (1219). See Puschmann, *Medical Education*, *p.*280 *f.*; and *CE*, *vol.x*, *p.*125.

[10] See White, *Warfare*, *vol.ii*, *p.*36.

[11] See Puschmann, *loc. cit.*

[12] So, for instance, by Pope Julius II to the Polish King Alexander in 1505; see Diepgen, *Die Theologie*, *p.*18 *f.*

[13] Canon 139 of the current Code prohibits clerics to practise medicine or surgery except by special dispensation; see S. Woywood, *A Practical*

(CHAPTER XX)

Commentary on the Code of Canon Law, 1926, *vol.i*, *p.*58. Priests defying this ban are "irregular from crime" if they thereby caused any death (*ib.*, *p.*528). But *cf. supra*, chpt.XVII (note 59).

14 T. J. Pettigrew, *On Superstitions Connected with the History and Practice of Medicine and Surgery*, 1844, *p.*34; quoted by Zimmels, *p.*2.

15 Diepgen, *op. cit.*, *p.*17 *f.*

16 Garrison, *Introduction*, *p.*169.

17 J. J. Walsh, *The Catholic Church and Healing*, 1928, *p.*83.

18 See McKenzie, *Infancy*, *p.*44.

19 Puschmann, *loc. cit.*

20 Garrison, *loc. cit.*

21 Diepgen (*loc. cit.*) regards this as the chief reason. See also Garrison, *loc. cit.*

22 According to T. C. Allbutt (*The Historical Relations of Medicine and Surgery to the End of the 16th Century*, 1905, *p.*22), "the sinister and perfidious '*ecclesia abhorret a sanguine*'" was first pronounced at Tours. The relevance of this doctrine to the clerical ban on surgery is also maintained by White (*op. cit.*, *p.*31 *f.*), Pettigrew (*loc. cit.*) and D. Riesman (*Medicine in Modern Society*, 1938, *p.*92). On the refusal of the Church from the earliest times to admit to the ministry men who had shed human blood, even apart from any guilt (*e.g.* a judge who pronounced a legitimate sentence of death), see Woywood, *op. cit.*, *p.*527). Diepgen (*loc. cit.*), however, does not regard this as the crucial reason for the ban, since it postdates by many centuries the earliest laws against bloodshed applicable to priests (first promulgated at the Synod of Lerida in 524 or 546). For a remote Jewish parallel, *cf. supra*, *p.* .

23 See *supra*, *p.*126.

24 See Samuel di Medina, rRaSHDaM, *Y.D.*, *no.*239; cited by Zimmels, *p.*263 (note 92).

25 For this reason, suggests Preuss (*p.*46), R. Yishmael did not himself participate in the anatomical experiments carried out by his disciples; see *supra*, *p.*135.

26 *E.g.*, the talmudic sages Chanina ben Dosa and his grandson, Chanina ben Chama, were both priests and physicians; see *Seder Hadoroth*, Karlsruhe, 1769, part *ii*, *p.*87b. But *cf.* Preuss, *p.*22.

27 In addition to the seven priestly rabbi-physicians in the Middle Ages listed by Zimmels (*p.*178 [note 64]), the following could be mentioned: In the 13th century: Solomon Cohen, Egyptian physician (see Friedenwald, *p.*176); Joseph Abraham Hacohen, physician to Ferdinand III (see Friedenwald, *p.*637); Don Judah ben Mons Hasohen, physician to Alphonso the Wise (see Friedenwald, *p.*637 *f.*); and Peretz Hacohen, author of *Sepher Ma'arkhoth 'Elokim* (see rRIVaSH, *no.*60). In the 14th century: Samuel Hacohen Astruc, body physician to the Algerian Sultan (see *JL*, *vol.i*, *p.*549). In the 15th century: Vital Cohen of Marseilles, appointed city physician of Toulon in 1440 (see Friedenwald, *p.*688). In the 16th century: Isaac Hacohen of Sienna (see Friedenwald, *p.*578); Joseph ben Joshua Hacohen, author of *'Emek Habakhah* and *Divrei Hayamim*, physician-in-ordinary to Andrea Doria, Doge of Genoa (see Friedenwald, *pp.* 600 and 687; and *JE*, *vol.vii*, *p.*266); Menachem Moses Cohen, communal physician at Cremone (see *MGWJ*, *vol.lxvi* [1922], *p.*205); and Eleazar Hacohen of Vitarbo ("*Theodorus de Sacerdotibus*"), papal physician (see Friedenwald, *p.*582). In the 17th century: Coen (exact name unknown), physician at the Moldavian court (see *JE*, *vol.iv*, *p.*140); Kalonymus Aaron (Clement) ben Samuel (Simon) Hacohen Cantarini and his brother Judah (Leon) Cantarini (see Friedenwald, *p.*606); several

other medico-rabbinical members of the Cantarini family (see *JE, vol.iii*, p.535 ff.); and Tobias Cohen, author of *Ma'asei Tuviah*, physician like his father and grandfather (see Friedenwald, *p.168*; and *JE, vol.iv, p.161 f.*). During these centuries, therefore, physicians of priestly stock, even among rabbis, were by no means uncommon.

28 Zimmels (*p.*19) suggests that observant priests were able to qualify as doctors "since dissection was not obligatory". But dissections could hardly have presented the only opportunity for a physician's contact with corpses or dying people.

29 Out of the 66 Jewish medical students who enrolled at the University of Frankfurt a/Oder between 1780 and 1810, there was apparently only one (Falk Kohen) of priestly descent; see L. Lewin, in *JJLG, vol.xvi* (1924), *p.*43 *ff.* At the University of Duisburg, we find one priest (Meyer Cohen of Duesseldorf) among the twenty Jewish medical students registered between 1708 and 1817; see A. Kober, "Juedische Studenten und Doktoranden der Universitaet Duisburg im 18. Jahrhundert", in *MGWJ, vol.lxxv* (1931), *p.*118 *ff.* Even to-day the usual proportion of Jews bearing the name "Cohen" alone (others, too, may be of priestly descent) is at least 2-3%; see *JE, vol.iv, p.*144. This bears out Lewin's statement (in *JJLG, vol.ix* [1911], *p.*395) that, because of the prohibition, he only rarely found priestly doctors.

30 The question how Elijah, as a priest, was permitted to touch the dead child was already raised by Tosaphoth (*Baba Metzi'a* 114b) who replied that as a prophet he knew the operation would be successful; hence, the saving of life justified the action. The argument was adduced to prove that in normal circumstances a priestly phyisician would not be permitted to defile himself for the sake of a dying person; see r*Beth Ya'akov*, no.130. But Zvi Hirsch Eisenstadt (*Nahalath Tzevi*, on *Y.D.*, ccclxx.1) rejected this reasoning, since in the case discussed by Tosaphoth the body was believed to be actually dead (hence the need for the prophetic assurance that the operation would succeed), whereas the dying may always be treated.

31 So Moses Schreiber, r*Hatham Sophe*r, *Y.D., no.*338; see *P.T., Y.D., ccclxx.*1. But Eisenstadt (*loc. cit.*) permits the practice even if other doctors are available. The attendance on the dying is also sanctioned by Z. H. Chajes (*Darkei Hahora'ah, no.*1; cited by Zimmels, *p.*182 [note 116]) and Daniel Tirni (*'Ikrei Dinim, Y.D., no.*35 [§32]). See also Grunwald, *Kol Bo, p.*223; *Sedei Hemed, s.v.* "*'Aveluth*", *no.*111; and *TE, vol.v, p.*398.

32 The sanction was first given by Isaac Samuel Reggio (in *Kerem Hemed, vol.v*; and *Hamelitz*, 1884, *no.*1), but it was strongly attacked by his contemporaries; see *e.g.*, B. H. Auerbach, *Nahal 'Eshkol*, 1867, part *i*, Introduction, *p.*xi *f.* In the 20th century Reggio's opinion was nevertheless supported (and further justified by the indispensable contribution of anatomical research to human health and life) by several mainly non-rabbinical scholars; see J. D. Eisenstein, *'Otzar Dinim Uminhagim*, 1917, *p.*453; and Grunwald, *Kol Bo, p.*81 *ff.*

33 *Glosses of RAVeD, Hil. Neziroth, v.*17. Cf. also r*RIVaSH, no.*94. Those utilising this source hold with Rozanes (*Mishneh Lemelekh, Hil. 'Avel, iii.*1) that Ibn Daud's statement (whereby all present-day priests, bing already defiled and incapable of purification, are no longer subject to the laws of defilement) implies the complete removal of the prohibition But Ezekiel Landau (*Dagul Mervavah*, on *Y.D.*, ccclxxii.2; see also *P.T., a.l.*, 9) suggests the suspension may only be meant to affect the penalty for the offence laid down in the Bible, but not the offence itself which remains biblically valid. This view is confirmed by Schreiber (*loc. cit.*)

who corroborates it by an explicit statement of Ibn Daud himself (in his *Tamim De'oth*, no.236[end]). On this controversy and the present-day status of priests in general, see also Loew, *Lebensalter, p.*114 *f.; JE, vol.iv, p.*144; *OY, vol.v, p.*259; Schalom Schachna, *Mishmereth Shalom,* 1930, part *ii, p.*46; and Grunwald, *loc. cit.*

[34] So Schreiber, *loc. cit.;* and various authorities cited by Schachna, *loc. cit.*

[35] So Judah Assad, r*MaHaRYA*, *O.H., no.*47; see also D. Hoffmann, r*Melamed Leho'il, O.H., no.*31; and *P.T., Y.D., ccclxx.*1.

[36] Schreiber, *loc. cit.*

[37] So Schreiber, *loc. cit.;* Abraham Samuel Benjamin Schreiber, r*Kethav Sopher, no.*16; and r*MaHaRYA, loc. cit. Cf.* Solomon Kluger, r*Uvahart Bahayim, no.*34; and Hoffmann, *loc. cit.* See Zimmels, *p.*182 (note 117).

[38] S. Kluger, r*Tuv Ta'am Vada'ath,* part *ii, no.*212; cited by Grunwald, *Kol Bo, p.*19.

[39] r*Duda'ei Hasadeh, no.*100; cited by Grunwald, *Kol Bo, p.*20. See also J. Meskin, in *Hapardes, vol.xxx, no.*2 (November 1955), *p.*5 *f.*

[40] Solomon Judah, r*Teshurath Shay, no.*559; cited by Grunwald, *Kol Bo, p.*19.

[41] Samuel Engel, r*MaHaRaSH,* part *iii, no.*27; and Meir Arik, in *Vayelakket Yoseph, vol.xiv, no.*74; cited by Grunwald, *Kol Bo, p.*20. *Cf.* also *Haposek,* 5704 (1944), *p.*662.

[42] See Gumbiner, *M.A., cccxi.*14; and Chajes, r*MaHaRaTZ, no.*22. *Cf. supra, chpt.*VIII (note 37).

[43] Hence the insistence on the burial of amputated limbs; see J. Reischer, r*Shevuth Ya'akov,* part *ii, no.*101; E. Landau, r*Noda Biyehudah,* part *ii, Y.D., no.*209; *P.T., Y.D., ccclxii.*1; and Hoffmann, *op. cit., Y.D., no.*118. Otherwise, there is no religious obligation to bury a severed limb; see A. Walkin, r*Zokan 'Aharon, no.*78. *Cf.* also Zimmels, *p.*116 *f.*

[44] r*Yad Remah, Y.D., no.*129.

APPENDIX

[1] See Robert Forbes, "The Medico-Legal Aspects of Artificial Insemination", in *Medico-Legal Review, vol.xii* (1944), *p.*139.

[2] The first experiments were carried out on a dog by the Italian physiologist, the Abbate Spallanzani, in 1780; see J. P. Greenhill, in Symposium on "Artificial Insemination", in *American Practitioner, vol.i, no.*5 (1947), *p.*227.

[3] *Ib.*

[4] See *The Report of a Commission Appointed by the Archbishop of Canterbury on Artificial Human Insemination,* 1948, *p.*13.

[5] By the year 1941 already, 3649 such children were known to have been born in the United States; see Schatkin, "Artificial Insemination and Illegitimacy", in *New York Law Journal, vol.cxiii, no.*148 (June 26, 1945). quoted in *The Report etc. p.*38. Other sources claim a much higher frequency of such inseminations; see *The Report etc., p.*12. In Israel it is estimated that there were tens, perhaps hundreds, of cases of A.I.D. by 1949; see A. H. Merzbach, "The Religious Physician and His Mission in the Jewish State", in *Dath Yisra'el Umedinath Yisra'el,* 1951, *p.*151. *Cf.* Akiba Joel, "Artificial Insemination in Israel", in *Hebrew Medical Journal, vol.xxvi,* part 2, (1953), *p.*190 *ff.*

[6] An indication of this difficulty was given in an American poll in 1941. Of the 30,000 physicians approached, 23,000—or more than three-fourths—did not answer at all. See J. Fletcher, *Morals and Medicine*, 1955, p.106.

[7] *Ontario Law Reports*, Orford v. Orford, 1921, *xlv*.15; see Forbes, *op. cit.*, p.144.

[8] Russell v. Russell, 1924, A.C., 721.

[9] See *American Practitioner*, *op. cit.*, p.277 *ff*. See also Fletcher, *op. cit.*, pp. 108 *f*. and 135 *f*.

[10] Parliamentary reply dated April 19, 1945.

[11] See H. U. Willink, in *The Practitioner*, *vol.clviii* (1947), p.349; *British Encyclopedia of Medical Practice*, suppl. 1950, p.287; and Fletcher, *loc. cit.*

[12] See Forbes, *loc. cit.* But in 1949 a nullity decree was granted on the grounds of the husband's incapacity to consummate the marriage, although it had produced a child through A.I.H. The verdict also rendered the child illegitimate. See *All England Law Reports*, Probate, Divorce and Admiralty Division, 1949, *vol.i*, p.141 *ff*.

[13] May 17, 1897. See A. Bonnar, *The Catholic Doctor*, 1948, p.87.

[14] Gerald Kelly, "Moral Aspects of Sterility Tests and Artificial Insemination", in *The Linacre Quarterly*, *vol.xvi*, nos. 1-2 (1949), p.35; and J. C. Heenan, "Artificial Human Insemination" (The Roman Catholic Church), in *Report of a Conference held under the auspices of the Public Morality Council*, 1948, p.18 *ff*.

[15] Gerald Kelly, *Medico-Moral Problems*, 1950, part *ii*, p.18 *ff*. See also sources cited in preceding note.

[16] *Ib*. For a full summary of the Catholic attitude, see also Fletcher, *op. cit.*, p.110 *ff*.

[17] *The Report etc.*, *op. cit.*, p.58. This is "the only thorough non-Roman study of this moral issue", according to Fletcher (*op. cit.*, p.122).

[18] *The Report etc.*, *loc. cit.* Cf. also G. L. Russell, in *Report of a Conference etc.*, *op. cit.*, p.50 *ff*.

[19] b*Hagigah* 15a; see Preuss, p.541.

[20] See *Lev. xxi*.13.

[21] Ploss and Bartels (*Woman*, *vol.ii*, p.651) consider the celebrated 12th century Arabic physician Averroes "of interest" because he was, apart from the Talmud, the first to contemplate a tub-pregnancy. For further details, see Preuss, p.541. Such a possibility was also recognised by Hai Gaon; see r*Teshuvoth Hage'onim*, ed. Mekitzei Nirdamim, no.25. Abraham Ibn Ezra (on *Gen. xxiv*.16), too, considered a virgin becoming pregnant feasible; see Isaac Elhanan Spector, r*'Eyn Yitzhak*, E.H., no.14.

[22] See Midrash *'Alpha Betha d'ben Sirah*, in J. D. Eisenstein, *'Otzar Midrashim*, 1928, p.43. L. Zunz (*Die gottesdienstlichen Vortraege der Juden*, 1909, p.105) regards this Midrash as a late composition. The source usually quoted in halakhic works is Jacob Molon Segal's *Likkutei MaHaRIL* (end). See also Zimels, p.211 (note 53).

[23] See Preuss, p.541; and Friedenwald, *vol.i*, pp. 363 and 386.

[24] So *He.M.*, *E.H.*, *i*.8; and Azulay, *Birkei Yoseph*, *i*.14.

[25] Lampronti, *Pahad Yitzhak*, *vol.ii*, p.30a.

[26] See *Deut. xxiii*.3. A Jewish child is illegitimate, and as such debarred from marriage with anyone except his like or a proselyte, only if born of an adulterous or incestuous union.

[27] So *TaZ*, *Y.D.*, cxcv.7, and *E.H.*, *i*.8; and Jacob Emden, r*She'ilath Yavetz*, part *ii*, no.97. These (and other) authorities hold that the duty of procreation cannot be fulfilled without the father's active and intimate association.

28 *Haggahoth SeMaK*; quoted in *TaZ, loc. cit.* For a similar 15th century precedent, see Simon Duran, r*TaSHBeTZ*, part *iii, no.*263.

29 So *B.S., E.H., i.*10; and *Birkei Yoseph, loc. cit.*

30 *Mishneh Lemelekh, Hil. 'Ishuth, xv.*4.

31 So, *e.g.*, Moses Schick, *Taryag Mitzvoth*, i; Solomon Schick, r*RaSHBaN, E.H., no.*8. *Cf.* Loew (*Lebensalter, p.*57 *ff.*), who construes the talmudic reference to a conception *sine concubito* as a sarcastic allusion to the Christian belief in the Immaculate Conception. But this view is opposed by Preuss (*p.*558), since the author of the talmudic statement (Ben Zoma, end of 1st century C.E.) lived at a time when the dogma of the Immaculate Conception was still unknown; *cf.* W. E. H. Lecky, *History of the Rise and Influence of the Spirit of Rationalism in Europe,* 1870, *vol.i, p.*213.

32 *Tzemah David*, ed. Offenbach, 1768, *p.*14b. *Cf.* also the refutation of the alleged birth of two talmudic savants under similar circumstances in *Seder Hadoroth*, Karlsruhe, 1769, part *ii, p.*71b *f.*

33 *Birkei Yoseph, loc. cit.*

34 Eybeschuetz, *Benei 'Ahuvah, 'Ishuth, xv.*6. So also Jacob Ettlinger, '*Arukh Lener*, on *Yevamoth* 12b.

35 *Lev. xviii.*20 (*cf.* Nachmanides, *a.l.*), where specific reference is made to giving one's "seed" to a neighbour's wife. *Cf.* also Rashi, *Lev. xx.*12.

36 J. L. Zirelsohn, r*Ma'arkhei Lev, no.*73.

37 So, *e.g.*, Abrahau Lurie, in *Haposek*, Heshvan-Kislev 5710 (1949); Obadiah Hadaya, in *No'am*, ed. M. S. Kasher, *vol.i*, 1958, *p.*137; and Solomon Zalman Auerbach, in *No'am, op. cit., p.*145 *ff.* See also Dov M. Krauser, in *No'am, op. cit., p.*122.

38 In the talmudic view, man enters into a partneship with God by perpetuating His creation through the propagation of the race (see b*Kiddushin* 30b; and *cf.* b*Yevamoth* 63b). Significantly, in Jewish law the obligation to marry derives specifically from the duty of procreation (*E.H., i.*1).

39 See authorities cited by Krauser, *op. cit., p.*120. On the levirate law, see *Deut. xxv.*5-9.

40 So Auerbach, *op. cit., p.*165; see also Krauser, *loc. cit.* The danger that the widespread practice of A.I.D. may result in incestuous marriages is not so remote when one considers that, as has been computed (M. Barton, K. Walker and B. P. Wiesner, "Artificial Insemination", in *British Medical Journal*, 1945, *vol.i, p.*40), one fecund donor submitting two specimens weekly could produce 400 children every week or 20,000 annually. Even if one discounts these figures as wildly exaggerated in practice, "the possibility of incest [being] plainly increased by A.I.D." is admitted even by its advocates (Fletcher, *op. cit., p.*130).

41 On these restrictions, see b*Kiddushin* 75a; Maimonides, *Hil. 'Issurei Bi'ah, xv.*23 and 33; and *E.H., iv.*31-36. While some authorities would impose a virtually complete marriage ban on such children (J. Weinberg, in *Hapardes, vol.xxi* [1951]), others hold that they would be debarred at least from marrying men of priestly descent (M. J. Breisch, r*Helkath Ya'akov, no.*24); see Krauser, *op. cit., p.*122. Although these disabilities may not exist if the donor was a non-Jew (r*Helkath Ya'akov, loc. cit.*; Auerbach, *op. cit., p.*161 *ff.*), the use of his semen for the insemination of a Jewess would meet with even graver moral objections (Auerbach, *op. cit.,* pp. 159 *ff.* and 165 *f.*); see also *No'am, op. cit., p.*124, in the name of an anonymous scholar).

42 See *supra, p.*183. While a few authorities would regard such a woman

as an adulteress and as such forbidden to live with her husband (r*Ma'arkhei Lev*, loc. cit.; Hadaya, op. cit., p.137), many hold that she would be subject to the usual restrictions applicable to pregnant women (B. Uziel, r*Mishpetei 'Uzi'el*, E.H., no.19; Eliezer Judah Waldenberg, r*Tzitz Eli'ezer*, part *iii*, no.27; see also Krauser, op. cit., p.121), or at least for three months prior to and following the insemination, so as to establish the paternity with certainty (Auerbach, op. cit., pp. 158 and 166).

43 Apart from the sources already cited in the preceding notes, numerous recent responsa have reached similar conclusions; see various contributors to discussion in *Tel Talpiyoth*, vol.*xxxviii* (1931), pp. 75 ff., 85 ff. and 93 f.; M. Kirschbaum, r*Menahem Meshiv*, part *ii*, no.26; David Obadiah, r*Yishmah Levav*, E.H., no.9; and especially summaries in *'Otzar Haposkim*, E.H., *i*.42; Meir Meiri, *'Ezrath Nashim*, vol.*iii*, 1955, p.319 ff.; Zvi Hirsch Friedman, in *Sepher Hayovel Hapardes*, 1951; and the excellent series of articles on the subject in *No'am*, op. cit., p.111 ff. Cf. Zimmels, p.66.

44 So r*RaSHBaN*, loc. cit.; and S. M. Holland, in *Haposek*, Shevat 5710 (1949). For this and other reasons the following are inclined to prohibit A.I.H. altogether if it involves masturbation: M. Z. Halevy of Lomza, r*Divrei Malki'el*, part *iii*, nos. 107 and 108; Uziel, loc. cit.; Hayim Fishel Epstein, r*Teshuvah Shelemah*, part *ii*, E.H., no.4; and Hadaya, op. cit., p.130 ff. See *No'am*, op. cit., p.113.

45 B.S., E.H., xxv.2; r*She'ilath Yavetz*, loc. cit., S. M. Schwadron, r*MaHaRSHaM*, part *iii*, no.268; E. Deitsch, r*Peri Hasadeh*, part *iii*, no.53; A. Wolkin, r*Zekan 'Aharon*, part *ii*, E.H., no.97; Joshua Baumel, r'*Emek Halakhah*, no.68; Weinberg, op. cit.; I. J. Weisz, r*Minhath Yitzhak*, no.50; and Israel Z'ev Minzberg, in *No'am*, op. cit., p.129.

46 See Meiri, loc. cit.; *'Otzar Haposkim*, loc. cit.; and *No'am*, op. cit., p.112. Cf. Zimmels, p.66. Some of the authorities mentioned in the preceding note will sanction such A.I.H. only if the marriage has proved barren for at least ten years.

47 See r*MaHaRSHaM*, loc. cit.; r*Zekan 'Aharon*, loc. cit.; r*Minhath Yitzhak*, loc. cit.; and Minzberg, loc. cit. Under such circumstances A.I.H. is completely prohibited according to r*Divrei Malki'el*, loc. cit.; Abraham Isaiah Karelitz *"Hazon 'Ish"* (see *Ha'ish Vehazono*, cited in *No'am*, op. cit., p.117); and Hadaya, op. cit., p.135.

48 See Samuel Rozin, "The Role of Seminal Plasma in Motility of Spermatozoa: Therapeutic Insemination with Husband's Spermatozoa in Heterologous Seminal Plasma" (Preliminary Report), in *Acta Med. Orient.*, vol.*xvii*, nos. 1-2 (1958), p.24 f. (This is an English version of a Hebrew article which appeared in *Harefuah*, vol.*liv*, no.5 [March 2, 1958], p.118 ff.)

ABBREVIATIONS

TALMUD AND RESPONSA.

(Small letters preceding talmudic tractate and title of responsa work)

b   Babylonian Talmud   m   *Mishnah*
j   Palestinian or Jerusalem Talmud   t   *Tosephta*
                    r   Responsa

CODES AND COMMENTARIES.

A.H.   *'Arukh Hashulhan*
Bah   *Beth Hadash*
B.S.   *Beth Shemu'el*
D.T.   *Darkei Teshuvah*, on *Yoreh De'ah*
E.H.   *'Even Ha'ezer*
(*Bi'ur*) *HaGRA* (Commentary of) Elijah
    of Vilna
H.e.M.   *Helkath Mehokek*
H.M.   *Hoshen Mishpat*
Hil.   Maimonides, *Yad Hahazakah, Hil-*
    khot
M.A.   *Magen 'Avraham* on *'Orah Hayim*

M.B.   *Mishnah Berurah*, on *'Orah Hayim*
O.H.   *'Orah Hayim*
P.M.   *Peri Megadim*
P.T.   *Pithhei Teshuvah*
S.A.   *Shulhan 'Arukh*
SHaKH   *Sifsei Kohen*
SMA   (*Sepher*) *Me'irath 'Enayim*
SMaG   *Sepher Mitzvoth Gadol*
S.T.   *Sha'arei Teshuvah*
TaZ   *Turei Zahav*
Tur   *Tur Shulhan 'Arukh*
Y.D.   *Yoreh De'ah*

RABBINICAL AUTHORS.

Many rabbinical works, particularly responsa and novellae, are known by abbreviations usually made up the first letters of the names of their authors (see *JE* vol. i, p.42). These are listed in full in the BIBLIOGRAPHY [A].

BOOKS.

Shortened titles are used for works frequently cited; see BIBLIOGRAPHY [B & C]

ENCYCLOPEDIAS.

For abbreviations used, see BIBLIOGRAPHY [D].

PERIODICALS.

For abbreviations used, see BIBLIOGRAPHY [E].

BIBLIOGRAPHY

A. HEBREW SOURCES.

(Except where otherwise stated, these sources are chronologically listed. The principal works are followed by the commentaries on them [indented]. These appear in the editions of the works to which they belong unless otherwise indicated.)

No dates are given for authors who lived during the past century.

1. BIBLE (WITH COMMENTARIES).

The Holy Bible (Authorised Version; for the Old Testament the translation of the Jewish Publication Society of America has been used).

Pentateuch, ed. Horeb, Berlin, 1928.

    Rashi (Solomon Yitzhaki, 1040-1105, France, Germany).

    Ibn Ezra (Abraham ibn Ezra, 1092-1167, Spain, S. France).

    Nachmanides (Moses ben Nachman, ca. 1195-1270, Spain).

    Bahyah (ben Asher, ca. 1260-1340, Spain), Amsterdam, 1726.

    'Akedath Yitzhak, by Isaac Arama (ca. 1420-1493, Spain, Turkey), Frankfurt a/o, 1785.

    Abarvanel (Isaac Abarvanel, 1437-1508, Portugal, Italy), Amsterdam, 1768.

    'Or Hahayim, by Hayim Atar (1696-1743, Morocco, Jerusalem), Vienna, 1929.

    Malbim (Meir Loeb ben Yechiel Michael, 1809-1879, Poland, Germany), Vilna, 1922.

    Torah Temimah, by Jacob Epstein, Vilna, 1904.

2. TARGUMIM.

Targum (Onkelos, probably 2nd century, C. E.), ed. Horeb; see *Pentateuch* above.

Targum Jonathan (probably later than 600), ed. Horeb; see *Pentateuch* above.

3. TALMUD (WITH COMMENTARIES AND NOVELLAE).

Mishnah. ed. Romm, Vilna, 1911.

    Maimonides, *Mishnah Commentary* (by Moses ben Maimon, 1135-1204, Spain, N. Africa), in *Babylonian Talmud,* ed, Romm, Vilna, 1895.

    Obadiah of Bartinura (2nd half of 15th century, Italy, Palestine).

    Novellae of Akivah Eger (1761-1837, Hungary, Posen).

    Tiph'ereth Yisra'el by Israel Lipschuetz (1782-1860, Germany).

Tosephta, with code of Alfasi, ed. Romm, Vilna, 1911.

    Hasdei David, by David Pardo (1719-1792, Italy, Jerusalem), Livorno, 1776.

    Minhat Bikkurim, by Samuel Avigdor of Slonimo.

    Hazon Yehezkel, by Yehezkel Abramsky, on t*Mo'ed,* vol i, Jerusalem, 1934.

Babylonian Talmud, ed. Romm, Vilna, 1895.

    R. Hananel (ben Kushiel, first half of 11th century, Tunis).

    Rashi (see *Bible* above).

    Tosaphoth (by various Franco-German authors, 12th-13th centuries).

    Novellae of RaMBaN (Nachmanides, see *Bible* above), Jerusalem, 1928.

(HEBREW SOURCES, Talmud)

Novellae of RaSHBA (Solomon ben Abraham Adreth, ca. 1235-1310, Spain), Warsaw, 1902.

Beth Habehirah, by Menahem Meiri (1249-1306, Provence), ed. A. Schreiber, Frankfurt, Jerusalem and New York, 1930.

Novellae of RaN (Nissim Gerondi, 1320-1380, Barcelona). New York, 1946.

Novellae of RITVA (Yomtov Ishbili, 1st half of 14th century, Spain), Muncasz, 1908.

Yam shel Shelomo, by Solomon Luria (1510-1573, Russia), Stettin, 1861.

MaHaRSHA (Samuel Edels, 1555-1631, Poland).

Kunteres Yom Hakippurim, by MaHaRaM ibn Habib (Moses ibn Habib, 17th century, Jerusalem), Pietrkow, 1912.

Shittah Mekubbetzeth, by Bezalel Ashkenazi (17th century, Egypt, Palestine), Warsaw, 1879.

Glosses of Yavetz (Jacob Emden, 1697-1776, Altona).

Kissei Rahamim on *Avoth d'Rabbi Nathan,* by Hayim Joseph David Azulay (1727-1806, Palestine, Italy), Ungvar, 1868.

Glosses of MaHaRaTZ Chajes (Zvi Hirsch Chajes, 1805-1855, Poland).

'Arukh Lener, on Yevamoth, by Jacob Ettlinger (1798-1871, Germany), Pietrkow, 1914.

RSHaSH (Samuel Strasson).

Melo Haro'im, by Jacob Zvi Jalisch, Warsaw, 1911.

Zikhron 'Avraham Mosheh, by Eliezer Duenner, Jerusalem, 1945.

Palestinian Talmud, ed. Romm, Vilna, 1922.

'Amudei Yerushalayim, by Israel Eisenstein.

4. MIDRASHIM AND ZOHAR.

Midrash Rabbah, ed. Romm, Vilna, 1923.

Tanhuma, ed. Horeb, Berlin, 1927; and ed. S. Buber, Vilna, 1913.

Mekhilta, Sifra and *Sifri,* ed. Malbim (see *Bible* above).

Sifri Zutta, ed. S. Horovitz, Breslau, 1917.

Pethikta Rabbathi, ed. M. Friedmann, Vienna, 1880.

'Avel Rabbathi, ed. M. Klotz, Berlin, 1890.

Tanna d'bei 'Eliyahu (Seder 'Eliyahu Rabbah and Zutta), ed. M. Friedmann, Vienna, 1902.

Yalkut, Vilna, 1898.

Shoher Tov (on *Psalms*), Warsaw, 1893.

Midrash Shemu'el (probably 11th century), Warsaw, 1893.

Midrash Temurah (probably 13th century), in J. D. Eisenstein, *'Otzar Midrashim,* New York, 1928.

Zohar, Amsterdam, 1800.

5. GEONICA.

Sh'iltoth d'Rabbi 'Ahai Gaon, Venice, 1546.

Teshuvoth Hage'onim, Livorno, 1869.

Likkutei Kadmoniyoth, ed. A. Harkavy, Petersburg, 1903.

Ginzei Schechter, ed. Louis Ginzberg, 2 vols., New York, 1928-9.

'Otzar Hage'onim, ed. B. Lewin (on *Shabbath*), Jerusalem, 1930.

6. CODES AND ALLIED WORKS (WITH COMMENTARIES)

Alfasi (Isaac Alfasi, 1013-1103, N. Africa, Spain), ed. Romm. Vilna, 1911.
> RaN (Nissim Gerondi, see *Talmud* above).
> *Shiltei Gibborim*, by Josua Boaz Baruch (d. 1557, Italy).

Maimonides, *Yad Hahazakah* (see *Talmud* above), Vilna, 1900.
> *Glosses of RAVeD* (Abraham ibn Daud, ca. 1125-1198. S. France).
> *Haggahoth Maimuni*, by Meir Hacohen (13th century, Germany).
> *Maggid Mishnah*, by Vidal of Tolosa (2nd half of 14th century, Spain).
> *Keseph Mishneh*, by Joseph Karo (see *Shulhan 'Arukh* below).
> *RaDBaZ* (David ibn Zimra, 1479-1598, Palestine N. Africa).
> *Lehem Mishneh*, by Abraham di Boton (1560-1609, Salonica).
> *Mishneh Lemelekh*, by Judah Rozanes (d. 1729, Turkey).
> *Benei 'Ahuvah*, by Jonathan Eybeschuetz (1690-1767, Moravia, Altona), Prague, 1819.

Maimonides, *Sepher Hamitzvoth*, Lemberg, 1860.
> *RaMBaN* (Nachmanides, see *Bible* above).

Sepher Ha'eshkol, by Abraham ben Isaac of Narbonne (ca. 1110-1178, S. France), Halberstadt, 1868.
> *Nahal 'Eshkol*, by Zvi Benjamin Auerbach.

Zikhron B'rith Larishonim (on laws of circumcision), by Jacob and Gershom Hagozer (12th century, Germany), ed. A. J. Glassberg, Berlin, 1892.

'Or Zaru'a by Isaac ben Moses of Vienna (ca. 1180-1260, Bohemia, Germany), Zitomir, 1862.

Torath Ha'adam, by Nachmanides (see above), Warsaw, 1840.

Mordecai (ben Hillel Ashkenazi, d. 1298, Germany), with Alfasi above.

Sepher Mitzvoth Gadol [*SMaG*] by Moses of Coucy (13th century, France), Muncacz, 1905.

Asheri (Asher ben Yechiel, ca. 1250-1327, Germany, Spain), with *Babylonian Talmud* above.
> *Kitzur Piskei HaROSH*, by Jacob ben Asher (see *Tur* below).
> *Korban Nethan'el*, by Nethanel Weil, (18th century, Germany).

Kaphtor Vapherah, by Eshtori Haparhi (ca. 1282-1357, Spain, Italy), ed. H. Edelmann, Berlin, 1852.

Likkutei Maharil, by Jacob Molin (1365-1427, Germany), Amsterdam, 1730.

Sepher Hahinnukh, by Aaron Halevy (early 14th century, Barcelona), Vilna, 1912.
> *Minhath Hinnukh*, by Joseph Babad.

Kol Bo, author uncertain (14th century?), Lemberg, 1860.

Tur (*Shulhan 'Arukh*), by Jacob ben Asher (ca. 1269-1343, Germany, Spain), Vilna, 1900.
> *Beth Yoseph*, by Joseph Karo (see *Shulhan 'Arukh* below).
> *Darkei Mosheh*, by Moses Isserles (see *Shulhan 'Arukh* below).
> *Beth Hadash* [*BaH*], by Joel Sirkes (1561-1640, Poland).
> *Perishah* and *Derishah*, by Joshua Falk (d. 1640, Poland).
> *Keneseth Hegedolah*, by Hayim Beneviste (d. 1673, Turkey), Constantinople, 1716.

'Issur Vehetter, by Jonah Ashkenazi (15th century, Germany; wrongly ascribed to Jonah Gerondi, 13th century), Ferara, 1555.

Halakhot Ketannoth, by Jacob Hagiz (1620-1674, Italy, Palestine), Venice, 1704.

'Eleh Hamitzvoth, by Moses Hagiz (1671-1750 Palestine), Warsaw, 1887.

Hokhmath 'Adam, by Abraham Danzig, Warsaw, 1908.

Binath 'Adam, by Abraham Danzig.

Hayei 'Adam, by Abraham Danzig, Warsaw, 1912.

7. THE SHULHAN 'ARUKH (WITH COMMENTARIES*) AND WORKS BASED ON IT.

Shulhan 'Arukh, by Joseph Karo (1488-1575, Turkey, Palestine), with Glosses by Moses Isserles (1510-1572, Poland), Lemberg, 1876; [Y.D.] ed. Romm, Vilna, 1911.

'Atereth Zekeinim, by Menahem Auerbach (17th century, Austria).

Ba'er Hetev, by Zechariah Mendel of Cracow (17th century, Poland).

Be'er Hagolah, by Moses Ribkes (d. 1671, Vilna).

Beth David, by David Katz of Bisteritz, Vacz, 1912.

Beth Lehem Yehudah, by Zvi Hirsch of Vilna (early 18th century, Poland).

Beth Me'ir, by Meir Posner (18th century, Danzig), Lemberg, 1860.

Beth Shemu'el [B.S.], by Samuel ben Uri (2nd half of 17th century, Poland),

Beth Ya'akov, by Jacob of Lissa (d. 1832, Poland).

Birkei Yoseph, by Hayim Joseph David Azulay (see Babylonian Talmud above), Livorno, 1774-6.

Bi'ur HaGRA, by Elijah of Vilna (1720-1797, Vilna).

Dagul Mervavah, by Ezekiel Landau (1737-1793, Prague).

Darkei Teshuvah [D.T.], by Zvi Hirsch Schapira, vol. i, Vilna, 1911; vol. ii, Muncacz, 1903; vol. iii, Szolyva, 1912; vol. iv, Pressburg, 1921.

Gilyon MaHaRSHA (Solomon Eger, son of Akivah Eger, see below).

Gur 'Aryeh Halevy (Aryeh Panzi of Mantua, 17th century, Italy).

'Ikrei Dinim, by Daniel Tirni (early 19th century Italy).

Kerethi Upelethi, by Jonathan Eybeschuetz (1690-1767, Moravia, Altona), Vienna, 1821.

Magen 'Avraham [M.A.], by Abraham Gumbiner (d. 1683, Poland).

Mishnah Berurah, and Bi'ur Halakhah, by Israel Meir Kagan, Warsaw, 1910.

Nahalath Tzevi, by Abraham Zvi Hirsch Eisenstadt (1813-1868, Russia).

Novellae of Akivah Eger (1761-1837, Hungary, Posen).

Pithhei Teshuvah [P.T.], by Eisenstadt (see Nahalath Tzevi above).

Peri Hadash, by Hezekiah Silva (d. 1689, Italy, Jerusalem).

Peri Megadim [P.M.], by Joseph Teumim (late 18th century, Poland, Frankfort), Warsaw.

Sepher Me'irath 'Enayim [SeMA], by Joshua Falk (d. 1614, Poland).

Sha'arei Teshuvah [S.T.], by Hayim Mordecai Margulies (d. 1818, Poland).

Shiyurei Berakhah, by Azulay (see Babylonian Talmud above), Salonica, 1814,

Siphsei Kohen [SHaKH], by Shabbatai Hacohen (1621-1662, Poland, Moravia),

Shulhan Gavoah, by Joseph Molko (18th century, Turkey), Salonica, 1757.

Turei Zahav [TaZ], by David Halevy (ca. 1586-1667, Russia),

Levush, by Mordecai Jaffe (1530-1612, Prague, Posen), Venice, 1620.

Tanya (Shulhan 'Arukh), by Shneur Zalman of Ladi (1746-1812, Poland), Zitomir, 1847-8.

---

* Alphabetically ordered.

(HEBREW SOURCES, *The Shulhan 'Arukh*)

'Arukh Hashulhan [*A.H.*], by Yechiel Michael Epstein, Warsaw, 1912-3; Vilna, 1923.

Kitzur Shulhan 'Arukh, by Solomon Ganzfried, ed. D. Feldmann, Leipzig, 1933.

Metzudath David, by David Feldmann.

Minhath Shabbath, by Samuel Hacohen Borstein, Warsaw, 1931.

'Oth Shalom (on laws of circumcision), by Hayim Eliezer Schapira, Beregszasz, 1921.

8. RESPONSA AND ALLIED WORKS.

(Alphabetically ordered)

'Ahi'ezer, by Hayim Ozer Grodzinski, Jerusalem, 1946.

'Akivah 'Eger (1761-1837, Hungary, Posen), New York, 1945.

'Arugath Habosam, by Moses Grunwald, Szolyva, 1912 (and later editions).

'Avodath Hagershuni, by Gershon Ashkenazi (d. 1693, Poland, Austria, Metz). Frankfurt, 1699.

BaH, by Joel Sirkes (1561-1640, Poland), Frankfurt, 1697.

Beth Hadash Hahadashoth, by Joel Sirkes (as above), Koretz, 1785.

Besamim Rosh, ascribed to Asheri (see *ROSH* below), Berlin, 1793.

Beth Ya'akov, by Jacob ben Samuel (2nd half of 17th century, Germany), Dyrenfurth, 1696.

Binyamin Ze'ev, by Benjamin ben Mattithiah (d. 1540, Turkey), Venice, 1539.

Binyan Tziyon*, by Jacob Ettlinger (1798-1871, Germany), Altona, 1868.

Bruna (*Israel,* 15th century Germany), Salonica, 1798.

Da'ath Kohen, by Abraham Isaac Kook (late Chief Rabbi of Palestine), Jerusalem, 1942.

Divrei Hayim, by Hayim Halberstam of Zanz (1793-1876, Poland), Bilgoraj, 1929.

Divrei Malki'el, by Malchiel Zvi Halevy of Lomza, Vilna, 1891-1901.

Duda'ei Hasadeh, by Eliezer Hayim Deitsch, Szeini, 1929.

'Eyn Yitzhak, by Isaac Elhanan of Kovno, Vilna, 1888.

'Ezrath Nashim, by Meir Meiri, vol. iii, London, 1955.

Hatham Sopher, by Moses Schreiber (1763-1839, Frankfort, Pressburg), Vienna, 1855.

Havath Ya'ir by Yair Bacharach (1639-1702, Germany) Lemberg, 1896.

Havatzeleth Hasharon, by Menahem Mannes Babad, Bilgoraj, 1931.

Helkath Ya'akov, by Mordecai Jacob Breisch, Jerusalem, 1951.

Hemdath Shelomo, by Solomon Zalman of Posen (d. 1839 Warsaw), Warsaw, 1836.

Heshiv Mosheh, by Moses Teitelbaum, Lemberg, 1886.

'Iggereth Bikkoreth, by Jacob Emden (1697-1776, Altona), Zitomir, 1868.

'Imrei No'am, by Joab of Deutschkreuz, Muncacz, 1884.

'Imrei Yosher, by Meir Arik, Muncacz, 1913.

Keneseth Yehezk'el by Ezekiel (Katzen) Ellenbogen (ca. 1670-1749, Altona), Altona, 1732.

Kethav Sopher, by Abraham Samuel Benjamin Schreiber (son of Moses Schreiber, see *Hatham Sopher* above), Pressburg, 1873-94.

Ko'ah Shor, by Isaac Schorr (d. 1776, Poland), Kolomea, 1888.

Levushei Mordekhai, by Mordecai L. Winkler, Budapest, 1922-8.

Ma'asei 'Avraham, by Nissim Abraham Ashkenazi, Smyrna, 1855.

---

* References in the notes are to part i, unless otherwise indicated.

Ma'arkhei Lev, by Judah Leib Zirelsohn, Kishinev, 1932.

Mahanei Hayim, by Hayim Sopher, Pressburg, 1882.

MaHaRaM Lublin (Meir ben Gedaliah, 1558-1616, Poland), Metz, 1764.

MaHaRaM Padua (Meir Katzenellenbogen, 1482-1565, Italy), Cracow, 1882.

MaHaRaM Rothenburg (Meir of Rothenburg, b. ca. 1220, Germany), ed. Mekitzei Nirdamim, Berlin, 1891.

MaHaRaM Shik (Moses Schick, 19th century, Hungary), [O.H.] Satmar, 1904; [Y.D.] Muncacz, 1881.

MaHaRaSH (Samuel Engel), Bardiov, 1926, and later volumes.

MaHaRaTZ Chajes (Zvi Hirsch Chajes, 1805-1855, Poland), Zolkova, 1849.

MaHaRIK (Joseph Kolon, ca. 1420-1480, France, Italy), Lemberg, 1796.

MaHaRIL Jacob Molin, 1365-1427, Germany), Cracow, 1881.

MaHaRIT (Joseph Trani, end of 16th century, Greece), Lemberg, 1861.

MaHaRSHaL (Solomon Luria, 1510-1573, Russia), Lemberg, 1859.

MaHaRSHaM (Solomon Mordecai Schwadron), Warsaw, 1902.

MaHaRYA (Yehudah Ya'aleh), by Judah Assad, Lemberg, 1873; Pressburg, 1880.

Mattei Levy, by Jacob Horovitz, part ii, Frankfurt, 1932.

Melamed Leho'il, by David Hoffmann, Frankfurt, 1926 and 1932.

Menahem Meshiv, by Menachem Kirschbaum, Lublin, 1936-8.

Milu'ei 'Even, by Elijah Klatzkin, Lublin, 1933.

*Minhath Yitzhak,** by Isaac Jacob Weisz, London, 1955.

Minhath Ele'azar, by Eleazar Hayim Schapira, Muncacz, 1902; Pressburg, 1930.

Mishpetei 'Uzi'el,* by Benzion M. Uziel (late Chief Rabbi of Palestine), Tel Aviv, 1935.

Nahalath Shiv'ah, by Samuel Halevy (17th century, Poland, Germany), Warsaw, 1884.

No'am, ed. M. M. Kasher, vol. i, Jerusalem, 1958.

Noda Biyehudah, by Ezekiel Landau (1737-1793, Prague), Vilna, 1904.

'Ohel Mosheh, by Moses Jonah Zweig, Jerusalem, 1949.

'Olath Shemu'el, by Samuel Florentin (18th century, Salonica), Salonica, 1776.

'Or Hame'ir, by Judah Meir Schapira, Pietrkow, 1926.

Panim Me'iroth, by Meir Ashkenazi of Eisenstadt (d. 1744, Hungary), Lemberg, 1889.

Pe'er Hador, by Maimonides (see *RaMBaM* below), Lemberg, 1859.

Parashath Mordekhai, by Mordecai Banet, Szeged, 1889.

Peri 'Asher, by Asher Gronis, Tel Aviv, 1946.

Peri Ha'aretz, by Israel Meir Mizrachi (late 17th century, Jerusalem), Constantinople, 1727.

Peri Hasadeh, by Eleazar Deitsch, Pacz, 1906.

Porath Yoseph, by Joseph Zweig, Bilgoraj, 1933.

RaDBaZ (David ibn Zimra, 1479-1589, Palestine, N. Africa), Warsaw, 1882.

RaMBaM (Moses ben Maimon, 1135-1204, Spain, N. Africa), ed. A. Freimann, Jerusalem, 1934.

*RaSHBA** (Solomon ben Abraham Adreth, ca. 1235-1310, Spain), Vienna, 1812.

RaSHBaN (Solomon Schick, Hungary), Satmar, 1905.

RaSHBaSH (Solomon ben Simon Duran, ca .1400-1467, Algiers), Livorno, 1742,

RaSHDaM (Samuel di Medina, ca. 1505-1589, Salonica), Lemberg, 1862.

---

*References in the notes are to part i, unless otherwise indicated

ReMA (Mose Isserles, 1510-1572, Poland), Amsterdam, 1711.
ReMaTZ (Meir Zvi Vitomir), Prezemysl, 1872.
RIVaSH (Isaac ben Sheshet Barfat, 1326-1408, Spain, N. Africa), Lemberg 1805.
ROSH (Asher ben Yechiel, ca. 1250-1327, Germany, Spain), Venice, 1607.
Rosh Mashbir, by Joseph Samuel Modena (early 18th century, Italy), Salonica, 1840.
Sha'arei De'ah, by Hayim Judah Loeb, Lemberg, 1878.
Shav Ya'akov, by Jacob Poppers (d. 1740, Germany), Frankfurt, 1742.
She'ilath Yavetz*, by Jacob Emden (1697-1776, Altona), Altona, 1739 and 1759.
Shemen Roke'ah, by Eleazar of Pielz (2nd half of 18th century, Poland), Nawidwahr, 1788.
Shevet Miyehudah, by Issar L. Unterman, Jerusalem, 1955.
Shevet Sopher, by Simchach Bunam Schreiber, Vienna, 1915.
Shevuth Ya'akov, by Jacob Reischer, (d. 1733, Metz), Lemberg, 1860.
Sho'el Umeshiv, by Joseph Saul Nathansohn, Lemberg, 1868 and 1890.
Sithri Umagini, by Sınai Schiffer, Tirnau, 1932-3.
Ta'alumoth Lev, by Elijah Chazan, Livorno, 1879.
TaSHBeTZ, by Simon ben Zemach Duran (1361-1444, Algiers), Amsterdam, 1739.
Terumath Hadeshen, by Israel Isserlein (ca. 1390-1460, Austria), Fuerth, 1778.
Teshurath Shay, by Solomon Judah Tabak, Szeged, 1905.
Teshuvah Me'ahavah*, by Elaezar Fleckeles 1754-1826, Prague), Kaschau, 1912.
Teshuvah Shelemah, by Hayim Fischel Epstein, Pietrkow, 1914.
Tuv Ta'am Vada'ath, by Solomon Kluger (d. 1869, Galicia), Podgorze, 1900.
Tzitz Eli'ezer, by Eliezer Judah Waldenberg, Jerusalem, 1954.
Yad Shalom, by David Ungar, Teltschau, 1911.
Zekan 'Aharon by Aaron Walkin, part ii, New York, 1951.
Zekher Simhah, by Simchah Bamberger, Frankfurt, 1925.

9. HALACHIC REFERENCE WORKS AND ENCYCLOPEDIAS.

Pahad Yitzhak, by Isaac Lampronti (1679-1756, Italy), ed. Mekitzei Nirdamim, Lyck, 1846.
Sedei Hemed, by Hayim Medini, Warsaw, 1903-7.
'Otzar Dinim Uminhagim, by Judah David Eisenstein, New York, 1917.
Mishmereth Shalom (on laws of mourning), by Shalom Schachna, Bilgoraj, 1930.
Kol Bo (on laws of mourning), by Yekuthiel Judah Grunwald, New York, 1947.
'Otzar Haposkim, Jerusalem, 1947-
Talmudic Encyclopedia [TE], Jerusalem, 1948.

10. PHILOSOPHICAL AND ETHICAL WORKS.

Guide of the Perplexed, by Maimonides (see *RaMBaM* above), Warsaw, 1872.
Hovoth Halevavoth, by Bachyah ibn Pekudah (1st half of 11th century, Spain), ed. A. Ziphroni, Jerusalem, 1928.
Sepher Hasidim, by Judah Hechasid (ca. 1200, Regensburg), Zitomir, 1897; and ed. J. Wisteniezki, Mekitzei Nirdamim, Berlin, 1891-93.
  Commentary, by Hayim Joseph David Azulay (see *Babylonian Talmud* above).
  Mishnath 'Avraham, by Abraham A. Price, Montreal, 1955.
Sepher Ba'alei Hanephesh, by Abraham ibn Daud (*RAVeD,* see *Codes* above), Berlin, 1762.

(HEBREW SOURCES, Philosophical and Ethical Works)

Shenei Luhoth Haberith [*SHeLaH*], by Isaiah Horovitz (ca. 1555-1625, Prague, Poland, Germany), Fuerth, 1764.

Kitzur SHeLaH, by Yechiel Michael Epstein (17th century, Russia), Fuerth, 1696.

Midrash Talpiyoth, by Elijah Hacohen of Ismir (d. 1729, Turkey), Smyrna, 1736.

Devash Lephi, by Hayim Joseph David Azulay (see *Babylonian Talmud* above), Livorno, 1801.

Hafetz Hayim, by Israel Meir Kagan, Frankfurt, 1925.

11. HISTORICAL WORKS.

Antiquities of the Jews, by Flavius Josephus (ca. 37-110, Jerusalem, Rome), German translation by H. Clementz, Berlin and Vienna, 1923.

Shevet Yehudah, by Solomon ibn Verga (ca. 1460-1554, Spain, Turkey), Lemberg, 1846.

Shalsheleth Hakabbalah, by Gedaliyah ibn Yachyah (16th century, Italy), Warsaw, 1877.

Pahad Yitzhak, by Isaac Hayim Cantarini ((1644-1723, Italy), Amsterdam, 1684.

Tzemah David, by David Gans (d. 1613, Prague), Offenbach, 1768.

Seder Hadoroth, by Yechiel Heilprin (1666-1746, Russia), Karlsruhe, 1769.

12. MEDICAL WORKS.

Doctor's Guide, by Isaac Israeli (ca. 830-932, N. Africa), German translation "Isak Israelis Propaedeutik fuer Aerzte", by David Kaufman, *Gesammelte Schriften*, Frankfurt, 1915, vol. iii.

Sepher Tzedah Laderekh (*The Poor Man's Medicine*), by Ahmad ben Abraham (Ibn Al Jezar, a pupil of Isaac Israeli), translated from the Arabic into Hebrew by Uri Barzel, in *Koroth*, vol. i, nos. 5-6, Jerusalem-Tel Aviv, 1955.

De Medico Hebraeo Anarratio Apologica (in Latin), by David de Pomis (1525-1588, Italy), Venice, 1588.

Curationum Medicinalium (in Latin), by Amatus Lusitanus (1511-1568, Portugal, Spain, Italy, Turkey), Venice, 1683 (cited as *Centuria*).

'Otzar Hahayim, by Jacob Zahalon (1630-1693, Italy), Venice, 1683.

Ma'asei Tuviah, by Tobias Cohen (1652-1729, Poland, Turkey), Venice, 1707.

'Aleh Teruphah, by Abraham ben Nansich (18th century, Hamburg), London, 1785.

13. PRAYER-BOOKS.

Siddur Beth Ya'akov, by Jacob Emden (1697-1776, Altona), Zitomir, 1880.

The Authorised Daily Prayer Book, with English translation by Simeon Singer, London, 1939.

14. HALACHIC PERIODICALS.

Tel Talpiyoth, ed. David Zvi Katzburg, Budapest.

Hapardes, ed. S. A. Pardes and S. Elberg, New York.

Haposek, ed. Hillel Posek, Tel Aviv.

B. MODERN JEWISH LITERATURE

(Works to which reference is made frequently are indicated in the notes by abbreviated titles. The references so used are marked by an asterisk following the shortened title.)

ABRAHAMS, Israel, *Jewish Life in the Middle Ages*, London, 1932.

—, *Hebrew Ethical Wills* (ed.), 2 vols., Philadelphia, 1926.

ADLER, Hermann, *Anglo-Jewish Memories*, London, 1909.

ADLER, S. "Die Entwickelung des Schulwesens der Juden zu Frankfurt a|M bis zur Emanzipation," in *JJLG*, vol. xix (1928).

APTOWITZER, Viktor, "Anteilnahme der physischen Welt an den Schicksalen des Menschen", in *MGWJ*, vols. lxiv and lxv (1920 and 1921).

—, "Observation on the Criminal Law of the Jews", in *JQR*, vol. xv (1924).

—, "The Status of the Embryo in the Jewish Law of Punishment" (Hebrew), in *Sinai*, vol. vi (1942).

ASAPH, Simchah, *Mekoroth Letoldoth Hahinnukh Beyisrae'el* (*Sources on the History of Education in Israel*), 4 vols., Tel Aviv, 1925-48.

ASHTOR-STRAUSS, E., "Saladin and the Jews", in *HUCA*, vol. xxvii (1956).

BAMBERGER, M. L., "Ueber Tierschutz nach den Lehren der Torah", in *Jeschurun*, vol. ii, (1915).

BARON, Salo Wittmayer, *A Social and Religious History of the Jews*, 3 vols., New York, 1937.

—, *The Jewish Community*, 3 vols. Philadelphia, 1942.

BELKIN, Samuel, *Philo and the Oral Law: The Philonic Interpretation of Biblical Law in Relation to the Palestinian Halakah*, Cambridge, Mass., 1940.

BERLINER, A., *Festschrift zum 70. Geburtstag*, ed, A. Freimann and M. Hildesheimer, Frankfurt, 1903.

BLAU, Ludwig, *Das altjuedische Zauberwesen*, Budapest, 1898.

BRECHER, Gideon, *Das Transcendentale, Magie und Magische Heilarten im Talmud*, Vienna, 1850.

CARMOLY, Eliakim, *Histoire des Médecins Juifs*, Brussels, 1844.

CASSUTO, J, "Aus dem aeltesten Protokolbuch der Portugiesisch-Juedischen Gemeinde in Hamburg", in *JJLG*, vols, vi-xiii (1908-1920).

CASTIGLIONI, Arturo, "The Contribution of the Jews to Medicine", in *The Jews**: *Their History, Culture and Religion*, ed. L. Finkelstein, vol. iii, Philadelphia, 1949.

CHAJES, Zvi Hirsch, *The Student's Guide through the Talmud*, ed. J. Schachter, Oxford, 1952.

DRACHMAN, Bernard, "The So-called 'Science Movements and their Relation to Judaism", in *Essays Presented to J. H. Hertz*, ed. I. Epstein, E. Levine and C. Roth, London, 1943.

EBSTEIN, Wilhelm, *Die Medizin im Neuen Testament und im Talmud*, Stuttgart, 1903.

EISLER, R., "Zur Terminologie und Geschichte der juedischen Alchemie", in *MGWJ*, vol. lxx (1926).

FRIEDENWALD* Harry *The Jews and Medicine*, 2 vols. Baltimore, 1944.

GEIGER, Abraham, *Urschrift* und Uebersetzungen der Bibel in ihrer Abwaengigkeit von der inneren Entwicklung des Judentums*, Breslau, 1857.

GINSBERG, Louis, *The Legends of the Jews*, 7 vols., Philadelphia, 1939.

GOLDZIHER, Ignaz, "Muhammedanischer Aberglaube ueber Gedaechtniskraft und Vergesslichkeit mit Parallelen aus der juedischen Litteratur", in *Berliner Festschrift*, Frankfurt, 1903.

GOODENOUGH, Erwin R., *The Jurisprudence of the Jewish Courts in Egypt*, New Haven, 1929.

GOSLAR, Max, "Biblische und Talmudische Quellen juedischer Eugenik", in *Hygiene und Judentum*, ed. H. Goslar, Dresren, 1930.

—, *Die Hygiene der Juden* (ed.), Dresden, 1911.

GUEDEMANN, Moritz, *Das juedische Unterrichtswesen waehrend der spanisch-arabischen Periode*, Vienna, 1873.

—, *Geschichte des Erziehungswesen und der Cultur der Juden in Frankreich und Deutschland*, Vienna, 1880.

—, "Ein Projekt zur Gruendung einer juedischen Universitaet aus dem 16. Jahrhundert", in *Berliner Festschrift*, Frankfurt, 1903.

GUTTMAN, Jacob, Die philosophischen Lehren des Isaak ben Salomon Israeli, Muenster, 1911.

GUTTMANN, Michael, *Das Judentum und seine Umwelt*, Berlin, 1927.

HEINEMANN, Isaak, *Die Werke Philos*, Berlin, 1910.

HIRSCH, W. *Rabbinic Psychology: Beliefs about the Soul in Rabbinic Literature of the Talmudic Period*, London, 1947.

HOFFMANN, David *Der Schulchan Aruch* und die Rabbinen ueber das Verhaeltnis der Juden zu den Andersglaeubigen*, Berlin, 1894.

—, "Mar Samuel", in *Jeschurun*, vol. ix (1922).

HOFMANN, W., "Zur Bewertung des Arztes und der Medizin in der juedischen Auffassung," in *Jeschurun*, vol. iv (1917).

JACOBSON, Jacob, "Die Stellung der Juden in den 1793 und 1795 von Preussen erworbenen Provinzen," in *MGWJ*, vol. lxv (1921).

JAKOBOVITS, Immanuel, "Artificial Insemination, Birth-Control and Abortion," in *The Hebrew Medical Journal*, vol. xxvi (1953).

—, "The Medical Treatment of Animals in Jewish Law," in *The Journal of Jewish Studies*, vol. vii (1956).

—, "Therapeutic Abortion" (Hebrew), in *Hapardes*, vol. xxx (1956).

—, "Euthanasia" (Hebrew), in *Hapardes*, vol. xxx (1956).

JUNES, Emile, "Etude sur la Circoncision Rituelle en Israel," in *Révue*, nos. 16 ff. (1953-4).

KAHANA, I., "Medicine in Halachic literature after the Compilation of the Talmud" (Hebrew), in *Sinai*, vol. xiv (1950).

KANTOR, Herman I., "History of Circumcision; Introduction of a New Instrument," in *Texas State Journal of Medicine*, 1953.

KATZENELSOHN, Judah L., *Hatalmud Veharephu'ah (Talmud and Medicine)*, Berlin, 1928.

KAUFMANN, D., *Gedenkbuch zur Erinnerung an David Kaufmann*, ed. M. Brann and F. Rosenthal, Breslau, 1900.

—, "Isak Israelis Propaedeutik fuer Aerzte," in *Gesammelte Schriften*, ed. M. Brann, vol. iii, Frankfurt, 1915.

KLEIN, Hermann, "Geburtenregelung. Eine halachische Abhandlung," in *Nachalath Zwi*, Berlin, vol. i (1931).

KOBER, Adolf, "Juedische Studenten und Dokotranten an der Universitaet Duisburg im 18. Jahrhundert," in *MGWJ*, vol. lxxxv (1931).

KRAUSS*, Samuel, *Talmudische Archaeologie*, 3 vols., Leipzig, 1910-2.

—, *Geschichte der juedischen Aerzte*, Vienna, 1930.

KURREIN, V., "Kartenspiel und Spielkarten im juedischen Schrifttume," in *MGWJ*, vol. lxvi (1922).

LANDAU, Richard, *Geschichte der juedischen Aerzte*, Berlin, 1895.

LAZARUS, Moritz, *Die Ethik des Judentums*, 2 vols., Frankfurt 1904-11.

(MODERN JEWISH LITERATURE)

LEIBOWITZ, Joshua, "On the Plague in the Ghetto at Rome in 1656" (Hebrew), Reprint from *Dappim Rephu'im*, 1943.

LEVY, Jacob, "Der Geburtenrueckgang—ein juedisches Problem," in *Jeschurun*, vol. xvii (1930).

—, "Geburtenstreik—die Frage der juedischen Ehe," in *Nachalath Zwi*, vol. i (1931).

—, "The Dissection of the Dead in Israel," in *Hama'yan*, vol. iii (1956).

LEWIN, B., "Zur Charakteristik und Biographie des R. Scherira Gaon," in *JJLG*, vol. viii (1910).

LEWIN, Louis, "Juedische Aerzte in Grosspolen," in *JJLG*, vol. ix (1911).

—, "Die juedischen Studenten an der Universitaet Frankfurt a/O," in *JJLG*, vols. xiv and xvi (1921 and 1924).

LEWIS, H. S., "Maimonides on Superstition," in *JQR*, vol. xvii (1905).

LOEW, Leopold, *Die Lebensalter* in der juedischen Litteratur*, Szegedin, 1875.

—, *Gesammelte Schriften*, ed. I. Loew, 3 vols., Szegedin, 1889-93.

MACE, David R., *Hebrew Marriage*, London, 1953.

MAIMON (FISCHMAN), J. L., *Sepher Hagra (Gaon Elijah of Vilna)*, 2 vols., Jerusalem, 1954.

MARGALITH, David, "Le Médecine et la Mouvement Hassidique," in *Révue*, no. 15 (1952).

MARX, Alexander, "The Scientific Work of Some Outstanding Mediaeval Jewish Scholars," in *Essays and Studies in Memory of Linda A. Miller*, ed. I. Davidson, New York, 1938.

MERZBACH, A. H., "The Religious Physician and his Mission in the Jewish State" (Hebrew), in *Dath Yisra'el Umedinath Yisra'el*, New York, 1951.

—, "La Circoncision", in *Révue*, no. 20 (1954).

MUNK, Saul, "Religionsgesetzliche Fragen die sich aus dem Gesetz zur Verhuetung von erbkranken Nachwuchses vom 14.7.33 ergeben", in *Nachalath Zwi*, vol. v (1935).

MUNTNER, Sussmann, "The Antiquity of Asaph the Physician and his Editorship of the Earliest Hebrew Book of Medicine", in *Bulletin of the History of Medicine*, vol. xxv (1951).

—, "Persian Medicine and its Relation to Jewish and Other Medical Science", in *The Hebrew Medical Journal*, vol. xxv (1952).

—, *The Problem of Dissection and Anatomical Science in Israel* (Hebrew), Jerusalem, 1955.

MUENZ, Isak, *Die juedischen Aerzte im Mittelalter*, Frankfurt, 1922.

NEUBURGER, Max, *Die Medizin im Flavius Josephus*, Vienna, 1919.

NEUFELD, E. *Ancient Hebrew Marriage Laws*, London, 1944.

NEUMAN, Abraham A., *The Jews in Spain*, 2 vols., Philadelphia, 1948.

PEREL, L., "La vie de l'anatomiste Hirschfeld", in *Révue*, on. 2 (1948).

PREIS, Karl, "Die Medizin im Sohar", in *MGWJ*, vol. lxxii (1928).

PREUSS, Julius, *Biblisch-Talmudische Medizin*, Berlin, 1911.

RABINOWITCH, I. M., *Post-Mortem Examinations and Jewish Law*, Montreal, 1945.

RABINOWITZ, Louis Isaac, *The Social Life of the Jews of Northern France in the XII-XIV Centuries as Reflected in the Rabbinical Literature of the Period*, London, 1938.

RITTER, Bernhard, *Philo und die Halachah*, Breslau, 1879.

ROTH, Cecil, *A History of the Jews in England*, Oxford, 1941.

—, *The Jewish Contribution to Civilization*, Oxford, 1943.

(MODERN JEWISH LITERATURE)

—, "The Qualifications of Jewish Physicians in the Middle Ages", in *Speculum*, vol. xxviii (1953).

—, "Elie Montalto et sa Consulation sur le Sabbat," in *REJ*, vol. xciv (1933).

SALTZBERG, Benzion, *Meshiv Kehalakhah, or On the Religious Duties of Physicians and Patients* (Hebrew), London, 1922.

SILBERSTEIN, M. D., "The Problem of Dissection and its Solution" (Hebrew), in *Dath Yisra'el Umedinath Yisra'el*, New York, 1951.

SIMON, I., "La Médecine legale dans la Bible et le Talmud", in *Révue*, no. 2 (1948).

—, "La gynécologie l'obsterique, l'embryologie et la puericulture dans la Bible et le Talmud", in *Révue*, no. 4 (1949).

—, "Le 'Serment Medicale' d'Assaph, Médicin Juif du VIIe Siècle," in *Révue*, no. 9 (1951).

—, "La Prière des Médecins de Jacob Zahalon", in *Révue*, no. 25 (1955).

SINGER, Charles, "Science and *Judaism**", in *The Jews**: *Their History, Culture and Religion*, ed. L. Finkelstein, vol. iii, Philadelphia, 1949.

STEINSCHNEIDER, Moritz, *Die Hebraeischen Uebersetzungen des Mittelalters, und die Juden als Dolmetscher*, Berlin, 1893.

STERN, A. *Die Medizin im Talmud*, Frankfurt, 1909.

STRACK, H. L., *Der Biutaberglaube in der Menschheit*, 1892.

—, *The Jew and Human Sacrifice*, transl. H. F. E. Blauchamp, London, 1909.

TERTIS, A., *Sepher Dam B'rith (On Circumcision)*, London, 1900.

TUCATZINSKY, J. M., "The Death Penalty According to the Torah in the Past and Present" (Hebrew). in *Hatorah Vehamedinah*, ed. S. Israeli, 4th series, Tel Aviv, 1952.

UNNA, Isak, "Christian Science", in *Jeschurun*, vol. ii (1915).

UNTERMAN, I. L., "The Law on the Saving of Life and its Definition" (Hebrew), in *Hatorah Vehamedinah*, ed. S. Israeli, 4th series, Tel Aviv, 1952.

WALLERSTEIN, L., "The Pioneer Role of Jews in Medicine", in *Commentary*, vol. xiv (1955).

WEISS, Isaac, *Dor Dor Vedorshav* (Hebrew), 5 vols., New York and Berlin, 1924.

WIESNER, L., "Kindersegen und Kinderlosigkeit im altrabbinischem Schrifttume", in *MGWJ*, vol. lrvi (1922).

WOHLGEMUTH, Joseph, "Vom Tier und seiner Wertung", in *Jeschurun*, vol. xiv (1927).

—, "Das Leid der Tiere", in *Jeschurun*, vol. xv (1928).

—, "Einfuehlung in das Empfindungsleben der Tiere", in *Jeschurun*, vol. xvi (1929).

ZEWIN, I. J., *Le'or Hahalakhah (In the Light of Jewish Law)*, Jerusalem, 1946.

ZIMMELS,* H. J., *Magicians, Theologians and Doctors: Studies in Folk-medicine and Folklore as Reflected in the Rabbinical Responsa (12-19th centuries)*, London, 1952.

C. GENERAL LITERATURE.

(Works to which reference is made frequently are indicated in the notes by abbreviated titles. The references so used are marked by an asterisk following the shortened title.)

1. REPORTS and ANONYMOUS WORKS.

A General Exposition of the General State of the Medical Profession, by "Alexipharmacus", London, 1829.

Address to the Public from Nature and Religion, against the unlimited Dissection of Human Bodies, London, 1829.

Artificial Human Insemination, Report of a Commission appointed by his Grace the Archbishop of Canterbury, London, 1948.

Artificial Insemination, Report of a Conference held under the auspices of the Public Morality Council, London, 1948.

The Healing Art, the Right Hand of the Church, by "Therapeutes", London, 1859.

Index Catalogue of the Library of the Surgeon-General's Office, U. S. Army, Washington.

Ethical and Religious Directives for Catholic Hospitals, issued by the Catholic Hospital Association of the United States and Canada, St. Louis, 1949.

Doctrine in the Church of England; The Report of the Commission on Christian Doctrine appointed by the Archbishops of Caterbury and York in 1922, London, 1950.

Premarital Health Examination Legislation. Analysis and Compilation of State Laws, U. S. Departmen of Health, Education and Welfare, Washington, 1954.

Lambeth Conference Reports, London, 1912, 1920, 1930 and 1958.

2. BOOKS and ARTICLES.

(References to ancient classics, and to the editions used, appear in the notes only.)

AHEARNE, P., "The Confessor and the Ogino-Knaus Theory", in *Irish Ecclesiastical Record,* vol. lxi (1943).

ALLBUTT, Thomas Clifford, *Science and Medieval Thought,* London, 1901.

—, *The Historical Relations of Medicine and Surgery to the End of the* 16th *Century,* London and New York, 1905.

—, *Greek Medicine* in Rome* (Fitzpatrick Lectures 1909-1910), London, 1921.

ALSTON, Mary N., "Attitude of the Church to Dissection before 1500", in *Bulletin of the History of Medicine,* vol xvi (1944).

BAAS, J. Hermann, *Grundriss der Geschichte der Medizin und des heilenden Standes,* Stuttgart, 1876.

—, *Outlines of the History of Medicin,* transl. H. E. Henderson, New York, 1889.

BARNES, Henry, "On Some Extracts from the Diaries of Bishop Nicholson", in *New York Medical Journal,* vol. lxxxii (1905).

BARUK, H., "Les Médecins allemands et l'experimentation médicale criminelle", in *Révue,* no. 7 (1950).

BAUMANN, E. D., "Antike Betrachtungen ueber Nutzen des Koitus", in *Janus,* vol. xliv (1940).

BONNAR, A., *The Catholic Doctor,* London, 1948.

BOUSCAREN, T. L., *Ethics of Ectopic Operations,* Milwaukee, 1944.

BROWNE, Edward Granville, *Arabian Medicine** (Fitzpatrick Lectures 1919-20), Cambridge, 1921.

(GENERAL LITERATURE, Books and Articles)

BUCK, Albert Henry, *The Growth of Medicine from the Earliest Times to about* 1800, New Haven, 1917.

BUCKLE, Henry Thomas, *History of Civilization in England*, 2 vols., London, 1857-61.

BUDGE, E. A. Wallis, *Syrian Anatomy, Pathology and Therapeutics; or "The Book of Medicines"*, 2 vols., London and Bombay, 1913.

BURK, S. B., "The Development of the Law of the Criminal Abortion", in *Medical Times*, 1929.

BURSHELL, P. L., *Ancient History of Medicine*, 1878.

CAMPBELL, Donald, *Arabian Medicine* and its Influence on the Middle Ages*, 2 vols., London, 1926.

—, "The Medical Curriculum of the Universities of Europe in the Sixteenth Century, with Special Reference to the Arabist Tradition", in *Science, Medicine and History*, ed. E. A. Underwood, Oxford, 1953.

CAPELLMANN, C., *Pastoral-Medizin*, Aachen, 1878, 1892 and 1904.

CASTIGLIONI, Arturo, *A History* of Medicine*, transl. E. B. Krumbhaar, New York and London, 1947.

CAWADIAS, Alexander P., "Male Eunuchism", in *Proceedings of the Royal Society of Medicine*, vol. xxxix (1946).

COLE, Rrancis Joseph, *A History of Comparatice Anatomy, from Aristotle to the 18th Century*, London, 1944.

CONNELL, F. J., "Birth-Control: The Case for the Catholic", in *Atlantic Monthly*, 1939.

—, "How soon may Embalming Begin?", in *American Ecclesiastical Review*, vol. cxviii (1948).

COWLES, E. S., *Religion and Medicine in the Church; Report for the Joint Commission on Christian Healing*, New York, 1925.

CUMSTON, Charles Greene, *An Introduction to the History of Medicine from the Pharaohs to the XVIIIth Century*, London, 1926.

CUNNINGHAM, B. J., *The Morality of Organic Transplantation*, 1946.

DAVIS, Henry, *Eugenics, Aims and Methods*, New York, 1930.

DEICHGRAEBER, K., "Die aerztliche Standesethik des Hippocratischen Eides", in *Quellen und Studien zur Geschichte der Nalurwissenschaften und Medizin*, vol. iii (1932).

DIEPGEN, P., *Die Theoldgic* und der aerztliche Stand*, Berlin, 1922.

—, "Die Bedeutung des Mittelsalters fuer den Fortschritt in der Medizin", in *Essays* on the History of Medicine*, ed. C. Singer and H. E. Sigerist, Oxford, 1924.

—, "Zur Frauenheilkunde im Byzantinischen Kulturkreis des Mittelsalters", in *Abhandlungen der Geistes- und Sozial-wissenschaftlichen Klasse*, 1950.

D'IRSAY, S., "Patristic Medicine", in *Annals of the History of Medicine*, vol. ix (1928).

DWORZECKI, M., "J'etons l'anathème contre la science criminelle Nazie", in *Révue*, no. 1 (1948).

DUNS, John, *The Life of Sir James Young Simpson*, Edinburgh, 1873.

EARENGEY, W. G. "Vountary Euthanasia", in *Medico-Legal and Criminological Review*, vol. viii (1940).

EBERS, George, *The Papyrus Ebers*, transl. B. Ebbell, Copenhagen and London, 1937.

EDELSTEIN, L., "Die Geschichte der Sektion in der Antike", in *Quellen und*

(GENERAL LITERATURE, Books and Articles)
Studien zur Geschichte der Naturwissenschaften und der Medizin, vol. iii (1932).
—, "Greek Medicine in Relation to Religion and Magic", in *Bulletin of the Institute of the History of Medicine,* vol. v (1937)
—,"The Hippocratic Oath", in *Supplements to the Bulletin of the History of Medicine,* 1943.
EHLINGER and KIMMING, *Ursprung und Entwickelungsgeschichte der Bestrafung der Fruchtabtreibung,* Munich, 1910.
EUKEN, Rudolf, "Paracelsus' Lehren von der Entwickelung", in *Beitraege zur Einfuehrung in die Geschichte der Philosophie,* Leipzig, 1906.
FINNEY, P. A., *Moral Problems in Hospital Practice,* 1935.
FLETCHER, Joseph *Morals and Medicine,* London, 1955.
FOSTER, Michael, *Lectures on the History of Physiology during the 16th-18th Centuries,* Cambridge, 1901.
FRANCIS, Henry Sayles, "Traditional Representation of Medicine and Healing in the Christian Hierarchy," in *Bulletin of the Medical Library Association,* vol. xxxii (1944).
FRAZER, James George, *Psyche's Task; a Discourse Concerning the Influence of Superstition on the Growth of Institutions,* London, 1913.
GALTON, Francis, *Inquiries into Human Faculty and Its Development,* London, 1883.
GARRISON, F. H., *An Introduction* into the History of Medicine,* Philadelphia, 1929.
GORDON, Henry Laing, *Sir James Young Simpson and Chloroform,* London, 1897.
GUTHRIE, Douglas, James, *A History of Medicine,* London, 1945.
HAAS, E., "Hippocrates und die Indische Medizin des Mittelalters," in *ZDMG,* vol. xxxi (1877).
HAGGARD, Howard Wilcox, *Devils,* Drugs and Doctors,* London, 1929.
—, *The Doctor in History,* New Haven and London, 1935.
HAEHNEL, R., "Der kuenstliche Abortus im Altertum," in *Sudhoff's Archiv fuer die Geschichte der Medizin,* vol. xxix (1936).
HAESER, Heinrich, *Lehrbuch der Geschichte der Medizin,* Jena, 1875.
HAMILTON, Mary Agnes, *Incubation, or the Cure of Disease in Pagan Temples and Christian Churches,* St. Andrews and London, 1906.
HARNACK, A., *Medizinisches* aus der aeltesten Kirchengeschichte,* Leipzig, 1902.
HARTMANN, Franz, *The Life of Philippus Theophrastus Bombast of Hohenhein, Known by the Name of Paracelsus,* London, 1896.
HIMES, Norman Edwin, "Medical History of Contraception," in *New England Journal of Medicine,* 1934 (separately reprinted).
—, "Soranus on Birth-Control," in *New England Journal of Medicine,* vol. ccv (1931).
HOBART, William Kirk, *The Medical Language of St. Luke,* Dublin and London, 1882.
HUMPHREYS, Justice, "Abortion—Should the Law be Reformed?", in *Medico-Legal and Criminological Review,* vol. vi (1938).
JAMES, R. R., "Licences to Practise Medicine and Surgery Issued by the Archbishops of Canterbury 1588-1775," in *Janus,* vol. xli (1937).
JONES, William Henry Samuel, *The Doctor's Oath,* Cambridge, 1924.
KELLY, Gerald, "Current Theology," in *Theological Studies,* vol. x (1949).
—, *Medico-Moral Problems,* St. Louis, 1950.
KLARMAN, A., *The Crux of Pastoral Medicine,* Ratisbon, 1912.

(GENERAL LITERATURE, Books and Articles)
KRUMBHAAR, E. B., "History of Autopsia and Its Relation to the Development
of Modern Medicine," in *Report of the Commission on Necropsies of the
American Hospital Association Bulletin, 1938.
LAWALL, Charles, *Four Thousands Years of Pharmacy,** Philadelphia and London.
1927.
LECKY, William Edward Hartpole, *History of the Rise and Influence of the Spirit
of Rationalism in Europe*, 2 vols., London, 1870.
—, *History of European Morals** from Augustus to Charlemagne*, 2 vols., London,
1911.
LITTRE, M. P. E., *Oevres Complètes d'Hippocrate* (ed.), Paris and London,
1839-61.
LUTHER, Martin, *Tischreden*, ed. Irmischer and ed. Koroker, Weimar, 1916.
—, *Werke*, ed. Weimar, 1901.
MACHER, M. L. *Pastoralheilkunde fuer Seelsorger*, 1860.
MACGILLIVRAY, *Moral Principles and Practice*, London, 1933.
MACKENZIE, D., *The Infancy** of Medicine: An Enquiry into the Influence of
Folk-lore upon the Evolution of Scientific Medicine*, London, 1927.
MACKINNEY, Loren M., "Medical Ethics and Etiquette in the Early Middle
Ages," in *Bulletin of the History of Medicine*, vol. xxvi (1952).
MACMURRICH, J. P., "Leonardo da Vinci and Vesalius," in *Medical Library
and Historical Journal*, vol. ix (1906).
MACNABB, Vincent, *Casti Connubii Encyclical Letter on Christian Marriage, with
Commentaries*, London, 1933.
MACNEILE, Alan Hugh, *The Gospel according to St. Matthew*, London, 1915.
MAGNUS, Hugo, *Religion und Medizin in ihren gegenseitigen Beziehungen*, 1902.
MASPERO, Gaston, *The Dawn of Civilisation: Egypt and Chaldea*, ed. A. H.
Sayce, London, 1910.
MASSEY, E., *A Sermon against the Dangerous and Sinful Practice of Inoculation*,
London, 1722.
MEYERHOF, Max, "Science and Medicine," in *Legacy of Islam*, ed. T. Arnold
and A. Guillaume, Oxford, 1931.
MEYER-STEINEG, T., *Geschichte des roemischen Aerztestandes*, Kiel, 1907.
MIGNE, Jacques Paul, *Patrologiae cursus completus* (ed.), *Series latina*, 221 vols.,
Paris, 1844-61. *Series Graeca*, 161 vols., Paris, 1857-66.
MILTNER, Theodor von, "Die Gesetzgeburg der Kulturvoelker zum Problem der
Fruchtabtreibung," in *Archiv fuer Gynaekologie*, vol. cxlii (1930).
MUELLER, Friedrich Max, *The Sacred Books of the East* (ed.), Oxford, 1880.
NEEDHAM, J., *A History of Embryology*, Cambridge, 1934.
NEUBURGER, Max, *Geschichte der Medizin*, Stuttgart, 1906.
—, *History** of Medicine*, transl. Ernest Playfair, vol. i, London, 1910.
—, "Zur Geschichte des Problems der Naturheilkraft," in *Essays** on the History
of Medicine*, ed. C. Singer and H. E. Sigerist, Oxford, 1924.
—, "Doctrine of the Healing Power of Nature throughout the Course of Time,"
in *Journal of the American Institute of Homeopathy*, vol. xxv (1932).
NITTIS, Savas, "The Hippocratic Oath in Reference to Lithotomy," in *Bulletin
of the History of Medicine*, vol. vii (1937).
—, "Hippocratic Ethics and Present-day Trends in Medicine," in *Bulletin of the
History of Medicine*, vol. xii (1942).
O'MALLEY, Austin and WALSH, James J., *Essays** in Pastoral Medicine*, New
York, London and Bombay, 1906.
O'RAHILLY, A., "Jewish Burial," in *Irish Ecclesiastical Record*, vol. lviii (1941).

— 377 —

(GENERAL LITERATURE, Books and Articles)

OSLER, William, *The Evolution* of Modern Medicine,* New Haven and and London, 1921.

OURSLER, Will, *The Healing Power of Faith,* Kingswood (Surrey), 1958.

PARK, Roswell, *An Epitome of the History of Medicine,* Philadelphia, New York and Chicago, 1897 and 1903.

PAYNE, Joseph Frank, *English Medicine in the Anglo-Saxon Times* (Fitzpatrick Lectures 1903), Oxford, 1904.

PETTIGREW, Thomas Joseph, *On Superstitions Connected with the History and Practice of Medicine and Surgery,* London, 1844.

PLOSS, Herman Heinrich, and BARTELS, Max, and Others, *Woman,** ed. E. J. Dingwall, 3 vols., London, 1935.

PUSCHMANN, Theodor, *Handbuch der Geschichte der Medizin,* 3 vols., Jena, 1902.

—, *A History of Medical Education* from the Most Remote to the Most Recent Times,* transl. Evan E. Hare, London, 1891.

RABINOWITCH, I. M., "Euthanasia," reprinted from *McGill Medical Journal,* Montreal, vol. xix (1950).

RASHDALL, Hastings, *The Universities* of Europe in the Middle Ages,* 3 vols. Oxford, 1936.

RIESMAN, David, *The Story of Medicine in the Middle Ages,* New York, 1935.

—, *Medicine in Modern Society,* Princeton, 1939.

—, "A Physician in the Papal Chair," in *Annals of the History of Medicine,* vol. v (1923).

RIVERS, William Halse Rivers, *Medicine, Magic and Religion* (Fitzpatrick Lectures 1915-16), London, 1924.

ROTH, M. *Andreas Vesalius Bruxellensis,* Berlin, 1892.

ROTH, R., "Indische Medizin," in *ZDMG,* vol. xxvi (1872).

SANFORD, A. E., *Pastoral Medicine: A Handbook for the Catholic Clergy,* New York, 1904.

SARTON, George, *Introduction to the History of Science,* vol. i, Baltimore, 1927.

—, *The History of Science and the New Humanism,* Cambridge, Mass., 1957.

SHAPER, J. K., "Premarital Health Examination," in *Public Health Reports,* Washington, no. lxix (May 1954).

SHARTEL, B., "Symposium on Sterilisation," in *American Practitioner,* vol. i (1947).

SIGERIST, Henry Ernest, *Great Doctors,* London, 1933.

—, *Civilisation* and Disease,* New York, 1944.

—, *Medicine* and Human Welfare,* New Haven and London, 1945.

—, "Die Geburt der abendlaendischen Medizin," in *Essays* on the History of Medicine,* ed. C. Singer and H. E. Sigerist, Oxford, 1924.

—, "The History of Medical Licensure," in *Journal of the American Medical Association,* vol. civ (1935).

SINGER, Charles, *The Evolution of Anatomy,** London, 1925.

—, *The Fasciculo di Medicina, Venice,* 1493 (ed.), 2 vols., Milan, 1925.

—, *From Magic to Science,* London, 1928.

—, "Galen as a Modern," in *Proceedings of the Royal Society of Medicine,* vol. xlii (1949).

—, and SIGERIST, Henry Ernest, *Essays* on the History of Medicine, Presented to K. Sudhoff on his 70th Birthday,* Oxford, 1924.

SMITH, Sidney, "The History and Development of Forensic Medicine," in *BMJ,* no. 4707 (1951).

(GENERAL LITERATURE, Books and Articles)
SPEERT, Harold, "Circumcision of the New-Born," in *Obstetrics and Gynecology*, vol. ii (1953).
STERN, Bernhard, *Medizin, Aberglaube und Geschlechtsleben in der Tuerkei*, 2 vols., Berlin, 1903.
STERN, B. J., *Should We be Vaccinated? A Survey of the Controversy*, New York and London, 1927.
—, *Society* and Medical Progress*, Princeton, 1941.
SUTHERLAND, Halliday Gibson, *Control of Life*, London, 1936 and 1944.
THORNDIKE, Lynn, *A History of Magic* and Experimental Science during the First 13 Centuries of Our Era*, 2 vols., London, 1932.
—, *Science and Thought in the 15th Century*, New York, 1930.
TIBERGHIEN, P., "Principles et conscience morale", in *Cashiers Laënnec*, 1946.
TOEPLY, Robert Ritter von, *Studien zur Geschichte der Anatomie im Mittelalter*, Leipzig and Vienna, 1898.
UNDERWOOD, E. Ashworth, *Science, Medicine and History. Essays on the Evolution of Scientific Thought and Medical Practice Written in Honour of Charles Singer*, (ed.)., 2 vols., Oxford, 1953.
VERING, A. M., *Handbuch der Pastoralmedizin*, 1835.
VIRCHOW, R., "Morgagni and the Anatomical Concept," in *Bulletin of the History of Medicine*, vol. vii (1939).
VORWAHL, H., "Die Beseelung des Menschen," in *Sudhoff's Archiv fuer die Geschichte der Medizin*, vol. xiii (1921).
WALL, Cecil, *The History of the Surgeon's Company*, 1745-1800, London, 1937.
WALSH, James J., *The Popes and Science:* History of the Papal Relations to Science during the Middle Ages and down to our own Time*, London, 1912.
—, *Religion and Health*, 1920.
—, *The Catholic Church and Healing*, London, 1928.
WESTERMARK, Edward Alexander, *The Origin and Development of the Moral Ideas,* 2 vols., London and New York, 1906.
—,*Christianity and Morals*, London, 1939.
WHERLI, G. A., "Das Wesen der Volksmedizin," in *Essays* on the History of Medicine*, ed. C. Singer and H. E. Sigerist, Oxford, 1924.
WHITE, Andrew Dickson, *A History of the Warfare* of Science with Theology in Christendom*, 2 vols., London and New York, 1896.
WITKOWSKI, G. J., *Le Mal qu'on a dit des Médicins*, Paris, 1884.
WICKERSHEIMER, E., "L'anatomie de Guido de Vigevano," in *Sudhoff's Archiv fuer die Geschichte der Medizin*, vol. vii (1914).
WINDLE, Bertram C. A., *The Church and Science*, London, 1920.
WITHINGTON, E. E., *Medical History from the Earliest Times*, London, 1894.
—, "The Asclepediadae and the Priests of Asclepius," in *Studies in the History and Method of Science*, ed. C. Singer, vol. ii, Oxford, 1921.
WOLFF, G., "Leichenbesichtigung und Untersuchung bis zur Carolina als Vorstufe gerichtlicher Sektion," in *Janus*, vol. xliii (1938).
WORCESTER, Elwood, and MACCOMB, Samuel, *Body, Mind and Spirit*, London, 1931.
WOYWOOD, A., *A Practical Commentary on the Code of Canon Law*, 2 vols., New York and London, 1926.
ZIMMERMAN, L. M., and HOWELL, K. M., "History of Blood-Transfusions," in *Annals of the History of Medicine*, vol. iv (1932).

D. ENCYCLOPEDIAS AND DICTIONARIES.

British Encyclopedia of Medical Practice, ed. Lord Horder, 12 vols., London, 1950-2.
Catholic Encyclopedia [CE], 15 vols., New York, 1907-12.
Encyclopedia Britannica [EB], 24 vols., Chicago, London and Toronto, 1953.
Encyclopedia of Religion and Ethics [ERE], ed. James Hastings, 12 vols., Edinburgh, 1908-21.
Encycyopedia Hebraica [HE], Jerusalem and Tel Aviv, 1949-
Jewish Encyclopedia [JE], ed. I. Singer, 12 vols., New York, 1901-6.
Juedisches Lexikon [JL], ed. G. Herlitz and B. Kirschner, 5 vols., Berlin, 1927-30.
'Otzar Yisra'el [OY], ed. J. D. Eisenstein, 10 vols., Berlin and Vienna, 1924.
Real-Encyclopaedie fuer Bibel und Talmud, by J. Hamburger [Hamburger,RE], part i, Strelitz, 1866 part ii, Leipzig, 1892. Supplements, Leipzig, 1886-97.
Talmudic Encyclopedia [TE], Jerusalem, 1947-
The Concise Oxford Dictionary, Oxford, 1940.
The Oxford Classical Dictionary, Oxford, 1949.
The Oxford English Dictionary, 12 vols., Oxford, 1933.
A Dictionary of Targumim, the Talmud Babli and Yerushalmi, and the Midrashic Literature, by Marcus Jastrow, Berlin, 1926.
Aruch Completum, by Alexander Kohut 8 vols,, Vienna and Berlin, 1926.
Neuhebraeisches und Chaldaeisches Woerterbuch ueber die Talmudim und Midraschim, by Jacob Levy, 4 vols., Leipzig, 1876-89.

E. PERIODICALS.

(Figures indicate year of foundation,)

1. JEWISH

Bikkurei Ha'ittim (1820), Vienna.
Commentary, (1945), ed. Elliot E. Cohen, New York.
Dappin Rephu'im, Israel.
Hame'asseph (1784), Koenigsberg.
Hamelitz (1871), St. Petersburg.
Hapardes (1926), ed. S. A. Pardes and S. Elberg, New York.
Hebraeische Bibliographie (1858). ed. M. Steinschneider, Berlin.
Hebrew Medical Journal, The (1927), ed. M. Einhorn, New York.
Hebrew Union College Annual [HUCA] (1924), Cincinnati.
Jahrbuch der Juedisch-Literarischen Gesellschaft [JJLG] (1903), Frankfort.
Jeschurun (1914), ed. J. Wohlgemuth, Berlin.
Jewish Chronicle (1841), London.
Jewish Quarterly Review [JQR] (1889-1908), ed. I. Abrahams and C.G. Montefiore, London. New Series (1909), Philadelphia and London.
Journal of Jewish Studies (1950), ed. A. Altmann, London.
Kerem Hemed (1833), Vienna.
Koroth, A Quarterly Journal Devoted to the History of Medicine and Science (1952), Jerusalem,
Monatsschrift fuer Geschichte und Wissenschaft des Judentums [MGWJ] (1851), Breslau.
Nachalath Zwi (1931), Berlin.
Révue des Etudes Juives [REJ] (1880), Paris.
Révue * *d'Histoire de la Medicine Hébraique* (1948), ed. I. Simon, Paris.
Sinai (1937), ed. J. L. Maimon (Fishman), Jerusalem.
Tel Talpiyoth (1892), ed. D. Z.Katzburg, Budapest.

2. GENERAL

Abhandlungen der Geistes- und Sozial-wissenschaftlichen Klasse, Berlin.
American Ecclesiastical Review.
American Journal of Surgery (1890), New York.
American Practitioner, Philadelphia.
Annals of the History of Medicine (1917), New York.
Archiv fuer Gynaekologie (1870), Berlin.
Atlantic Monthly.
British Medical Journal [*BMJ*], London.
Bulletin of the History of Medicine, Baltimore; continued as *Bulletin of the History of Medicine,* Baltimore.
Bulletin of the American Library Association (1911), Baltimore.
Cahiers Laënnec (1935), Paris.
Irish Ecclesiastical Record, Maynooth.
Isis (1913), Brussels.
Janus (1896), Amsterdam, Paris.
Journal of the American Institute of Homeopathy, New York.
Journal of the American Medical Aseociation (1883), Chicago.
Lancet (1823), London.
MacGill Medical Journal, Montreal.
Medical Library and Historical Journal (1903), Brooklyn, New York.
Medical Times, New York.
Medico-Legal and Criminological Review (1933), London.
New England Journal of Medicine (1928), Boston.
New York Medical Journal (1865), New York.
Obstetrics and Gynecology, New York.
Proceedings of the Royal Society of Medicine (1913), London.
Quellen und Studien zur Geschichte der Naturwissenschaften und der Medizin.
Speculum, A Journal of Mediaeval Studies (1925), Cambridge, Mass.
Sudhoff's Archiv fuer Geschichte der Medizin (1907), Leipzig.
Texas State Journal of Medicine (1905), Austin.
Theological Studies (1939), St. Louis.
Zeitschrift der Deutschen Morgenlaendischen Gesellschaft [*ZDMG*] (1847), Leipzig.